CELL INJURY AND PROTECTION IN THE GASTROINTESTINAL TRACT

CELL INJURY AND PROTECTION IN THE GASTROINTESTINAL TRACT

From Basic Sciences to Clinical Perspectives 1996

Editors

Gy. Mózsik *(Pécs, Hungary)*

L. Nagy *(Pécs, Hungary)*

A. Pár *(Pécs, Hungary)*

K.D. Rainsford *(Sheffield, UK)*

 SPRINGER-SCIENCE+BUSINESS MEDIA, B.V.

Library of Congress Cataloging-in-Publication Data is available.

ISBN 978-94-010-6268-8   ISBN 978-94-011-5392-8 (eBook)
DOI 10.1007/978-94-011-5392-8

Printed on acid-free paper

Printed by Antony Rowe Ltd, Chippenham, Wiltshire

CONTENTS

III. CELL INJURY AND PROTECTION IN SMALL INTESTINE AND IN THE LARGE BOWEL

IV. CELL INJURY AND PROTECTION IN THE LIVER AND IN THE PANCREAS

V.   CELL INJURY AND PROTECTION OF THE PREMALIGNANT STATUS AND MALIGNANT DISEASES IN THE GASTROINTESTINAL TRACT

FOURTH INTERNATIONAL SYMPOSIUM ON CELL INJURY AND PROTECTION IN THE GASTROINTESTINAL TRACT: from Basic Sciences to Clinical Perspectives

October 8–11, 1995
Pécs, Hungary

PREFACE

The phenomenon of 'gastric cytoprotection' was discovered by Jacobson and Chaudhury (Gastroenterology. 1978;74:59) and was internationally accepted and evaluated by Robert et al. (Gastroenterology. 1979;77:433–443.

The First, Second and Third International Symposium on Gastrointestinal Cytoprotection were organized in Pécs in 1983, 1987 and 1991. These meetings were successful and all the scientific material was published in the journal, Acta Physiol. Hung. (1984;64:34; 1988; 1992) and edited as books by the Akadémiai Kiadó, Budapest (1984; 1988; 1992).

The Fourth International Symposium on 'Cell Injury and Protection in the Gastrointestinal Tract: from Basic Sciences to Clinical Perspectives' was held in October 8–11, 1995 (Pécs, Hungary), under the auspices of the Hungarian Academy of Sciences, Hungarian Society of Gastroenterology (Section of Nutrition and Metabolism, Research Forum), International Union of Pharmacology, International Brain–Gut Society, Standing Committee of Ulcer Research and Medical University of Pécs. Our principal aims are the same as they have been for 12 years.

International Scientific Committee:

A. Bertelli (Milano, Italy)
M. Beinborn (Hannover, Germany)
L. Buéno (Toulouse, France)
F. Capasso (Naples, Italy)
M. Dell Tacca (Pisa, Italy)
S. Evangelista (Florence, Italy)
E. Ezer (Budapest, Hungary)
J. Fehér (Budapest, Hungary)
T. Gaginella (Madison, USA)
M. Garamszegi (Pécs, Hungary)
K. Gyires (Budapest, Hungary)
I. Hermecz (Budapest, Hungary)
M. Jablonská (Prague, Czech Republic)

M. Kitajima (Tokyo, Japan)
J. Lonovics (Szeged, Hungary)
L. Nagy (Pécs, Hungary)
A. Németh (Pécs, Hungary)
S. Okabe (Kyoto, Japan)
C.J. Pfeiffer (Blacksburg, USA)
M. Papp (Budapest, Hungary)
P. Sikiric (Zagreb, Croatia)
I. Simek (Olomuc, Slovak Republic)
L. Simon (Szekszárd, Hungary)
N. Sato (Tokyo, Japan)
J. Stachura (Krakow, Poland)
S. Szabo (Irvine, USA)

The scientific main programmes of these series of symposia changed from time to time following the international scientific trends.

The main programmes of the *First Symposium* were: 1. Gastric and intestinal cytoprotection; 2. Hepatoprotection; 3. Pancreatic protection. For the *second* one: 1. Gastrointestinal mucosal 'cytoprotection'; 2. Liver 'cytoprotection'; 3. Pancreatic 'cytoprotection'; 4. Free radicals and scavangers; 5. Computer approach to cytoprotection. For the *third* one: 1. Basic, central, peripheral and cellular mechanisms of gastrointestinaol cytoprotection; 2. Esophagal protection; 3. Gastric protection; 4. Small intestinal injury and protection; 5. Large bowel injury and protection; 6. Liver injury and protection; 7. Pancreas injury and protection.

The main scientific programmes of the *Fourth International Symposium on 'Cell Injury and Protection in the Gastrointestinal Tract'* are: 1. General mechanisms of gastrointestinal injury and protection; 2. Cell injury and protection in the stomach; 3. Cell injury and protection in the small intestine and in the large bowel; 4. Cell injury and protection in the liver and pancreas; 5. Cell injury and protection of the premalignant status and malignant diseases in the gastrointestinal tract.

The presented papers are published in this book.

The abstracts of this meeting were published in *Digestive Diseases and Sciences*, and we record appreciation of the Editor of that journal for their publication.

Some of the papers published here have appeared in *Inflammopharmacology* 1996;4:331–398.

ORGANIZERS
Gy. Mózsik (*Pécs, Hungary*)
L. Nagy (*Pécs, Hungary*)
A. Pár (*Pécs, Hungary*)
K.D. Rainsford (*Sheffield, UK*)

INFLAMMOPHARMACOLOGY

Basic and clinical studies on inflammation and its pharmacological control

Aims and Scope

The journal *Inflammopharmacology* publishes papers on all aspects of inflammation and its pharmacological control, emphasizing comparisons of (a) different inflammatory states, and (b) the actions, therapeutic efficacy and safety of drugs employed in the treatment of inflammatory conditions. The comparative aspects of the types of inflammatory conditions include gastrointestinal disease (e.g. ulcerative colitis, Crohn's disease), parasitic diseases, toxicological manifestations of the effects of drugs and environmental agents, and arthritic conditions. Inflammopharmacology covers all the major aspects of the experimentally-induced clinical pathology, its biochemistry and cell biology, as well as the clinical and experimental pharmacology and toxicology of therapeutic agents. The emphasis on comparative aspects of the actions of drugs is intended to highlight their efficacy and toxicity profiles as well as the variability in their clinical response and safety.

ISSN 0925-4692

In summary the journal covers:

- Experimental development of in vitro systems and in vivo animal models
- Assay methodologies
- Biochemical, immunological and pharmacological studies
- Clinical pharmacology and therapeutics
- Drug-induced side-effects — their incidence and mechanisms
- Comparative drug studies and trials
- Novel approaches towards the therapy of inflammatory conditions, including brief but carefully conducted reports on therapies with as yet undefined materials (e.g. natural products, immunological agents) which may be considered as giving leads or encouragement to others to further purify or define the active ingredients and explore their actions.

The journal publishes peer-reviewed unsolicited papers, reviews, short communications, letters to the editor, drug status reports, editorials and short summaries of hypotheses, and supplements.

Editor-in-Chief: **KD Rainsford**   *See overleaf for further details*

Subscription price, per volume (4 issues): NLG 451.00 inclusive of postage

ORDER FORM
Please fill in the order form and send to your regular subscription agent or to: Kluwer Academic Publishers, PO Box 322, 3300 AH Dordrecht, The Netherlands.
USA and Canada: Kluwer Academic Publishers, PO Box 358, Accord Station, Hingham, MA 02018-0358, USA
Japan: Maruzen Co. Ltd, Subscription Department, PO Box 5050, Tokyo Int 100-31, Japan
India: Allied Publishers Subscription Agency, 13/14 Asaf Ali Road, Delhi 110002, India

..... Please enter .... 1997 Institutional subscriptions to *Inflammopharmacology*

..... Please enter .... 1997 Private subscriptions to *Inflammopharmacology*

..... Please send me a free sample copy of *Inflammopharmacology*

ORDERS BY INDIVIDUALS MUST BE PREPAID

..... Payment enclosed to the amount of ....

OR I authorise you to charge my credit account:

    Card:...................... Number:..

    Expiry date:.................... Signature:.......................................

OR Please invoice me

Name [please print]...

Address..

....

....

PRIVATE JOURNAL SUBSCRIPTIONS SHOULD BE SENT TO THE PUBLISHERS

**KLUWER
ACADEMIC
PUBLISHERS**

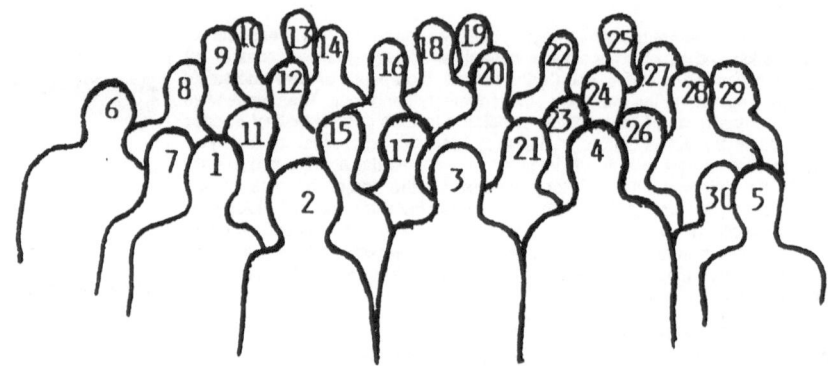

PARTICIPANTS

1. A. Pár (Pécs, Hungary)
2. E. Rőth (Pécs, Hungary)
3. K.D. Rainsford (Sheffield, UK)
4. Gy. Mózsik (Pécs, Hungary)
5. P. Sikiric (Zagreb, Croatia)
6. J. Szabó (Pécs, Hungary)
7. K. Kalmár (Pécs, Hungary)
8. L. Nagy (Pécs, Hungary)
9. P. Csere (Pécs, Hungary)
10. Cs. Kövesdy (Pécs, Hungary)
11. V. Nosálová (Bratislava, Slovak Republic)
12. E. Ezer (Budapest, Hungary)
13. Á. Vincze (Long Beach, USA)
14. P. Del Soldato (Naples, Italy)
15. B. Bódis (Pécs, Hungary)

16. O.M.E. Abdel-Salam (Pécs, Hungary)
17. M. Gué (Toulouse, France)
18. G. Sütő (Pécs, Hungary)
19. A. Cziráki (Pécs, Hungary)
20. Gy. Rumi (Pécs, Hungary)
21. K. Gyires (Budapest, Hungary)
22. K. Kálmán (Pécs, Hungary)
23. S. Giljanovic (Zagreb, Croatia)
24. E. Kiszelly (Budapest, Hungary)
25. A. Debreceni (Pécs, Hungary)
26. D. Erceg (Zagreb, Croatia)
27. I. Szabó (Pécs, Hungary)
28. V. Simicevic (Zagreb, Croatia)
29. M. Veljaca (Zagreb, Croatia)
30. M. Jablonská (Prágue, Czech Republic)

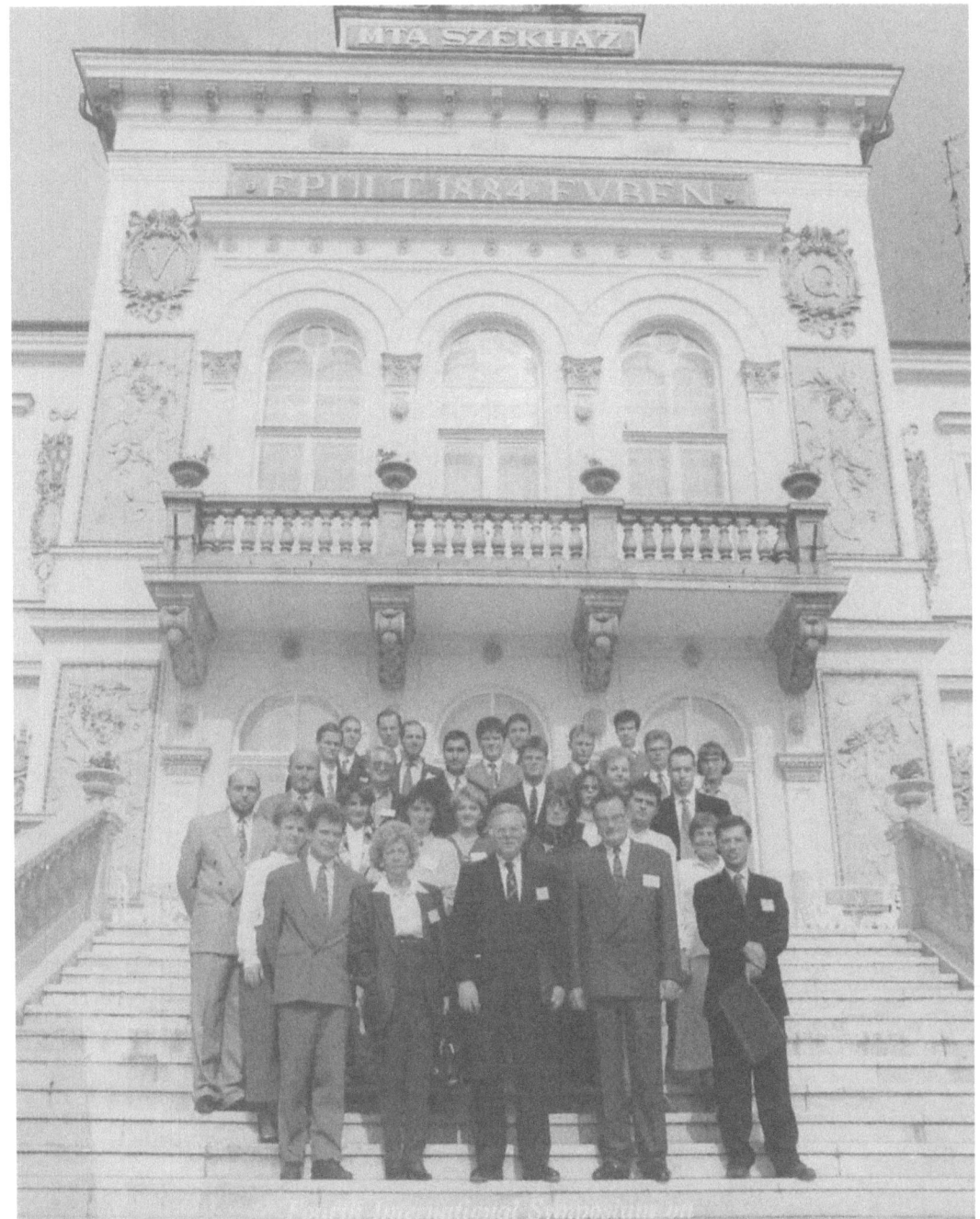

Fourth International Symposium on
Cell Injury and Protection in the Gastrointestinal Tract:
From Basic Sciences to Clinical Perspectives
October 8-11, 1995
Pécs, Hungary

G Mózsik et al. Cell Injury and Cytoprotection in the GI Tract. 1–7.

EMERGING RESEARCH IN GASTROINTESTINAL DISEASES

K.D. RAINSFORD

Division of Biomedical Sciences, Sheffield Hallam University, Pond Street, Sheffield, S1 1WB, UK

ABSTRACT

Upper gastrointestinal (GI) ulceration from drugs and stress, as well as inflammatory bowel diseases (IBD) are relatively common GI pathologies which have an appreciable morbidity and mortality. Furthermore, the role of environmental, genetic and nutritional factors in the aetiology of various cancers and other GI disorders emphasizes the importance of research into these and other GI conditions. Each of these pathologies has multiple mechanisms. Recent studies examining the effects of these agents or conditions on the development of acute GI ulceration have highlighted: (1) vascular injury and factors mediating this, among them eicosanoids, endothelins and nitric oxide, (2) leucocyte adhesion, infiltration and activation, (3) neuro-inflammatory reactions, (4) altered production of cytokines, and (5) enteric flora, including *Helicobacter pylori*. Longer term (chronic) injury involves not only these acute phenomena but also alterations in growth factors and stem cells and the occurrence of complex immuno-inflammatory reactions. In IBD, these alterations are driven by altered T-cell populations and pathological organisms (e.g. *Mycobacterium paratuberculosis* in Crohn's disease). An impressive array of strategies have and are being developed to prevent these conditions. Most have focussed on manipulating the mediators, cytokines, growth factors and cells participating in the pathology of these states. For the NSAIDs, procedures have been developed which minimize the occurrence of gastroduodenal mucosal injury (e.g. cyclo-oxygenase-II specific drugs; carboxyl and alkyl nitrite esters; compounds with prostaglandin analogues, micronutrients or other anti-ulcer drugs). Some specific agonists, antagonists or enzymes regulators participating in these reactions have been developed which have impressive actions in animal and human models. However, in some conditions, multivalent drugs may prove more successful, reflecting the multiplicity of factors and cells involved in GI pathologies.

Keywords: gastrointestinal; ulcer; anti-ulcer drugs; anti-inflammatory drugs; *Helicobacter pylori*; inflammatory bowel diseases

INTRODUCTION

The case for research into gastrointestinal (GI) functions in health and disease is compelling (Table 1). It has long been recognized that the relatively high incidence of gastrointestinal (GI) ulceration arises from a variety of causes, among them stressful conditions, ulcerogenic drugs, infections, smoking and high intake of alcohol. While the incidence of peptic ulcer disease continues to be high, the trend is, overall, towards a decline (despite some fluctuations in reported statistics in some countries), except in individuals above 65 years of age where the incidence is increasing [1]. Silent, or asymptomatic, peptic ulcer disease which is evident in about 10% of peptic ulcer patients is of particular importance because it often has a fatal outcome [2]. Gastric and other GI cancers, while continuing to decrease in incidence, still have a rather poor prognosis [3]. Recognition of the major role of diet and *Helicobacter pylori* now affords a basis for their prevention [3]. The inflammatory bowel diseases (IBDs) of the lower

TABLE 1
The case for gastrointestinal research

---

1. High prevalence of GI diseases exists from:
   – Upper GI ulcers from stress, ethanol, drugs, infections
   – Inflammatory bowel diseases – ulcerative colitis and Crohn's disease
   – Irritable bowel syndrome
   – Parasitic diseases of intestinal tract.

2. Nutritional disorders abound worldwide attributable to heritable, nutritional and
   environmental variables.

3. Environmentally related conditions lead to abnormal functions, cancer, etc.

Thus, there is a need to develop greater understanding of these conditions, the normal states of
health, and procedures and therapies to restore health more effectively than we can today!

---

intestinal tract, ulcerative colitis, Crohn's disease and irritable bowel syndrome have a
complex aetiology [4]. The incidence of IBDs appears to be increasing, though it is not
certain if this is not a consequence of improved efficiency in their diagnosis [4]. A
variety of nutritional disorders of complex genetic and environmental origin compli-
cate further the clinical picture of GI disease. Finally, it is important to know not only
the mechanisms underlying all these conditions but also how the GI mucosa protects
itself from injury or insult, such as that from the potentially irritating and noxious
substances we consume.

The recognition of the continuing need for GI research, especially that devoted to
the study of the mechanisms of ulcerogenesis, as well as the prevention and cure of
these conditions, is evidenced by strong international support for this meeting, the
fourth in the series.

Examination of the recent trends and discoveries reveals some remarkable developments (Table 2). A brief overview of these major trends will be given in this paper,
together with some critical issues which have been raised, and some indications of
where research may be expected to go in the near future.

INFECTIOUS AETIOLOGIES IN GI DISEASES

The importance of understanding the roles of infectious agents in the pathogenesis of
certain GI inflammatory/ulcer diseases has been appreciated in the last decade or so
with studies on: (a) *Helicobacter pylori* in peptic/duodenal ulcer disease and gastric
malignancies, (b) the suggested role of mycobacterial or other bacterial species in the
development of Crohn's disease, and (c) the influence of enteric bacteria in the
pathogenesis of intestinal ulcer induced by drugs such as the NSAIDs, and their
actions in other conditions.

TABLE 2
The impact of molecular and cell biology for research on GI diseases

---

Genes for enzymes, macromolecules and receptors cloned and expressed,
e.g. – Cyclo-oxygenases
    – Nitric oxide synthases
    – Prostanoid/leukotriene receptors
    – Neurotransmitters
    – *H. pylori*
    – Mucus
    – Unique molecules from infectious organisms
    – Leucocyte markers, adhesion molecules
    – Cytokines, growth factors

These give tools and targets for:
    – Understanding fundamental and practical (applied) approaches
    – Development of therapies

Helicobacter pylori – role in gastroduodenal ulcers and gastric malignancies

H. pylori must be the pathogenic organism of the decade as evidenced by the research and clinical interest reflected by the substantial numbers of publications which have appeared in the form of original studies and reviews on this bacterium [5,6]. *H. pylori* is probably the most common of the bacterial infections in humans throughout the world [5,6]. It is endemic in Western populations aged 50–60 years [5,6] and probably more prevalent in younger aged groups in Eastern countries (of the former Soviet group) [7]. Patterns of distribution in the world may be due to transmission being faecal–oral in the Third World and oral–oral in the First World [8]. *H. pylori* is now well-recognized as a major aetiological agent in the pathogenesis of gastroduodenal (peptic) ulceration, chronic type-B gastritis, gastric carcinoma and MALT-associated lymphoma, as well as in Ménétrier's disease [5,6].

The modern techniques of molecular and cell biology, microbiology and immunology have all given powerful insight into the mechanisms underlying the pathogenic actions of *H. pylori* [6,8,9]. Some of these findings have been surprising. For example, the fact that there are specific molecules on the surface of the organism, adhesins, that go through cleverly orchestrated changes, but whose specific interaction, predominantly, is with receptors on surface epithelial cells (and no others in the mucosa) of primates bearing the *bis*-fucosyl-glycoproteins containing blood group Le[b] antigens [9].

Despite the impressive knowledge of the molecular basis of infection and the success of the so-called 'triple therapies' based on combinations of bismuth salts, metronidazole (or other macrolide antibiotics) and amoxycillin, or combinations of antibiotics with omeprazole or related drugs, there is a still need to develop more effective, longer-lasting treatments, without the problems of antibiotic resistance, and which have fewer side-effects than those encountered at present [5,6,8]. Various approaches involving development of antagonists to the adhesin–fucosyl–glycoprotein mucous cell receptor interactions have been initiated [8,9] in order to lead to reduced tropism [9] of *H. pylori* for mucous cells. Immunization, including use of IgA-like antibodies which appear to react with the 120-kDa protein of *H.pylori* [10], may also be a useful strategy.

More fundamentally, we need to know if other organisms that exist in the gastroduodenal region, e.g. *Gastropirillum (=Helicobacter) hominis* which has been reported occasionally [11], may contribute to the pathogenesis of peptic ulcer, non-ulcer dyspepsia (the role for *H. pylori* for which is controversial at present [5,6]), and gastric cancer. The transmission of *Gastrospirillum* spp. and other micro-organisms present in the gastrointestinal tract of domestic pets has also yet to be considered in relation to the development of upper GI ulceration and dyspepsia in humans.

The role of *H. pylori* in the pathogenesis of NSAID-induced ulcers has been considered at length [5,12]. The consensus has been expressed that these may be considered independent, non-additive risk factors for mucosal ulceration [5]. However, the underlying acid stimulatory actions of some NSAIDs and the gastrinaemia induced by *H. pylori* infection [12,13] raises the question of whether or not there are subtle acid-related factors in the pathogenesis of ulcer disease from both these agents when there is, as frequently encountered, overlap in associations. Where there are strong neutrophil-associated inflammatory reactions as in duodenitis or where there is gastric metaplasia, it appears, paradoxically, that NSAIDs may be associated with decreased mucosal pathology [14]. This is both puzzling and intriguing; is this a reflection of the anti-inflammatory actions of the NSAIDs? It is important that this should be understood and exploited therapeutically. Could the low ulcerogenic, possibly pro-drug, NSAIDs be usefully employed in these inflammatory states, and in what doses? Maybe only relatively low doses of these drugs have to be given for substantial benefit without development of the mucosal ulcerative reactions?

Mycobacterial aetiology in Crohn's disease

The association of *Mycobacterium paratuberculosis* infection with Crohn's disease has been one of the most difficult challenges in GI diseases [15–18]. Indeed, it has been described rather euphemistically by one of the experts in this field as 'a tricky customer' [15]. An example of how modern molecular biological techniques have helped in advances in knowledge of this disease has come with the recognition of IS900, a 1.45-kb DNA insertion element repeated 18–20 times in the genomic sequence of *M. paratuberculosis* [15]. This genomic sequence has enabled the organism to be identified, when hitherto it was regarded as being difficult to do so because it is a slow-growing species requiring unique culture conditions. No doubt with further advances in molecular techniques it will be possible to more accurately define the conditions for infection and occurrence of this putative aetiological agent in Crohn's disease [18]. Other aetiological agents have been proposed (e.g. *Listeria* spp., measles virus or vaccines) but the evidence for these is unconvincing. Enteric microbial overload may play a role, especially in the development of initial immune suppression [18].

MOLECULAR GENETICS AND AETIOPATHOGENESIS OF IBDs

The familial association of IBDs, reinforced by demonstration of increased incidence of both Crohn's disease and ulcerative colitis in monozygotic twins, is quite compelling evidence for an inherited component in the aetiology of both these diseases [17,19]. As for many aetiological associations in IBD, the evidence, while tantalizing, is not definitive [17]. Genetic markers, such as HLA class II antigens and cytokine polymorphisms, have provided interesting data and may well prove additional factors in the predisposition to IBD [17,20]. Of the HLA associations observed, that for the DR2 system is relatively strong [20]. Within this system, however, there appear to be variations that may be due to ethnic origins (e.g. high frequency of DRB1.1502 alleles in Japanese and Jewish patients with ulcerative colitis but not in white non-Jewish subjects) [20]. These studies and the lack of convincing information on other genetic associations that have been proposed give support for further research in these fields.

NSAID- AND ETHANOL-ASSOCIATED GASTROINTESTINAL ULCERATION

The evidence for the association of NSAIDs and ethanol in the aetiology of upper GI ulceration and gastritis/duodenitis is now substantial [21–24]. What is less clear is the association of some NSAIDs with inflammatory enteropathy in the post-duodenal region of the intestine. While a substantial number of case reports have appeared implicating certain NSAIDs, especially those with delayed- or slow-release formulations and those exhibiting enterohepatic recirculation, the incidence of NSAID-associated enteropathy (ulcers, perforations, 'diaphragm-like' strictures) in rheumatic patients taking these drugs for long-term pain relief is not known. The difficulty of diagnosing enteropathic conditions contributes to the lack of definitive data on the incidence of these states. Clearly, there is a major need for improvements in the techniques for diagnosis of these conditions. The hope that magnetic resonance imaging (MRI) techniques could be used to diagnose enteropathic conditions has not yet been fully realised though undoubtedly progress could be forthcoming with improvements in the use of imaging agents as well as developments in computational methods to capture images more rapidly (so overcoming problems arising from peristaltic movement). Analysis at higher resolution will no doubt lead to major technical advances in the application of MRI techniques for non-invasive diagnosis of intestinal ulceration as well as IBDs.

A variety of approaches is currently being developed to overcome the problem of GI ulceration from NSAIDs. Ultimately, each of these new drugs or modifications will have to be measured against bench standards, i.e. existing NSAIDs or paracetamol, that show low ulcerogenicity. For example, azapropazone, etodolac, ibuprofen and nabumetone all have lower ulcerogenicity than many of the established NSAIDs (aspirin, indomethacin, piroxicam) [21–23]. While there have been a few reports of azapropazone producing a high frequency of upper GI injury, these are from relatively few cases and, in the case–control matching, the possibility exists that there are high statistical errors from these few cases. Ibuprofen has a low incidence of GI ulceration and is extensively used, but it may be that, being a drug of first choice in treating rheumatic patients, the drug is not taken by patients with more advanced disease who are taking other anti-rheumatic or other drugs that may interact with ibuprofen (or for that matter other comparable NSAIDs), so promoting the risk of GI or other side-effects [21–24].

Among the newer NSAIDs are the COX-2-selective drugs that are intended to selectively inhibit production of prostaglandins in inflamed sites but spare the production of gastric and renal prostaglandins that are necessary for physiological functions and (in the GI tract) mucosal protective mechanisms [25]. We await the results of long-term studies with these new COX-2 selective agents in rheumatic patients with much interest.

The development of so-called nitric oxide (NO)-donating NSAIDs was based on an interesting concept that NO protects against the vascular injury produced by NSAIDs in the mucosa. Chemically, these drugs are butyl nitrate esters of NSAIDs and it is difficult to envisage how NO is produced from the hydrolysis of the butyl nitrate moiety. If, as might be suspected, nitrate is produced, then there could be safety concerns since nitrates are known to be associated with gastric cancer. Also, it is difficult to envisage how the butyl nitrate esters could be superior to simple alkyl or other esters of carboxylate NSAIDs since these are well known to be appreciably less ulcerogenic than the corresponding NSAIDs [22,23]. There is also a puzzling feature why butyl nitrate esters should be advantageous since systemic production of the NSAIDs (from which they are produced) would be expected to show appreciable blood levels of the drug such that the systemic mode of ulceration could occur. Clearly, these and many other questions remain to be answered.

CONCLUSIONS

There are many areas of GI research which require investigation. The field is evolving, exciting and full of new promise and innovation.

REFERENCES

1. Gilinsky NH. Peptic ulcer disease in the elderly. Gastroenterol Clin N Am. 1990;19:255–71.
2. Corinaldesi R, De Giorgio R, Paternicõ A, Stanghellini V. Asymptomatic peptic ulcer disease. Is it worth looking for? Drugs. 1991;41:821–4.
3. Hencerson BE, Ross RK, Pike MC. Toward the primary prevention of cancer. Science. 1991;254:1131–8.
4. Monteiro E, Tavarela Veloso F, eds. Inflammatory bowel diseases. New insights into mechanisms of inflammation and challenges in diagnosis and treatment. Lancaster: Kluwer Academic Publishers; 1995.
5. Walsh JH. Unanswered questions about Helicobacter pylori. Ailment Pharmacol Ther. 1995;9 (Suppl. 1):31–7.
6. Hung RH, Tytgat GNJ, eds. Helicobacter pylori. Basic Mechanisms to Clinical Cure. Dordrecht, Boston, London: Kluwer Academic Publishers; 1994.

7. Matysiak-Budnik T, Megraud F. *Helicobacter pylori* in eastern European countries: what is the current status? Gut. 1994;35:1683–6.
8. Misiewicz JJ. Current insights in the pathogenesis of *Helicobacter pylori* infection. Eur J Gastroenterol Hepatol. 1995;7:701–3.
9. Borén S, Normark S, Falk P. *Helicobacter pylori*: molecular basis for host recognition and bacterial adherence. Trends Microbiol. 1994;2:221–8.
10. Crabtree JE, Taylor JD, Wyatt JI, et al. Mucosal IgA recognition of *Helicobacter pylori* 120kDa protein, peptic ulceration, and gastric pathology. Lancet. 1991;338:332–5.
11. Mazzucchelli L, Wilder-Smith CH, Ruchti C, Meyer-Wyss B, Merki HS. *Gastrospirillum hominis* in asymptomatic, healthy individuals. Dig Dis Sci. 1993;38:2087–9.
12. Taha AS, Russell RI. *Helicobacter pylori* and non-steroidal anti-inflammatory drugs: uncomfortable partners in peptic ulcer disease. Gut. 1993;34:580–3.
13. El-Omar EM, Penman ID, Ardill JES, Chittajallu RS, Howie C, McColl KEL. *Helicobacter pylori* infection and abnormalities of acid secretion in patients with duodenal ulcer disease. Gastroenterology. 1995;109:681–91.
14. Taha AS, Dahill S, Nakshabendi I, Lee FD, Sturrock RD, Russell RI. Duodenal histology, ulceration, and *Helicobacter pylori* in the presence or absence of non-steroidal anti-inflammatory drugs. Gut. 1993;34:1162–6.
15. Sanderson JD. Environmental factors – bacterial infection: Crohn's disease and *Mycobacterium paratuberculosis*. In: Monteiro E, Tavarela Veloso F, eds. Inflammatory bowel diseases. New insights into mechanisms of inflammation and challenges in diagnosis and treatment. Dordrecht, Boston, London: Kluwer Academic Publishers; 1995:86–90.
16. Travis SPL. Mycobacteria on trial: guilty or innocent in the pathogenesis of Crohn's disease? Eur J Gastroenterol Hepatol. 1995;7:1173–6.
17. Jewell DP. Pathogenesis of Crohn's disease: the environment revisited. Eur J Gastroenterol Hepatol. 1995;7:383–4.
18. Sartor RB, Rath HC, Sellon RK. Microbial factors in chronic intestinal inflammation. Curr Opin Gastroenterol. 1996;12:327–33.
19. Farmer RG, Michener WM. Association of inflammatory bowel diseases in families. Front Gastrointest Res. 1986;11:17–26.
20. Satsangi J, Jewell DP. Genetic markers in inflammatory bowel disease. Curr Opin Gastroenterol. 1996;12:322–6.
21. Rainsford KD, Quadir M. Gastrointestinal damage and bleeding from non-steroidal anti-inflammatory drugs. 1. Clinical and epidemiological aspects. Inflammopharmacology. 1995;3:169–90.
22. Rainsford KD. Mechanisms of gastrointestinal toxicity of non-steroidal anti-inflammatory drugs. Scand J Gastroenterol. 1988;24 (Suppl. 163):9–16.
23. Rainsford KD. Mechanisms of gastrointestinal ulceration from non-steroidal anti-inflammatory drugs. In: Rainsford KD, Velo GP, eds. Side-effects of anti-inflammatory drugs – 3. Lancaster: Kluwer Academic Publishers; 1992:97–114.
24. Rainsford KD. Mode of action, uses and side-effects of anti-rheumatic drugs. In: Rainsford KD, ed. Advances in anti-rheumatic therapy. Boca Raton: CRC Press; 1996:59–111.
25. Rainsford KD. Introduction to advances in anti-rheumatic therapy. In: Rainsford KD, ed. Advances in anti-rheumatic therapy. Boca Raton: CRC Press; 1996:1–10.

Section I

GENERAL MECHANISMS OF GASTROINTESTINAL INJURY AND PROTECTION

G Mózsik et al. Cell Injury and Cytoprotection in the GI Tract. 11–24.
© 1997 Kluwer Academic Publishers.

ANALYSES OF PATHOGENIC ELEMENTS INVOLVED IN GASTRIC LESIONS INDUCED BY INDOMETHACIN IN RATS

K. TAKEUCHI*, S. KATO, K. TAKEHARA AND Y. ASADA

Department of Pharmacology and Experimental Therapeutics, Kyoto Pharmaceutical University, Misasagi, Yamashina, Kyoto 607, Japan
*Correspondence

ABSTRACT

Gastric lesions induced by non-steroidal anti-inflammatory drugs (NSAIDs) are considered to involve multiple pathogenic elements, such as deficiency of prostaglandins (PGs), gastric hypermotility, neutrophil activation and luminal acid. The present study was performed to examine the effects of these elements, either alone or in combination, on the rat gastric mucosa and to investigate which element may be most closely associated with gastric ulcerogenic response to NSAID. The following treatments were employed to express various pathogenic elements: a low dose of indomethacin to cause PG deficiency; 2-deoxy-D-glucose (2DG) to induce gastric hypermotility and acid secretion; histamine to induce acid hypersecretion; and n-formyl-Met-Leu-Phe (fMLP) to elicit neutrophil activation. When rats which had been fasted for 18 h were subjected to each treatment alone and killed 4 h later, only 2DG caused slight macroscopic damage in the gastric mucosa. Indomethacin showed over 90% inhibition of the mucosal PG generation, and fMLP increased the myeloperoxidase activity to 4 times greater than normal values, yet neither of these treatments alone caused any damage in the stomach. The combined treatments of indomethacin with 2DG or histamine caused severe lesions in the stomach or the duodenum, respectively, whereas fMLP did not modify or potentiate the mucosal ulcerogenic propensity to other treatments. We conclude that (1) among various pathogenic components both gastric hypermotility and PG deficiency are crucial for induction of gross damage in the rat stomach; gastric hypermotility is by itself sufficient to induce mild damage in the mucosa, while PG deficiency is prerequisite for later extension of damage to severe lesions, and (2) the neutrophil activation alone is not ulcerogenic in the gastric mucosa or does not potentiate the ulcerogenic effect of other elements.

Keywords: indomethacin, gastric lesion, pathogenesis, gastric motility, prostaglandin, neutrophil

INTRODUCTION

Non-steroidal anti-inflammatory drugs (NSAIDs), such as indomethacin, cause haemorrhagic mucosal injury in the stomach of man and experimental animals [1]. The pathogenic mechanisms of these lesions are considered to involve multiple elements, such as deficiency of endogenous prostaglandins (PGs), neutrophil activation, gastric hypermotility, microcirculatory disturbances, oxygen free radicals, and luminal acid [2–8]. However, as these components closely interact with each other, it would be difficult to determine which pathogenic element is of prime importance in the ulcerogenic response to NSAIDs. Indeed, neutrophil activation is caused by alteration of arachidonic acid metabolism, such as PG deficiency [9]; gastric hypermotility leads to microcirculatory disturbance, resulting in enhancement of the neutrophil adherence

This paper was presented at the Symposium on 'Cell injury and protection in the gastrointestinal tract: from basic science to clinical perspectives', October 8–11, 1995, Pécs, Hungary.

to the vascular endothelium [8]; and the production of oxygen radicals is brought about by neutrophil–endothelium cell interaction as well as haemodynamic alterations due to gastric hypermotility [8,10].

In the present study, we employed different treatments to express various pathogenic elements involved in the ulcerogenic response to indomethacin, such as PG deficiency, neutrophil activation, gastric hypermotility and acid secretion, and examined the effect of these treatments, either alone or in combination, on the rat gastric mucosa. We investigated the components which may be most closely associated with the ulcerogenic action of indomethacin in the stomach.

MATERIALS AND METHODS

Male Sprague–Dawley rats, weighing 250–300 g (Charles River, Shizuoka, Japan), were used in all experiments. The animals were kept in individual cages with raised mesh bottoms and deprived of food but allowed free access to tap water for 18 h prior to experiments. All studies were carried out using 4–9 rats under unanaesthetized conditions, unless otherwise specified.

General protocols

Animals were divided into 10 groups as follows: control; indomethacin at 25 mg/kg sc; indomethacin at 5 mg/kg sc; 2-deoxy-D-glucose (2DG; 200 mg/kg + 100 $mg\,kg^{-1}\,h^{-1}$ iv); histamine (8 $mg\,kg^{-1}\,h^{-1}$ iv); n-formyl-Met-Leu-Phe (fMLP; 80 $\mu g\,kg^{-1}\,h^{-1}$ iv); indomethacin plus 2DG; indomethacin plus histamine; fMLP plus 2DG; fMLP plus histamine. In the above treatments, a low dose of indomethacin (5 mg/kg) was used to cause PG deficiency (inhibition of cyclo-oxygenase activity) [5], 2DG to increase both gastric acid secretion and motility [11], histamine to increase acid secretion, and fMLP to activate neutrophils [12]. Indomethacin was given sc as a single injection, while fMLP and histamine were infused iv during a test period. 2DG was first given as a single iv injection (200 mg/kg) followed by a continuous iv infusion (100 $mg\,kg^{-1}\,h^{-1}$). In the combined treatment, indomethacin (5 mg/kg) was given sc 30 min before the onset of iv infusion of 2DG or histamine, while fMLP was continuously infused iv during a test period, starting 30 min before the onset of 2DG or histamine infusion.

Macroscopic evaluation of gastric mucosa

The animals were killed under deep ether anaesthesia 4 h after the various treatments. The stomachs were removed, inflated by injecting 8 ml of 2% formalin, immersed in 2% formalin for 10 min to fix the gastric wall, opened along the greater curvature and examined for lesions under a dissecting microscope with a square grid (× 10). The area (mm^2) of each lesion was measured, summed per stomach and used as a lesion score. The person measuring the lesions did not know the treatments given to the animals.

Measurement of mucosal prostaglandin levels

PG levels in the gastric mucosa were measured 4 h after administration of indometha-cin (5 and 25 mg/kg sc) or the onset of 2DG infusion (200 mg/kg + 100 mg $kg^{-1} h^{-1}$). Under ether anaesthesia, the stomachs were quickly removed, opened along the greater curvature, and rinsed with ice-cold saline. To separate the mucosal layer, the corpus mucosa was placed between two glass slides squeezed with rubber-band and placed in hexane-frozen dry ice and acetone [13]. After the sample was frozen, these glasses were separated, the mucosa was collected, weighed, and put into 5 ml of 100% methanol containing 10^{-4} mol/L sodium meclofenamate to prevent any further formation of PG. After homogenization, each sample was processed for extraction and chromatography of PGs [14], and levels of PGE_2 were determined by radioimmunoassay using rabbit anti-PGE_2 serum.

Measurement of myeloperoxidase activity

Myeloperoxidase (MPO) activity in the gastric mucosa was measured at 4 h after various treatments, according to the method of Castro et al. [15]. Under deep ether anaesthesia, the rats were killed, the stomachs removed, opened along the greater curvature and rinsed with cold saline. The corpus mucosa was separated, weighed and homogenized in phosphate buffer. The homogenized samples were subjected to freeze and thaw three times, and centrifuged at 2000 rpm for 10 min at 4°C. After adding 5 μl of 0.3% H_2O_2 to the supernatant, changes in absorbance at 475 nm of each sample were monitored on a Hitachi recorder (Model 200-100, Mito, Japan) connected to the spectrophotometer. MPO activity (μmol/L H_2O_2 min^{-1}(g protein)$^{-1}$) was obtained from the slope of the reaction curve.

Measurement of gastric motility

Gastric motility was determined using a miniature balloon according to the previously published method [5,8]. Briefly, under ether anaesthesia, the balloon and the support catheter were placed into the stomach through an incision of the forestomach. The animals were kept in Bollman cages, and gastric motility was monitored on a Hitachi recorder (Model 056, Mito, Japan) using a pressure transducer (Narco Telecare, Model 151-T, Houston, TX, USA) and a polygraph device (San-ei, Model 6M-72, Tokyo, Japan) after complete recovery from anaesthesia. After basal motility had stabilized well, the animals were subjected to various treatments, and the motility was measured for 4 h thereafter. Quantitation of gastric motility was performed by measuring the amplitude of each contraction (clear spike) over a 10-min period, determining the mean for this period from these values and by calculating the mean ± SE for each time period from 4–5 different rats.

Determination of acid secretion

Acid secretion was measured in urethane-anaesthetized rats according to the previously published paper [16]. The animals were anaesthetized with urethane (1.25 g/kg ip). An acute gastric fistula prepared by means of a polyethylene tube was implanted in the forestomach. Another polyethylene tube was inserted into the stomach from the pylorus through a slit in the duodenum, and was held in place by a ligature around the pylorus. The stomach was then perfused at a flow rate of 1 ml/min with saline that was gassed with 100% O_2, heated at 37°C and kept in a reservoir. Acid secretion was measured at luminal pH 7.4 using a pH-stat method (Hiranuma Comtite-7, Tokyo, Japan) and by adding 100 mmol/L NaOH to the reservoir.

Preparation of drugs

Drugs used were indomethacin, fMLP (Sigma, St Louis, MO, USA), 2DG, histamine (Nacalai Tesque, Kyoto, Japan), meclofenamate (Warner-Lambert, Tokyo, Japan), urethane (Tokyo Kasei, Tokyo, Japan) and anti-PGE_2 rabbit serum (Pasteur Institute, Marnes, France). Indomethacin and meclofenamate sodium were suspended in saline with a drop of Tween 80 (Wako, Osaka, Japan), while other agents were dissolved in saline. Each agent was prepared immediately before use and given ip or sc in a volume of 0.5 ml per 100 g body weight; iv in a dose of 0.1 ml per 100 g body weight; and infused iv in a volume of 1.2 ml/h.

Statistics

Data are presented as the mean $\pm$ SE from 4–9 rats per group. Statistical analyses were performed using a two-tailed Dunnett's multiple comparison test, and values of $p < 0.05$ were regarded as significant.

RESULTS

Effect of various treatments on gastric and duodenal mucosa

Single treatment

Subcutaneous administration of indomethacin at 25 mg/kg produced multiple lesions in the gastric mucosa within 4 h without any damage in the duodenum. Characteristically, the damage was located parallel to the long axis of the stomach and consisted mostly of haemorrhagic lesions, the lesion score being 23.1 ± 4.7 mm^2. In contrast, a low dose of indomethacin (5 mg/kg sc) did not induce any visible damage in either the stomach or the duodenum (Figure 1). Likewise, any macroscopic damage was not provoked after iv infusion of fMLP (80 μg kg^{-1} h^{-1}) or histamine (8 mg kg^{-1} h^{-1}) for 4 h. On the other hand,

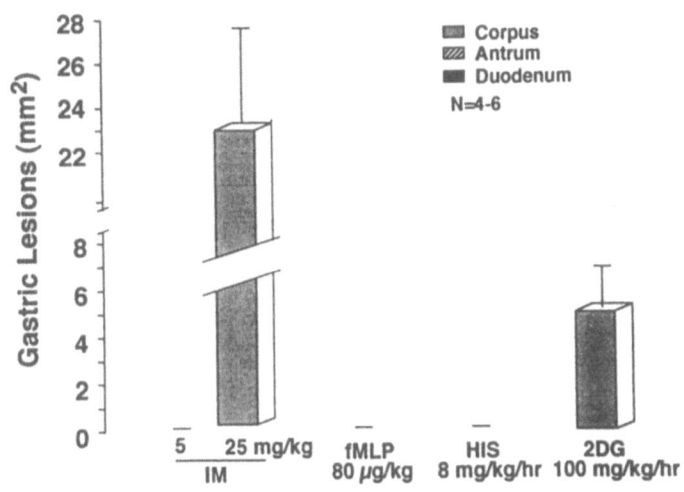

Figure 1. Effects of indomethacin (5 and 25 mg/kg sc), fMLP (80 µg kg^{-1} h^{-1} iv), histamine (8 mg kg^{-1} h^{-1} iv) and 2DG (200 mg/kg + 100 mg kg^{-1} h^{-1} iv) on the rat gastric mucosa. The animals were subjected to the above treatments and were killed 4 h later. Data are presented as the mean $\pm$ SE from 4–6 rats; IM, indomethacin; HIS, histamine

iv infusion of 2DG (200 mg/kg + 100 mg kg^{-1} h^{-1} iv) induced apparent damage in the stomach, the lesion score being 5.4 $\pm$ 1.3 mm^2. The damage induced by 2DG was mostly non-haemorrhagic lesions but localized in the corpus mucosa along the mucosal foldings, similar to the lesions induced by a high dose of indomethacin.

Combination treatment

As shown in Figure 2, the additional treatment of fMLP did not cause any potentiation of the ulcerogenic effect of 2DG in the gastric and duodenal mucosa; some damage was found in the stomach but the severity of the lesions was not significantly different from that caused by 2DG alone. However, in the presence of a low dose of indomethacin, 2DG produced severe haemorrhagic lesions in the same areas of the stomach as observed after treatment with 2DG alone; the damage consisted mostly of haemorrhagic lesions, the lesion score being 29.6 $\pm$ 5.9 mm^2. In this group, some damage was also found in the duodenum, in 2 of 6 animals. On the other hand, when histamine was administered in combination with a low dose of indomethacin, severe haemorrhagic lesions were induced in the duodenum with some damage in the stomach. The lesion score in the duodenum and the stomach was 41.3 $\pm$ 6.2 mm^2 and 8.2 $\pm$ 3.1 mm^2, respectively. The addition of fMLP to histamine, however, did not cause any visible lesions in the stomach or the duodenum.

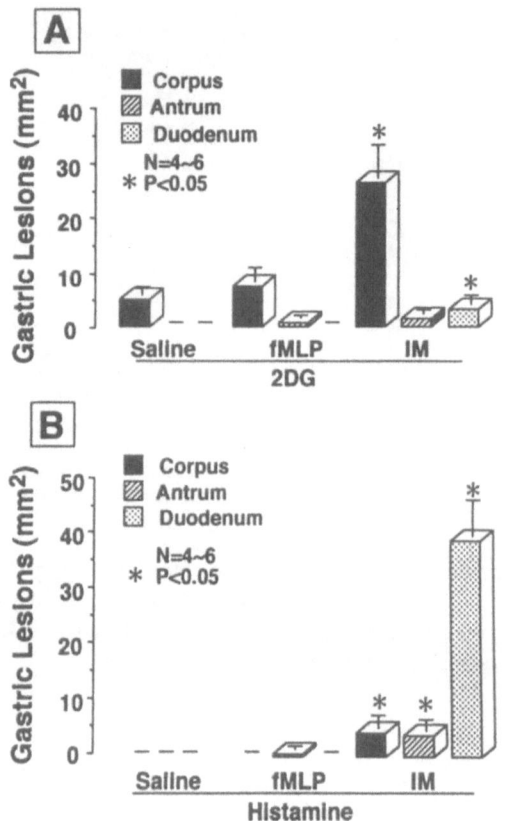

Figure 2. Effects of 2DG (**A**; 200 mg/kg + 100 mg kg^{-1} h^{-1} iv) and histamine (**B**; 8 mg kg^{-1} h^{-1} iv), either alone or in combination with indomethacin (5 mg/kg sc) or fMLP (80 µg kg^{-1} h^{-1} iv), on rat gastric mucosa. The animals were subjected to the above treatments and were killed 4 h later. Data are presented as the mean ± SE from 4–6 rats. *Statistically significant difference from saline, at $p < 0.05$

Effects of various treatments on biochemical aspects and functions in the gastric mucosa

Prostaglandin levels

Levels of PGE$_2$ in the normal rat gastric mucosa were 333.3 ± 41.7 ng/g tissue. Subcutaneous administration of indomethacin significantly reduced the PGE$_2$ levels in the corpus mucosa at both 5 and 25 mg/kg, the inhibition being 93.0% and 94.2%, respectively (Figure 3). Intravenous infusion of 2DG (200 mg/kg + 100 mg kg^{-1} h^{-1}) for 4 h did not significantly alter mucosal PG biosynthesis, and the levels of PGE$_2$ were 419.4 ± 83.9 ng/g tissue, which were not statistically significant from those in control

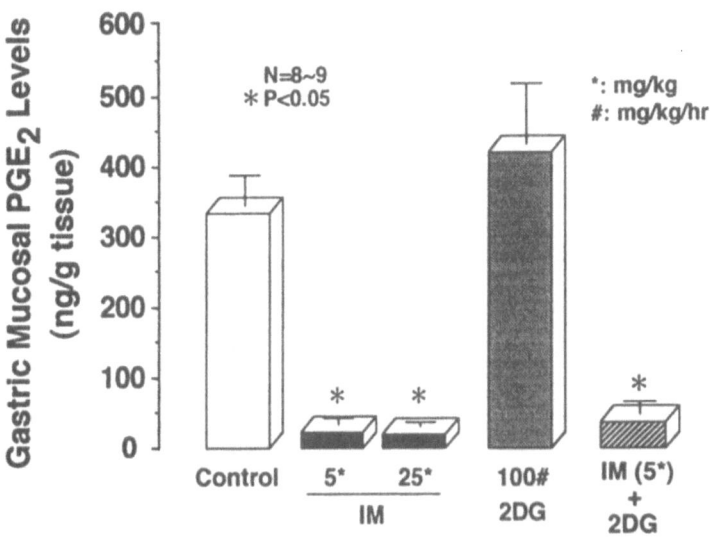

Figure 3. Effects of indomethacin (5 and 25 mg/kg sc) and 2DG (200 mg/kg + 100 mg kg^{-1} h^{-1} iv), either alone or in combination, on mucosal PGE$_2$ levels in rat stomachs. Animals were subjected to the above treatments, and PGE$_2$ levels were measured 4 h after treatment. Values are presented as the mean $\pm$ SE from 8–9 rats per group. *Statistically significant difference from control, at $p < 0.05$

animals. However, the combined treatment of a low dose of indomethacin with 2DG infusion markedly decreased the PGE$_2$ levels to the same degree observed in the animals given indomethacin alone (23.4 $\pm$ 8.3 ng/g tissue).

Myeloperoxidase activity

MPO activity in the normal stomach was 29.6 $\pm$ 8.7 μmol/L H$_2$O$_2$ min^{-1} (g protein)$^{-1}$. As expected, iv infusion of fMLP (40 and 80 μg kg^{-1} h^{-1}) increased MPO activity in a dose-related manner, and, at 80 μg kg^{-1} h^{-1} this activity reached significantly higher levels, the values being 100.2 $\pm$ 22.3 μmol/L H$_2$O$_2$ min^{-1} (g protein)$^{-1}$ (Figure 4). The mucosal MPO activity also responded to iv infusion of 2DG (200 mg/kg + 100 mg kg^{-1} h^{-1}) by a significant increase 4 h after the treatment, but was not significantly changed in response to histamine (8 mg kg^{-1} h^{-1}). On the other hand, sc administration of indomethacin at a low dose (5 mg/kg) did not significantly affect the mucosal MPO activity but, at a high dose (25 mg/kg), significantly increased the MPO activity, reaching values about 6 times greater than basal levels (172.0 $\pm$ 18.5 μmol/L H$_2$O$_2$ min^{-1} (g protein)$^{-1}$.

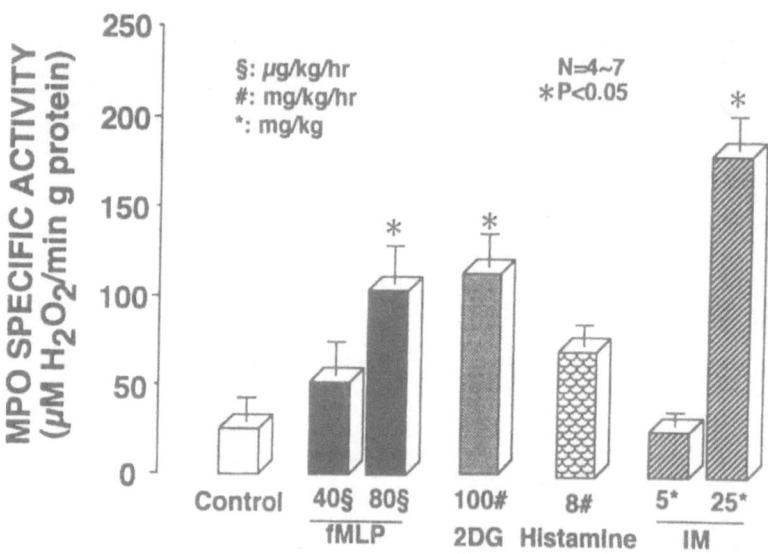

Figure 4. Effects of indomethacin (5 and 25 mg/kg sc), fMLP (40 and 80 $\mu g\,kg^{-1}\,h^{-1}$ iv), 2DG (200 mg/kg + 100 mg $kg^{-1}\,h^{-1}$ iv) and histamine (8 mg $kg^{-1}\,h^{-1}$ iv) on myeloperoxidase (MPO) activity in the rat gastric mucosa. Animals were subjected to the above treatments, and the MPO activity was determined 4 h after treatment. Data are presented as the mean $\pm$ SE from 4–7 rats. *Statistically significant difference from control, at $p < 0.05$

Gastric motility

The stomachs of control animals contracted at a frequency of $10.2 \pm 2.8/10$ min with an amplitude of 16.8 ± 1.9 cm H_2O. Subcutaneously administered indomethacin at 25 mg/kg induced a marked enhancement of gastric motility, whereas, at 5 mg/kg, this agent did not significantly affect the motor activity of the stomach (not shown). The motility also progressively increased after the onset of 2DG infusion (200 mg/kg + 100 mg $kg^{-1}\,h^{-1}$), reached the plateau level 40 min later, and remained elevated thereafter (Figure 5). The enhanced gastric motor activity caused by 2DG was significantly augmented in the presence of a low dose of indomethacin. On the other hand, iv infusion of fMLP (80 $\mu g\,kg^{-1}\,h^{-1}$) alone did not affect gastric motility and did not significantly modify the enhanced motor activity in response to 2DG treatment.

Acid secretion

In normal rat stomachs under urethane anaesthesia, acid secretion was increased in response to histamine (8 mg $kg^{-1}\,h^{-1}$ iv) from 5.3 ± 1.8 $\mu Eq/15$ min to the plateau value of 38.9 ± 6.2 $\mu Eq/15$ min within 75 min and remained elevated during the test period

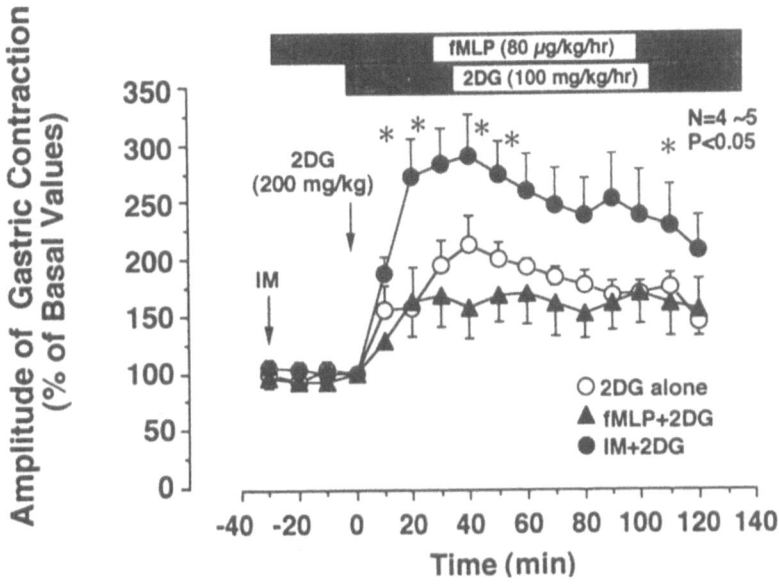

Figure 5. Effects of indomethacin (5 mg/kg sc) and fMLP (80 µg kg^{-1} h^{-1} iv) on gastric motility response induced by 2DG (200 mg/kg + 100 mg kg^{-1} h^{-1} iv) in rats. Gastric motility was measured using a miniature balloon placed in the glandular part of the stomach. Data are expressed as % of basal values and represent the mean ± SE of values determined every 10 min from 4–5 rats. *Statistically significant difference from 2DG alone, at $p < 0.05$

(Figure 6). Intravenous infusion of 2DG (200 mg/kg + 100 mg kg^{-1} h^{-1} iv) also increased acid secretion from 3.6 ± 0.8 µEq/15 min to the maximal values of 16.2 ± 4.8 µEq/15 min within 90 min. Coadministration of indomethacin (5 mg/kg sc) slightly potentiated the acid secretory response to histamine or 2DG but the overall results were not significantly different from those obtained by histamine or 2DG alone. On the other hand, iv infusion of fMLP (80 µg kg^{-1} h^{-1}) by itself had no effect on acid secretion and did not modify the acid secretory response caused by histamine or 2DG.

DISCUSSION

Pathogenesis of gastric lesions induced by NSAIDs such as indomethacin is considered to involve multiple components including PG deficiency, neutrophil activation, gastric hypermotility, and luminal acid [3–8]. In the present study, these pathogenic components involved in the ulcerogenic response to indomethacin were expressed by other means, such as low dose of indomethacin to induce PG deficiency, fMLP to induce neutrophil activation, 2DG to induce gastric hypermotility and acid secretion, and histamine to induce acid hypersecretion, and we examined the effects of these elements, both alone and in combination, on the gastric mucosa.

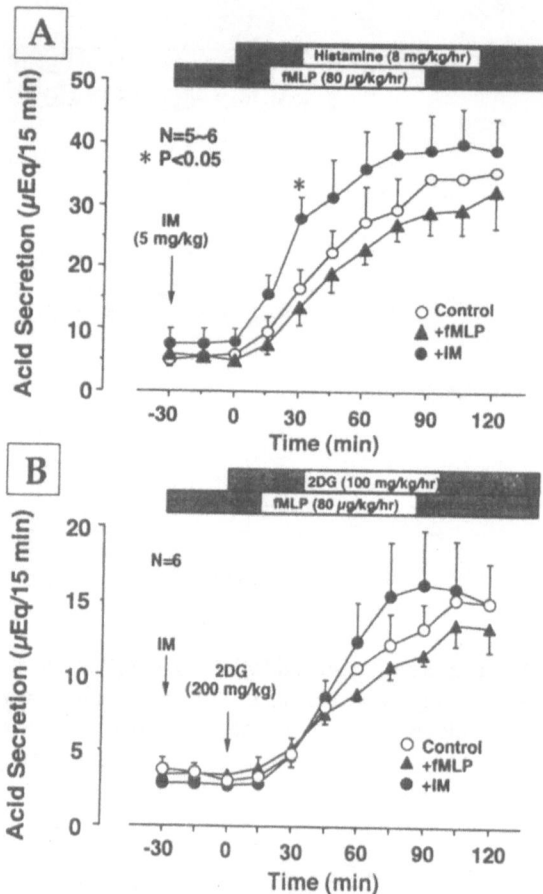

Figure 6. Effects of indomethacin (5 mg/kg sc) and fMLP (80 µg kg^{-1} h^{-1} iv) on acid secretory response induced by 2DG (A; 200 mg/kg + 100 mg kg^{-1} h^{-1} iv) or histamine (B; 8 mg kg^{-1} h^{-1} iv) in anaesthetized rats. Acid secretion was determined in saline-perfused stomachs using pH-stat method and by adding 100 mmol/L NaOH. Data are presented as the mean $\pm$ SE of values determined every 15 min from 6 rats

Firstly, when the animals were given these treatments alone, mild damage was observed only in the case of 2DG treatment. Other treatments, including indomethacin (low dose), fMLP or histamine, did not by themselves cause visible damage to the gastric and duodenal mucosa. These results suggest that either PG deficiency, neutrophil activation or acid secretion alone is not sufficient for induction of gross damage in the gastroduodenal mucosa, but that gastric hypermotility, as induced by 2DG, is by itself sufficient to induce damage in the gastric mucosa. Here, 2DG did not have any effect on mucosal PG biosynthetic activity. Thus, these results with 2DG distinguish the motility effect from PG deficiency and indicate that muscle has a role in the pathogenetic mechanism of indomethacin-induced gastric lesions. In this study, a significant increase in MPO activity was observed 4 h after 2DG treatment, similar to the case after treatment with fMLP which is known to activate neutrophils both *in vivo* and *in vitro* [16]. Garrick et al. [17] reported that high-amplitude contractions during cold–restraint stress results in a temporal restriction of blood flow to the mucosa and decreases mucosal resistance to injury. Yamaguchi [18] monitored gastric mucosal haemodynamics and motility simultaneously and found oscillatory changes in the haemodynamics during gastric hypercontraction induced by water-immersion stress. Indomethacin at an ulcerogenic dose also induced oscillatory changes in mucosal blood flow associated with gastric hypercontraction [8]. In addition, such microcirculatory disturbances are known to enhance neutrophil adhesion to the vascular endothelium [9]. Thus, the increase in MPO activity caused by 2DG may be secondary to gastric hypermotility changes and is not a cause of lesion induction during 2DG treatment.

Secondly, when the above pathogenic elements were combined, severe haemorrhagic lesions were observed mainly in the stomach after 2DG treatment in the presence of a low dose of indomethacin and in the duodenum after histamine treatment in the presence of a low dose of indomethacin. Gastric mucosal damage induced by 2DG was markedly potentiated and became haemorrhagic in the presence of a low dose of indomethacin, which, by itself, had little or no effect on acid secretion or gastric motility, and did not induce any visible damage in the stomach. This dose of indomethacin (5 mg/kg), however, reduced mucosal PG levels to the same extent as an ulcerogenic dose (25 mg/kg), resulting in PG deficiency in the gastric mucosa. These findings, together with our previous paper [11] led to the inference that PG deficiency may be strongly associated with the process by which damage develops into haemorrhagic lesions. On the other hand, it is well known that PG deficiency causes duodenal HCO_3^- secretory impairment and induces duodenal damage in the presence of acid hypersecretion [19]. The present results with histamine are in agreement with our previous paper demonstrating the induction of duodenal lesions induced by indomethacin plus histamine [19]. In addition, these results also suggest that the pathogenic elements involved in duodenal lesions are different from those in gastric lesions. As shown in this study, histamine induces acid hypersecretion without any effect on gastric motility, and 2DG induces gastric hypermotility and acid secretion. It is assumed that the pathogenesis of gastric mucosal lesions may be associated more closely with gastric motility than with acid secretion.

Neutrophil infiltration into a tissue as reflected by MPO activity is a hallmark of inflammation. Neutrophils have been implicated as culprits in the damage associated with NSAIDs [6,7]. These cells are recruited to a site of injury by the chemotoxins and participate in amplifying the inflammatory response by releasing several chemotoxins and by producing further tissue injury through the release of reactive oxygen metabolites. Many studies, including ours, show that gastric lesions induced by NSAIDs are prevented by decreasing the number of neutrophils by antineutrophil serum or by inhibiting the neutrophil–endothelium cell interaction with a monoclonal antibody against the CD18 adhesion molecule [6–8]. In the present study, however,

TABLE 1
Summary of effects of treatments on various parameters

	Lesion		PG	Motility	Acid Secretion	MPO Activity
	Stomach	Duodenum				
Indomethacin (IM) (5 mg/kg)	–	–	↓	–	–	–
2-Deoxy-D-Glucose (2DG) (200 mg/kg + 100 mg/kg/hr)	+	–	–	↑↑	↑↑	↑
Histamine (His) (8 mg/kg/hr)	–	–	–	–	↑↑	–
fMLP (80 µg/kg/hr)	–	–	NT	–	–	↑↑
2DG + IM	++++	+	↓	↑↑	↑↑	↑
2DG + fMLP	+	–	NT	↑↑	↑↑	↑↑
His + IM	+	++++	↓	–	↑↑	–
His + fMLP	–	–	NT	–	↑↑	↑↑

In this study, indomethacin (5 mg/kg) was used to inhibit cyclo-oxygenase activity, 2DG to induce gastric hypermotility and acid hypersecretion, histamine to induce acid hypersecretion, and fMLP to induce neutrophil activation.

–, absence; +, slight damage; ++++, severe damage; ↓, decrease; ↑, slight increase; ↑↑, marked increase; NT, not tested. The shaded areas indicate changes in various parameters associated with development of gastric or duodenal lesions

additional treatment with fMLP did not cause any macroscopically visible lesions in the presence of histamine nor did it modify the ulcerogenic effect of 2DG. Even the combined treatment of fMLP plus a low dose of indomethacin did not cause any damage in the gastroduodenal mucosa. The dose of fMLP is sufficient to cause neutrophil activation and increase mucosal MPO activity to several times greater than normal levels. On the basis of these results, it is assumed that the co-existence of neutrophil activation with other elements, except gastric motility, is not sufficient to induce gross damage in the stomach. These results are, in part, consistent with the recent findings by Santucci et al. [20] who showed that although G-CSF (granulocyte colony stimulating factor) markedly increased MPO activity, it significantly prevented indomethacin-induced gastric lesions, and suggested that no relationship exists between MPO activity and ulcerogenic response. Because indomethacin at an ulcero-genic dose induces the sequential events at the early stage of lesion formation during gastric hypercontraction, the microcirculatory disturbances due to abnormal mucosal compression of the gastric wall, followed by lipid peroxidation and increased vascular permeability [8], the neutrophil-related events may be involved in these processes associated with gastric hypermotility. Indeed, the increase in MPO activity as well as lesion formation induced by the ulcerogenic dose of indomethacin were prevented when the enhanced gastric motility response was inhibited by atropine [8,21].

In conclusion, the present results taken together with previous studies [5,8,1] suggest that, among various pathogenic elements, both gastric hypermotility and PG deficiency are crucial for induction of gross damage in the rat stomach; gastric hypermotility is by itself sufficient to induce damage in the mucosa, while PG deficiency may be a prerequisite for later extension of damage to haemorrhagic lesions; and neutrophil activation alone is not ulcerogenic in the gastric mucosa and does not potentiate the ulcerogenic effect of other factors (Table 1).

REFERENCES

1. Robert A. Prostaglandins and the gastrointestinal tract. In: Johnson LR, Cristensen J, Grossman MI, Jacobson ED, Shuktz SG, eds. Physiology of the Gastrointestinal Tract. New York: Raven Press; 1981:1407–34.
2. Whittle BJR. Temporal relationship between cyclooxygenase inhibition, as measured by prostacyclin biosynthesis, and the gastrointestinal damage induced by indomethacin in the rat. Gastroenterology. 1981;80:94–8.
3. Mersereau WA, Hinchey EJ. Role of gastric mucosal folds in formation of focal ulcers in the rat. Surgery. 1982;91:150–5.
4. Takuechi K, Ueki S, Okabe S. Importance of gastric motility in the pathogenesis of indomethacin-induced gastric lesions in rats. Dig Dis Sci. 1986;31:1114–21.
5. Ueki S, Takeuchi K, Okabe S. Gastric motility is an important factor in pathogenesis of indomethacin-induced gastric mucosal lesions in rats. Dig Dis Sci. 1988;33:209–16.
6. Wallace JL, Keeman CM, Granger DN. Gastric ulceration induced by non-steroidal anti-inflammatory drugs is a neutrophil-dependent process. Am J Physiol. 1990;259:G462–7.
7. Wallace JL, Granger DN. Pathogenesis of NSAID gastropathy; are neutrophils the culprits? Trends Pharmacol Sci. 1992;13:129–31.
8. Takeuchi K, Ueshima K, Hironaka Y, Fujioka Y, Matsumoto J, Okabe S. Oxygen free radicals and lipid peroxidation in the pathogenesis of gastric mucosal lesions induced by indomethacin in rats. Digestion. 1991;49:175–84.
9. Asaka H, Kubes P, Wallace JL, Granger DN. Indomethacin-induced leukocyte adhesion in mesenteric venules; role of lipoxygenase products. Am J Physiol. 1992;262:G903–8.
10. Grisham MB, Hernandez LA, Granger DN. Xanthin oxidase and neutrophil infiltration in intestinal ischemia. Am J Physiol. 1986;251:G567–74.
11. Okada M, Niida H, Takeuchi K, Okabe S. Role of prostaglandin deficiency in pathogenetic mechanism of gastric lesions induced by indomethacin in rats. Dig Dis Sci. 1989;34:694–702.
12. Perianin A, Gaudry M, Marquetty C. Protective effect of indomethacin against chemotactic deactivation of human neutrophils induced by formylated peptide. Biochem Pharmacol. 1988;37:1693–8.
13. Arakawa T, Nakamura H, Chono S, Yamada H, Kobayashi K. Prostaglandin E_2 in the rat gastric mucosa; establishment of assay procedure and effects of non-steroidal anti-inflammatory compounds. Jpn J Gastroenterol. 1980;77:8–15.
14. Orcyk GP, Berhrnam HR. Ovulation blockade by aspirin or indomethacin; in vitro evidence for a role of prostaglandins in gonadotropin secretion. Prostaglandins. 1972;1:3–20.
15. Castro GA, Roy SA, Stockstill RD. Trichinella spiralis: peroxidase activity in isolated cells from the rat intestine. Exp Parasit. 1974;36:307–15.
16. Takeuchi K, Ohuchi T, Okabe S. Endogenous nitric oxide in gastric alkaline response in the rat stomach after damage. Gastroenterology. 1994;106:367–74.
17. Garrick T, Buack S, Bass P. Gastric motility is a major factor in cold–restraint-induced lesion formation in rats. Am J Physiol. 1986;250:G191–9.
18. Yamaguchi T. Relationship between gastric mucosal hemodynamics and gastric motility. Jpn J Gastroenterol. 1989;25:299–305.

19. Takeuchi K, Furukawa O, Tanaka H, Okabe S. A new model of duodenal ulcers induced in rats by indomethacin plus histamine. Gastroenterology. 1986;90:636–45.
20. Santucci L, Fiorucci S, Di Matteo FM. Role of tumor necrosis factor α release and leukocyte margination in indomethacin-induced gastric injury in rats. Gastroenterology. 1995;108:393–401.
21. Takeuchi K, Takehara K, Okabe S. Analyses of pathogenic elements involved in gastric lesions induced by nonsteroidal antiinflammatory drugs in rats. Gastroenterology (Abstract). 1995;106:A-917.

G Mózsik et al. Cell Injury and Cytoprotection in the GI Tract. 25–32.

NO-NSAID: A NOVEL CLASS OF ANTI-INFLAMMATORY DRUGS WITH REDUCED GASTROINTESTINAL AND RENAL TOXICITY

P. DEL SOLDATO[1*], G. CIRINO[2] AND J.L. WALLACE[3]

[1]NicOx Ltd, London, UK; [2]Department of Experimental Pharmacology, via Domenico Montesano 49, 80131 Naples, Italy; [3]Department of Pharmacology and Therapeutics, University of Calgary, Calgary, Alberta, T2N 4N1, Canada
*Correspondence

ABSTRACT

While non-steroidal anti-inflammatory drugs remain among the most widely used medications, their long-term use is associated with significant adverse effects, such as gastric ulceration, bleeding and perforation, as well as in increased risk of bleeding from pre-existing peptic ulcers. Several strategies have been taken to develop NSAIDs that are less toxic. Many such strategies have failed to make a significant impact on NSAID-related adverse effects. Two new approaches have been taken recently which show great promise. One is based on producing selective inhibitors of inducible cyclo-oxygenase that have been shown to spare the gastrointestinal tract. A second approach is the linking of standard NSAIDs to a nitric-oxide-releasing moiety. The studies so far conducted on this class of compounds have shown greatly reduced gastrointestinal toxicity. Here we report on the experimental evidence so far published on the good tolerability of this class of compounds in the stomach and kidney.

Keywords: cyclo-oxygenase, nitric oxide, kidney damage, gastrointestinal damage, non-steroidal anti-inflammatory drugs

Non-steroidal anti-inflammatory drugs (NSAIDs) are among the most commonly used drugs [1]. They are prescribed mainly for their anti-inflammatory and analgesic properties but are also used in over-the-counter preparations for their antipyretic effects with the only exception of aspirin that is also used for its antithrombotic effect [2]. However, NSAID use is limited by their significant untoward effects on the gastrointestinal tract [3] and, to a lesser extent, the kidneys [4]. Like the beneficial effects of NSAIDs, the gastric and renal toxicity is mainly related to the ability of these agents to suppress prostaglandin synthesis, through inhibition of the enzyme cyclo-oxygenase [5]. Prostaglandins play an important role in the gastrointestinal tract in that they mediate several components of the mucosal defence, such as blood flow, mucus, bicarbonate secretion and mucosal immunocyte function. In the kidney, prostaglandins play an important role in modulating flow, particularly in individuals with renal or hepatic impairment.

Recently, it has been shown that neutrophils have a role in the pathogenesis of NSAID-induced gastric injury [6]. Indeed, it has been suggested that interactions between neutrophils and the vascular endothelium are critical in the genesis of mucosal injury, and represent a potential target for gastroprotective drugs [7]. NSAIDs can promote adhesive interactions between neutrophils and endothelium by suppressing endothelial production of prostacyclin, a potent inhibitor of neutrophil activation and

---

This paper was presented at the Symposium on 'Cell injury and protection in the gastrointestinal tract: from basic science to clinical perspectives', October 8–11, 1995, Pécs, Hungary.

adherence [8,9]. On the other hand, endothelial nitric oxide may counteract the effects of suppression of prostacyclin synthesis by NSAIDs and therefore prevent the development of mucosal injury.

Over the past few decades, a number of strategies have been taken to reduce gastrointestinal injury caused by NSAIDs. These include coating the NSAIDs to prevent absorption in the stomach, parenteral administration, and formulation of pro-drugs that require hepatic metabolism for the cyclo-oxygenase activity to be unmasked. Modifications of this type have not yet been proven to have a significant impact on the incidence of severe adverse reactions to NSAIDs [10]. Recently, two novel approaches have been taken to develop NSAIDs that are devoid of adverse effects in the gastrointestinal tract and kidney. One approach is the development of selective inhibitors of the inducible form of cyclo-oxygenase (COX) namely COX-2 [11]. Another approach is based on the linking of a nitric-oxide-releasing moiety to an NSAID [12].

This chapter will focus on the latter approach and give an update of the more recent experimental evidence.

NITRIC-OXIDE-RELEASING NSAIDs

Based on the evidence suggesting that reduced gastrointestinal blood flow and activation of neutrophils play critical roles in the pathogenesis of NSAID-induced gastric injury, and on the observations that nitric oxide is capable of increasing gastric blood flow, inhibiting neutrophil adherence and protecting the gastric mucosa against damage induced by an irritant, we have proposed that the inclusion of a nitric-oxide-releasing moiety into the structure of NSAIDs would reduce their toxicity. Moreover, if this derivatization did not interfere with the ability of the NSAID to suppress COX activity, then all the beneficial effects of the NSAIDs should be retained. We have tested this hypothesis by using nitric-oxide-releasing derivatives of flurbiprofen, ketoprofen and diclofenac (Figure 1) obtained by inserting a nitroxybutylester group on the carboxyl group. We will refer to this class of compounds as NO-NSAIDs.

ANTI-INFLAMMATORY ACTIVITY

The anti-inflammatory activities of diclofenac, flurbiprofen, ketoprofen and their nitrated derivatives, nitrofenac, nitroflurbiprofen and nitroketoprofen, have been tested in the rat carrageenin paw oedema test. All three NO-NSAIDs retained their anti-inflammatory activity in this test [13–15]. Figure 2 shows the effect of nitrofenac, diclofenac and of a dimeric form of diclofenac in which there is another molecule of diclofenac in the place of the NO-releasing moiety (Figure 1). As can be seen, nitrofenac and diclofenac were equally active in this test. However, when esterification on the carboxyl group was carried out by using another molecule of diclofenac, the anti-inflammatory activity was strongly diminished. Furthermore, nitrofenac and diclofenac are equally active in a model of chronic inflammation [16].

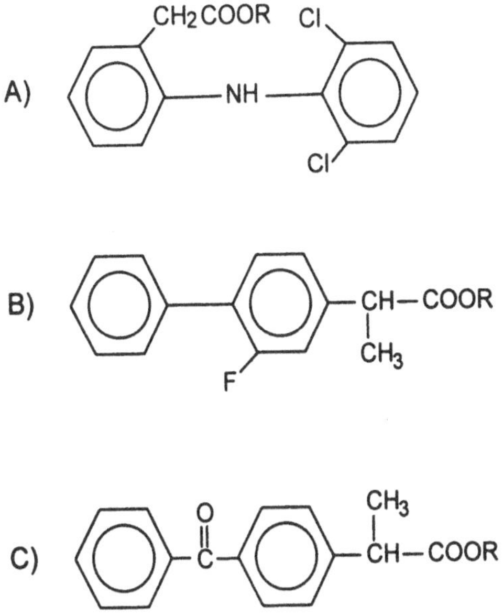

Figure 1. Structure of diclofenac (A), flurbiprofen (B) and ketoprofen (C). Nitrofenac, nitroflurbiprofen and nitroketoprofen were obtained by inserting a nitroxybutylester group, $R = (CH_2)_4-ONO_2$. The dimeric form of diclofenac is obtained by inserting another molecule of diclofenac in R

ANTITHROMBOTIC ACTIVITY

An enhanced antithrombotic activity has been described for nitrofenac and nitro-flurbiprofen [14,17]. Indeed, both drugs are able to inhibit human or rabbit platelet aggregation induced by thrombin or collagen in vitro significantly more actively than the parent compounds. Both NO-NSAIDs, when tested in a rat in-vivo model of platelet aggregation, produced more activity than diclofenac and flurbiprofen, respectively [14,17]. Indeed, both derivatives were able to reduce, in a dose-dependent manner, platelet aggregation induced by collagen more effectively than the parent drugs. This increased activity has been shown to be related to increased release in vivo of nitrite, which did not produce any change in systemic blood pressure in anaesthetized rats [13,14].

GASTROINTESTINAL DAMAGING PROPERTIES

Gastrointestinal damaging properties of nitrofenac, nitroflurbiprofen and nitroketoprofen have been evaluated in comparison with the parent drugs in a model of gastric mucosal injury. Drugs were administered to rats fasted overnight, and, 5 h later, the rats were killed and the extent of haemorrhagic gastric damage was evaluated. All three NO-NSAIDs caused no damage to the gastric mucosa while the parent drugs

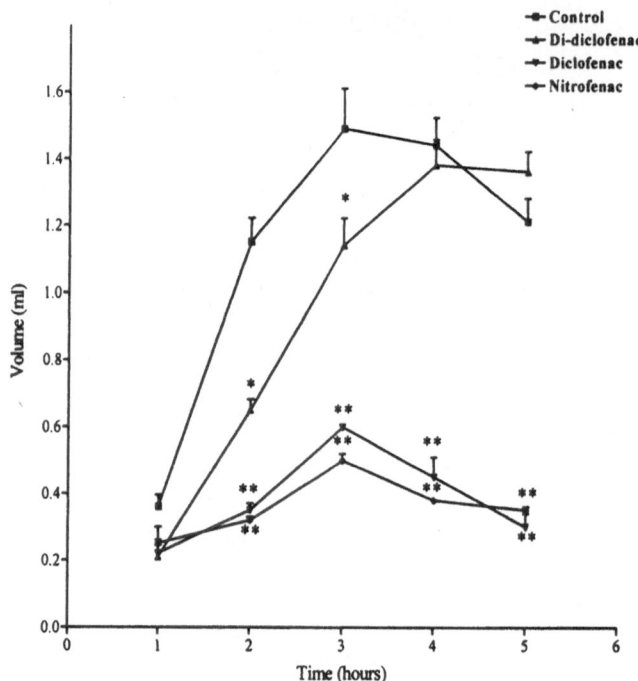

Figure 2. Effect of diclofenac, nitrofenac and di-diclofenac on rat carrageenan paw oedema. Asterisks denote significant differences between treated groups versus the control group ($*p < 0.05$, $**p < 0.001$). Nitrofenac and diclofenac were not significantly different. However, both compounds were significantly different from di-diclofenac at 3, 4 and 5 hours ($p < 0.001$)

produced significant damage [13–15]. In order to determine whether the effect was due to lack of effect of NO-NSAIDs on COX, pieces of the corpus region of gastric mucosa were excised, after the damage was scored, and incubated in vitro for determination of prostaglandin E_2 biosynthetic capacity. All three NO-NSAIDs inhibited production of PGE_2 to the same extent [13–15] implying that NO-NSAIDs have a reduced gastrointestinal toxicity but keep their anti-inflammatory properties and potency.

As we have already mentioned, there is compelling evidence for a role of neutrophils in the pathogenesis of experimental NSAID gastropathy and it is now clear that NSAID-induced leucocyte adherence could contribute to gastric mucosal injury. A reduction of gastric blood flow following NSAID administration has been reported by many groups [18–20] and it has been shown to occur after the appearance of 'white thrombi' in the gastric circulation [19]. Administration of flurbiprofen elicits significant leucocyte adherence to mesenteric postcapillary venules in vivo in the rat within 30 min of its administration. Conversely, nitroflurbiprofen does not induce significant adherence. Interestingly, in rats that received nitroflurbiprofen, there was a significant increase in vessel diameter of $16.6 \pm 5.4\%$ with no change in systemic blood pressure [13].

RENAL TOXICITY

While standard NSAIDs reduce gastric blood flow, NO-NSAIDs do not [13]. Thus, it seems possible that NO-NSAIDs may also have a sparing effect on renal blood flow. We have therefore examined the effect of systemic administration of an NSAID (diclofenac) vs an NO-NSAID (nitrofenac) on renal blood flow in both healthy and cirrhotic rats. Renal blood flow was measured by laser Doppler flowmetry. The left kidney of anaesthetized rats was exposed, covered with plastic film to prevent desiccation, then the laser Doppler was positioned such that it was in contact with the outside surface of the kidney. Basal blood flow was recorded for 15 min, then either diclofenac (20 mg/kg) or nitrofenac (30 mg/kg, equimolar doses) were administered intravenously ($n = 6$–8 per group). Systemic arterial blood pressure was recorded throughout the experiment. In a separate group of experiments, rats received diclofenac or nitrofenac, as above, or vehicle and were anaesthetized 30 min later. A blood sample was drawn from the descending aorta for determination of blood thromboxane A_2 synthesis, using a sensitive and specific ELISA assay for TXB_2. The data derived from these experiments provide evidence of bioavailability of the two drugs, and confirmation of their effects on cyclo-oxygenase activity.

Cirrhosis was induced by bile duct ligation, with the experiments being performed 28 days later. Only rats with histologically proven cirrhosis of the liver were used in the experiments. Control rats received a sham operation. Experiments identical to those described above were then performed. Neither diclofenac nor nitrofenac significantly affected systemic arterial blood pressure at any time in the experiments, in either healthy or cirrhotic rats. However, diclofenac did have significant effects on renal blood flow. As shown in Figure 3, diclofenac administration to healthy rats resulted in a steady decline in renal blood flow which reached a maximum at the 30-min point. Renal blood flow gradually recovered to basal levels over the final 30 min of the experiment. It should be noted that the measurement of blood thromboxane synthesis confirmed that nitrofenac and diclofenac had equivalent effects on cyclo-oxygenase activity, each reducing thromboxane synthesis by 75% compared with vehicle-treated rats. Diclofenac also produced a significant decrease in renal blood flow in the cirrhotic rats. As shown in Figure 4, blood flow decreased within minutes of administration of diclofenac, being significantly depressed at both the 15- and 30-min points. On the other hand, renal blood flow was preserved in the nitrofenac-treated group. Indeed, renal blood flow increased significantly above basal levels during the final 15 min of the experiments, although this was not associated with any significant change in systemic blood pressure. These studies demonstrate that, in acute studies in both healthy and cirrhotic rats, a standard NSAID causes a significant decrease in renal blood flow. Conversely, an NO-releasing NSAID derivative (nitrofenac), while still significantly inhibiting systemic cyclo-oxygenase activity, did not decrease renal blood flow. These effects were observed despite a lack of effect on systemic blood pressure.

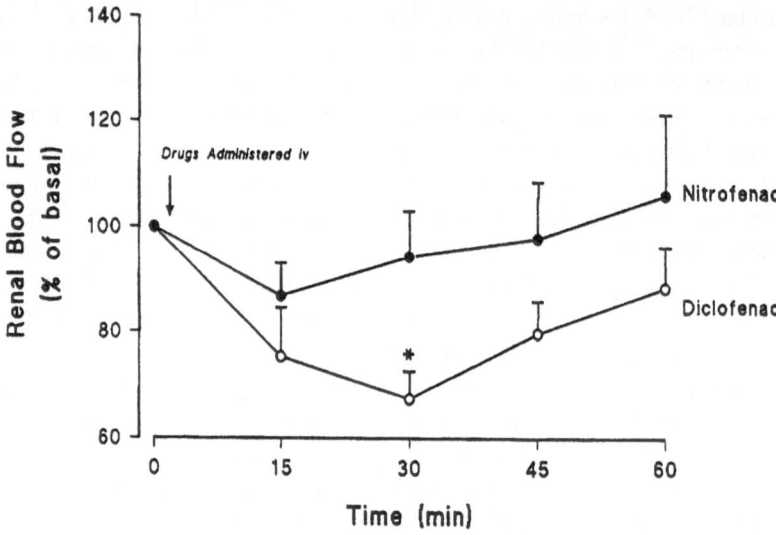

Figure 3. Renal blood flow in healthy rats. Asterisks denote significant differences between the two groups (*$p < 0.05$)

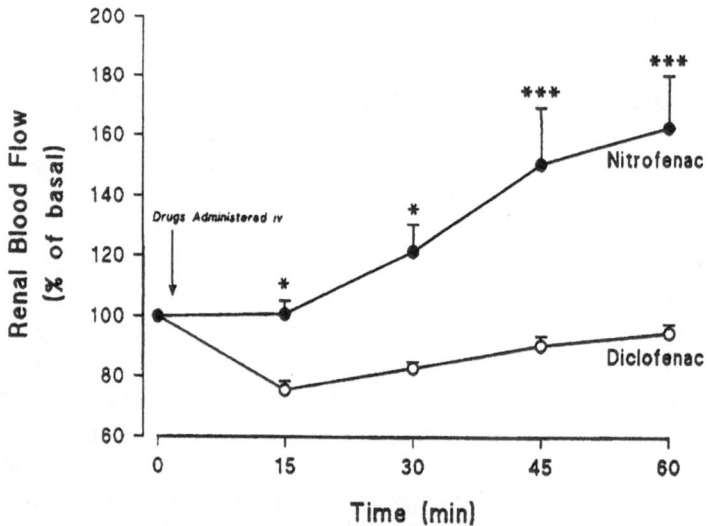

Figure 4. Renal blood flow in rats with secondary biliary cirrhosis. Asterisks denote significant differences between the two groups (*$p < 0.05$, ***$p < 0.001$)

CONCLUSIONS

The addition of a nitroxybutylester group to flurbiprofen, ketoprofen and diclofenac markedly reduces their ulcerogenic properties without altering their effectiveness as anti-inflammatory agents or cyclo-oxygenase inhibitors. Therefore, the NO-NSAIDs represent a novel class of compounds which retain the desired effect of the parent NSAID but produce markedly less toxicity in the gastrointestinal tract. Furthermore, here we have shown experimental data suggesting that these compounds may spare renal blood flow. Unlike selective inhibitors of COX-2, the NO-NSAIDs are capable of inhibiting platelet thromboxane synthesis and, therefore, platelet aggregation. For these reasons, the NO-NSAIDs may represent an alternative to existing anti-inflammatory NSAIDs. Indeed, due to their reduced gastrointestinal and renal toxicity, they could be used in therapy where normal NSAIDs, even though producing beneficial effects, are limited by their untoward effects.

REFERENCES

1. Garner A. Adaptation in the pharmaceutical industry, with particular reference to gastrointestinal drugs and diseases. Scand J Gastroenterol. 1992;27:83–9.
2. Patrono C. Aspirin as an antiplatelet drug. N Engl J Med. 1994;107:173–9.
3. Soll AH, Weinstein WM, Kurata J, McCarthy D. Nonsteroidal anti-inflammatory drugs and peptic ulcers diseases. Ann Intern Med. 1991;114:307–19.
4. Segasothy M, Samad SA, Zulfigar A, Bennet WM. Chronic renal diseases and papillary necrosis associated with long-term use of nonsteroidal anti-inflammatory drugs as the sole predominant analgesic. Am K Kidney Dis. 1994;24:17–24.
5. Vane JR. Inhibition of prostaglandin synthesis as a mechanism of action of aspirin-like drugs. Nature New Biol. 1971;231:232–5.
6. Wallace JL, Granger DN. The pathogenesis of NSAID gastropathy – are neutrophils the culprits? Trends Pharmacol Sci. 1992;13:129–31.
7. Wallace JL. Gastric ulceration: critical events at the neutrophil–endothelium interface. Can J Physiol Pharmacol. 1993;71:98–102.
8. Wallace JL, Keenan CM, Granger DN. Gastric ulceration induced by non steroidal anti-inflammatory drugs is a neutrophil-dependent process. Am J Physiol. 1990;259:G462–7.
9. Wallace JL, Afors K-E, McKnight GW. A monoclonal antibody against the CD18 leukocyte adhesion molecule prevents indomethacin-induced gastric damage in the rabbit. Gastroenterology. 1991;100:878–83.
10. Graham DY. The relationship between nonsteroidal anti-inflammatory drug use and peptic ulcer disease. Gastroenterol Clin N Am. 1990;19:171–82.
11. Vane JR, Botting RM. New insights into the mode of action of anti-inflammatory drugs. Inflamm Res. 1995;44:1–10.
12. Wallace JL, Cirino G. Gastrointestinal-sparing NSAIDs on the horizon? Trends Pharmacol Sci. 1995;15:405–6.
13. Wallace JL, Reuter B, Cicala C, McKnight W, Grisham MB, Cirino G. Novel nonsteroidal anti-inflammatory drug derivatives with markedly reduced ulcerogenic properties in the rat. Gastroenterology. 1994;107:173–9.
14. Wallace JL, Reuter B, Cicala C, McKnight W, Grisham MB, Cirino G. A diclofenac derivative without ulcerogenic properties. Eur J Pharmacol. 1994;257:249–55.
15. Reuter BK, Cirino G, Wallace JL. Markedly reduced intestinal toxicity of a diclofenac derivative. Life Sci. 1994;55:PL1–8.
16. Cuzzolin L, Conforti A, Donini M, Adami A, Del Soldato P, Benoni G. Effects of intestinal microflora, gastrointestinal tolerability and antiinflammatory efficacy of diclofenac and nitrofenac in adjuvant arthritic rats. Pharmacol Res. 1994;29:89–97.

17. Cirino G, Cicala C, Mancuso F, Baydoun AR, Wallace JL. Flurbinitroxybutylester: a novel antiin-flammatory drug has enhanced antithrombotic activity. Thromb Res. 1995;79:73–81.
18. Ashley SW, Sonnenschein LA, Cheung LY. Focal gastric mucosal blood flow at the site of aspirin-induced ulceration. Am J Surg. 1985;149:53–9.
19. Kitahora T, Guth PH. Effect of aspirin plus hydrochloric acid on the gastric mucosal microcirculation. Gastroenterology. 1987;93:810–17.
20. Gana TJ, Huhlewych R, Koo J. Focal gastric mucosal blood flow in aspirin-induced ulceration. Ann Surg. 1987;205:399–403.

GASTRIC MUCOSAL PREVENTIVE EFFECTS OF PROSTACYCLIN AND β-CAROTENE, AND THEIR BIOCHEMICAL EFFECTS IN RATS TREATED WITH ETHANOL AND HCl AT DIFFERENT DOSES AND TIME INTERVALS AFTER ADMINISTRATION OF NECROTIZING AGENTS

Gy. MÓZSIK*, O.M.E. ABDEL-SALAM, B. BÓDIS, O. KARÁDI, Á. KIRÁLY, G. SÜTŐ, Gy. RUMI, I. SZABÓ AND Á. VINCZE
First Department of Medicine, Medical University of Pécs, Ifjúság út, H-7643 Pécs, Hungary
*Correspondence

This paper was first published in: Inflammopharmacology. 1996;4:361–378.

ABSTRACT

Prostacyclin (PGI$_2$) and β-carotene have a key role in gastric mucosal defence against endogenous or exogenous noxious agents. Prostacyclin has appreciable protective effects on the gastrointestinal (GI) mucosa, while β-carotene (as one of the retinoid compounds) has oxyradical scavenging properties.

Aims: The aims of these studies were to evaluate the biochemical mechanisms involving energy metabolism of:

1. Gastric mucosal damage affected by oral administration of 0.6 mol/L HCl (representing an acid-dependent model) and 96% ethanol (EtOH) (as a non-acid-dependent model);

2. PGI$_2$-induced (ED$_{50}$ = 5 μg/kg po) and β-carotene-induced (ED$_{50}$ = 1 mg/kg po) gastroprotection on the gastric mucosal damage produced by HCl and EtOH at different times and doses.

Methods: Sprague–Dawley rats were used. After 24 h starvation (with tap water ad libitum), gastric mucosal damage was induced by oral administration of 1 ml 0.6 mol/L HCl or 96% EtOH. Rats were pretreated with oral saline, PGI$_2$ (5 and 50 μg/kg) and β-carotene (1 and 10 mg/kg) and killed at 0, 1, 5, 15, 30 and 60 min after administration of the necrotizing agents. The number and severity of gastric mucosal lesions, measurement of adenosine triphosphate (ATP), adenosine diphosphate (ADP), adenosine monophosphate (AMP), lactate (enzymatically), and cyclic adenosine monophosphate (cAMP) by RIA were carried out at different time intervals after the necrotizing agents were administered. The ratio of ATP/ADP, adenylate pool (ATP+ADP+AMP) and 'energy charge' [(ATP+0.5 ADP)/(ATP+ADP+AMP)] were calculated.

Results: The results showed that:

1. The mucosal damage (number and severity) reached about 50% of that obtained 60 min after administration of the necrotizing agents in both models;

This paper was presented at the Symposium on 'Cell injury and protection in the gastrointestinal tract: from basic science to clinical perspectives', October 8–11, 1995, Pécs, Hungary.

2. PGI$_2$ prevented in the early period (0–15 min), while β-carotene inhibited in the later period (15–60 min) the gastric mucosal damage produced by EtOH and HCl;

3. The ATP–ADP transformation was decreased in the first (early; 0–15 min) by PGI$_2$ and in the late period (15–60 min) by β-carotene;

4. ATP–cAMP transformation was increased in the early period by PGI$_2$ and in the late phase by β-carotene;

5. No significant change was obtained in the 'energy charge' and lactate by PGI$_2$ or β-carotene administration;

6. The changes in adenine nucleotides were the same in the EtOH or HCl models with and without treatment with PGI$_2$ and β-carotene; however, the mucosal protective action of PGI$_2$ and β-carotene, and the energy metabolism, differed significantly dependent on dose and time after administration of EtOH and HCl.

Conclusions:

1. The development of gastric mucosal damage and its prevention can be discriminated into early and late phases;

2. The early phase of gastric mucosal damage can be prevented by PGI$_2$, and the late phase by β-carotene;

3. The β-carotene effect only partly depends on its presumptive scavenging properties; and

4. PGI$_2$ prevents the development of gastric mucosal damage, while β-carotene stimulates the repair mechanisms.

Keywords: acid-dependent gastric ulcer; non-acid-dependent gastric ulcer; prostacyclin; β-carotene; cellular energy systems; early and late phase of gastric mucosal damage; repair mechanisms

INTRODUCTION

Peptic ulcer disease (PUD) is a common disorder affecting about 10% of the total population. The disorder is heterogeneous since drugs (non-steroidal anti-inflammatory drugs, reserpine, etc.), chemicals (weak acids, alcohol, etc.) and different diseases (such as chronic pulmonary obstruction, liver cirrhosis, Zollinger–Ellison syndrome, etc.) are all involved in its aetiology [1–6]. Further, in about 80% of patients with PUD, no obvious cause can be found and this is referred to as 'genuine ulcer'.

In spite of the considerable research in humans and in animal models to evaluate the possible mechanisms of peptic ulcer disease, the precise aetiology is still poorly understood. In animal models, gastric mucosal damage can be induced in a very short time (1 h) by the application of different chemicals, such as concentrated ethanol (96%), acid (0.6 mol/L HCl), 2 mol/L NaOH and concentrated saline (25% NaCl) [2]. Mucosal damage reaches about 50% of the 1 h value after administration of necrotizing agents. The changes in gastric mucosal biochemistry (obtained before and after macroscopic appearance of mucosal damage) might give an explanation for its development (0–15 min) and for the insufficient recovery (15–60 min).

In the present study, the mucosal protective effects of PGI$_2$ and β-carotene were examined in both acid-dependent (0.6 mol/L HCl) and non-acid-dependent (96% EtOH) gastric ulcer models. The PGI₂- and β-carotene-induced changes of gastric mucosa were evaluated at various doses and times after administration of necrotizing agents. Prostacyclin represents the mucosal protecting natural agent, while β-carotene is a typical nutritional compound having scavenging properties [7–14].

MATERIALS AND METHODS

The experiments were performed on male CFY Sprague–Dawley rats, weighing 180–210 g body weight. The animals were fasted for 24 h before the experiments but allowed tap water freely.

The studies were initiated at 8.00 am according to the protocol illustrated in Figure 1. The gastric mucosal damage was produced by oral administration of 1 ml of 96% ethanol or 0.6 mol/L HCl. The control animals received 1 ml of saline or oleum helianthin orally before the administration of the necrotizing agents. PGI₂ (Chinoin, Budapest; 5 and 50 µg/kg, po) and β-carotene (Hoffmann La Roche, Geneva; 1 and 10 mg/kg, po) were given 30 min before administration of the necrotizing agents. PGI₂

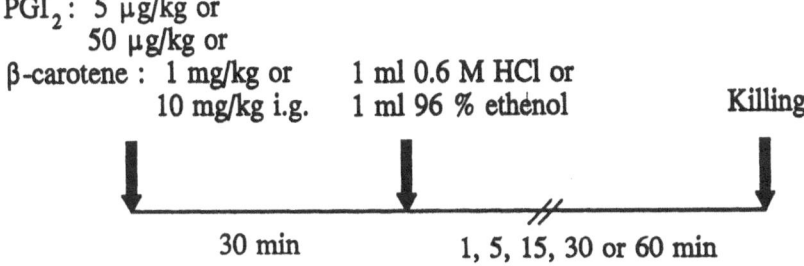

Measurement:
- number of mucosal lesions,
- severity of mucosal lesions,
- ATP, ADP, AMP level of mucosa (enzymatically measured),
- cAMP (by RIA),
Calculations of:
- ATP / ADP ratio,
- Adenylate pool (ATP+ADP+AMP),
- "Energy charge" (ATP+0.5ADP) / (ATP+ADP+AMP)

Figure 1. Experimental protocol used for evaluation of the PGI₂- and β-carotene-induced gastric mucosal protection in rats treated with ethanol (EtOH) and HCl

was dissolved in physiological saline (untreated rats received saline) or oleum helianthin (untreated rats received the oleum helianthi). The protective agents (PGI$_2$ or β-carotene) or their vehicles (saline or oleum helianthi) were given in 1 ml volume 30 min before administration of the necrotizing agents. The animals were sacrificed at 0, 1, 5, 15, 30 and 60 min after administration of EtOH and HCl, when the number and severity of gastric mucosal lesions were noted and tissue levels of ATP, ADP, AMP, cAMP and lactate were measured from the total homogenate of the scraped gastric mucosa. The protein was measured by the method of Lowry et al. [15].

The ratio of ATP/ADP, adenylate pool (ATP+ADP+AMP) and 'energy charge' [(ATP+0.5 ADP)/((ATP+ADP+AMP)] [16] were calculated. The ATP, ADP, AMP were expressed as nmol/mg protein, cAMP as pmol/mg protein and lactate as mmol/mg protein (mean ± SEM). The ulcer severity was calculated using a semiquantitative scale [3].

Statistical methods

The unpaired Student's t-test was applied for the statistical analysis of the data on the number of mucosal lesions and changes in adenine nucleotides. Mann–Whitney test was used for statistical evaluation of changes in ulcer severity. Comparisons were made between:

1. Results obtained in ethanol- and HCl-treated rats at time 0 min vs. different times (control group) (denoted by +);

2. Results obtained at the same time of measurement between untreated (pathological control) vs. treated groups (denoted by *)

The results were taken to be significant when the $p < 0.05$.

RESULTS

The number and severity of gastric mucosal lesions induced by 96% ethanol and 0.6 mol/L HCl were reduced by PGI$_2$ at an early time (0–15 min), and by β-carotene at a later time (15–60 min) after administration of the necrotizing agents (Figures 2–5).

The tissue levels of ATP were decreased 15 min after administration of EtOH (Figure 6) or HCl (Figure 7), followed by a progressive increase up to 60 min. Prostacyclin further decreased the tissue level of ATP in both models compared with ethanol alone, while β-carotene increased its level (Figures 6 and 7).

The gastric mucosal ADP was higher, compared with the control, in the early (0–15 min) phase; thereafter, it increased in the late period (15–60 min) dose-related in both EtOH- and HCl-treated rats produced by PGI$_2$. No similar changes were found in these models after β-carotene treatment (Figures 8 and 9).

The ratio of ATP/ADP decreased after PGI$_2$ administration, while its value was

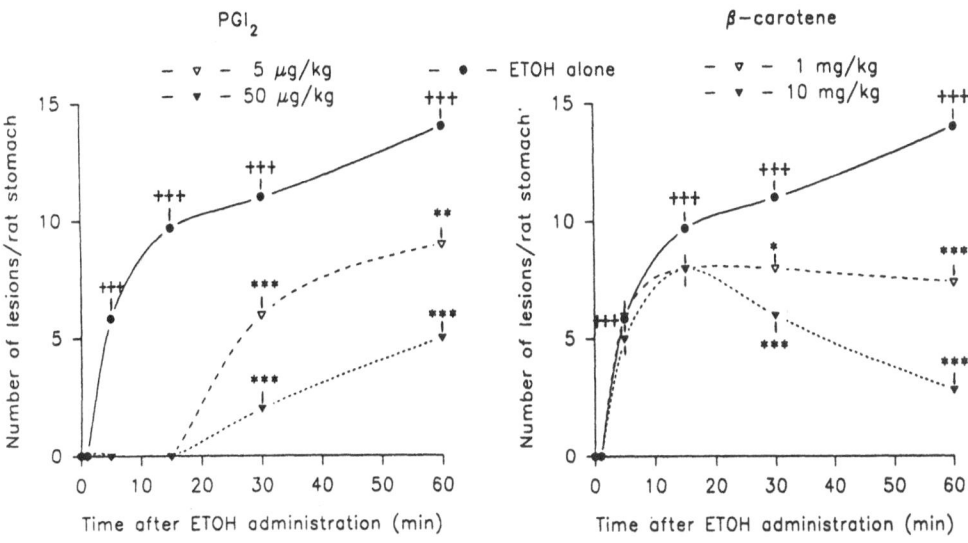

Figure 2. PGI₂-induced (5 and 50 µg/kg ig) and β-carotene-induced (1 and 10 mg/kg ig) decrease in number of ethanol-induced (96%, 1 ml ig) gastric mucosal lesions, related to dose and time after ethanol administration. The results are expressed as means ± SEM, n = 12. Statistical analyses were carried out (*left*) between results obtained after administration of necrotizing agents at 0 min (control) vs. results at different times (denoted by +), and (*right*) between the results in untreated (pathological control) and treated (PGI₂ and β-carotene) groups at the same time (denoted by *) p values: + or * = p < 0.05; ++ or ** = p < 0.01; +++ or *** = p < 0.001

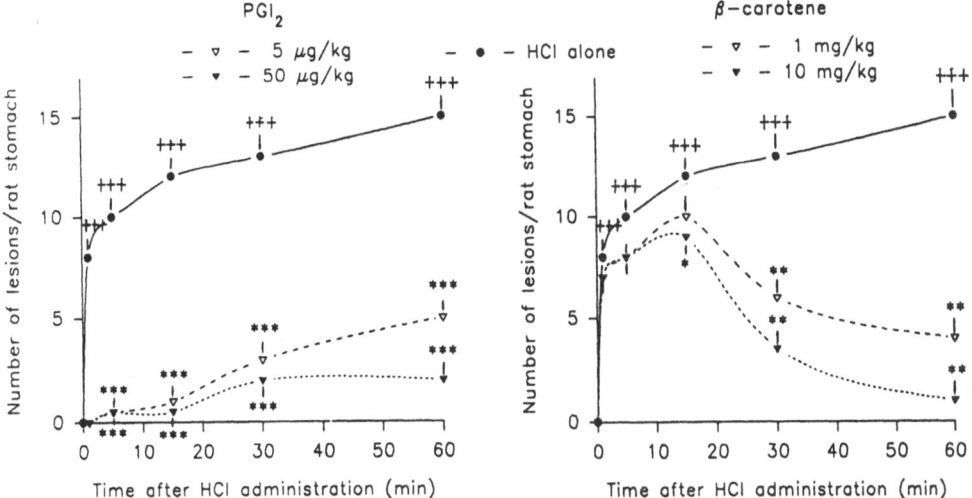

Figure 3. PGI₂-induced (5 and 50 µg/kg ig) and β-carotene-induced (1 and 10 mg/kg ig) decrease in the number of HCl-induced gastric mucosal lesions related to dose and time after HCl administration. See Figure 1 for further explanation

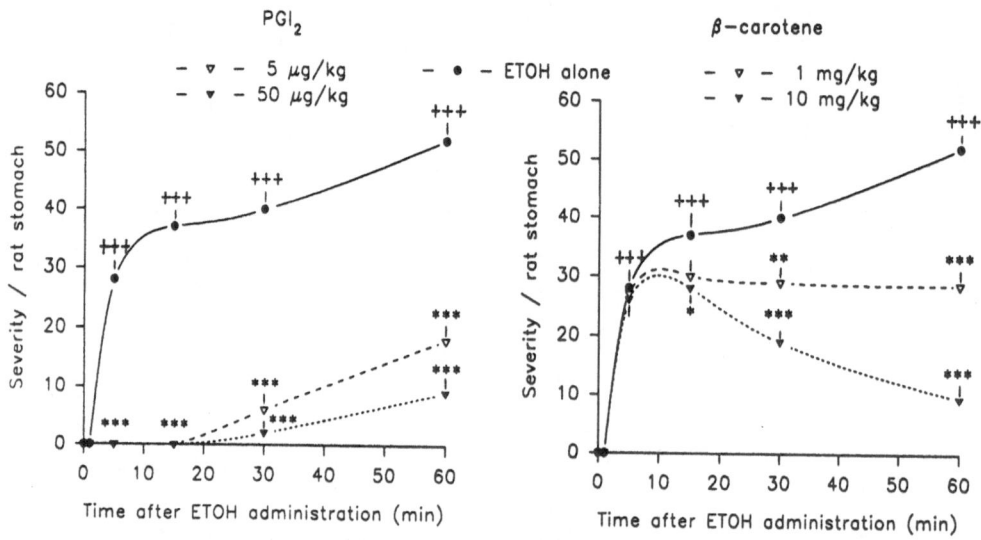

Figure 4. PGI₂-induced (5 and 50 μg/kg ig) and β-carotene-induced (1 and 10 mg/kg ig) decrease in the severity of EtOH-induced gastric mucosal damage in relation to dose and time after EtOH administration. See Figure 1 for further explanation

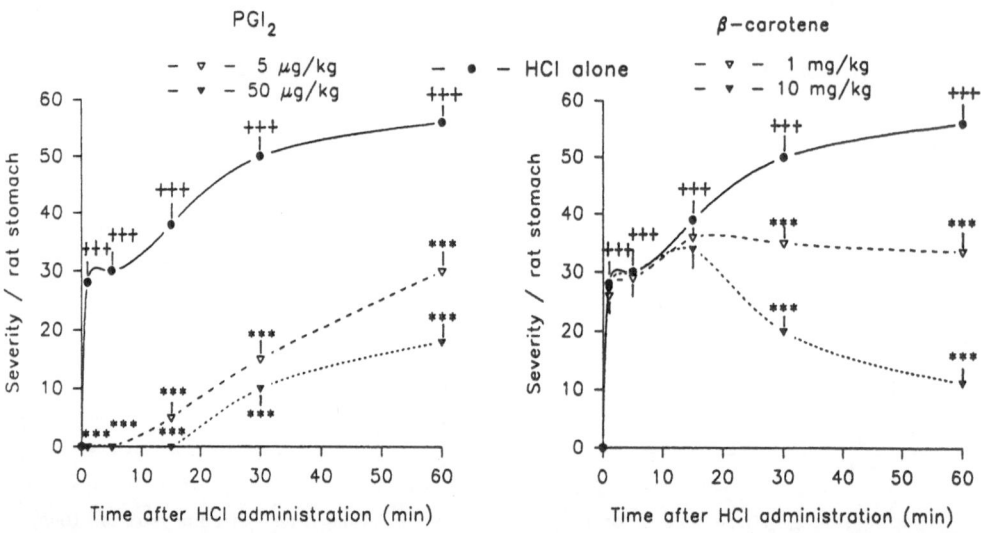

Figure 5. PGI₂-induced (5 and 50 μg/kg ig) and β-carotene-induced (1 and 10 mg/kg ig) decrease in the severity of HCl-induced gastric mucosal damage in relation to dose and time after HCl administration. See Figure 1 for further explanation

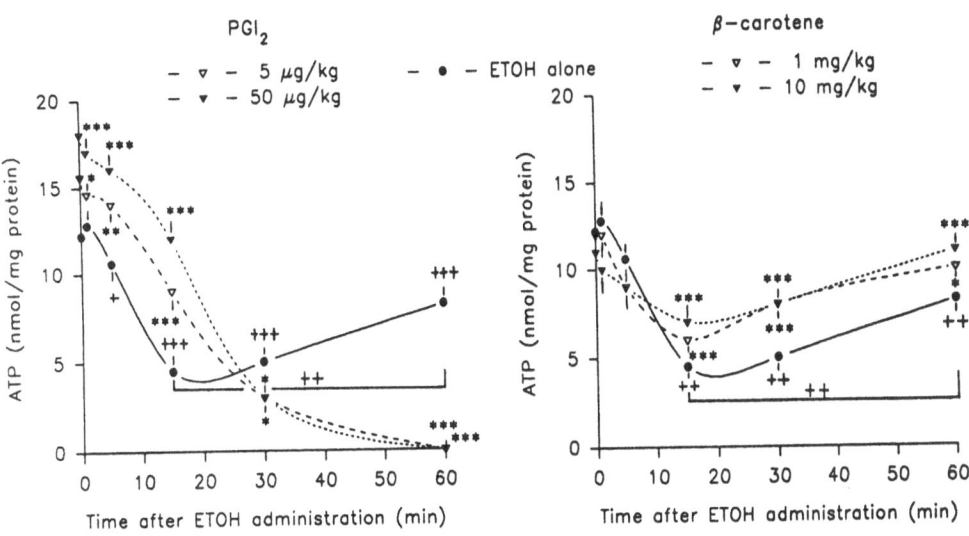

Figure 6. PGI₂-induced (5 and 50 µg/kg ig) and β-carotene-induced (1 and 10 mg/kg ig) changes in the gastric mucosal ATP of EtOH-treated rats in relation to dose and time after EtOH administration. See Figure 1 for further explanation

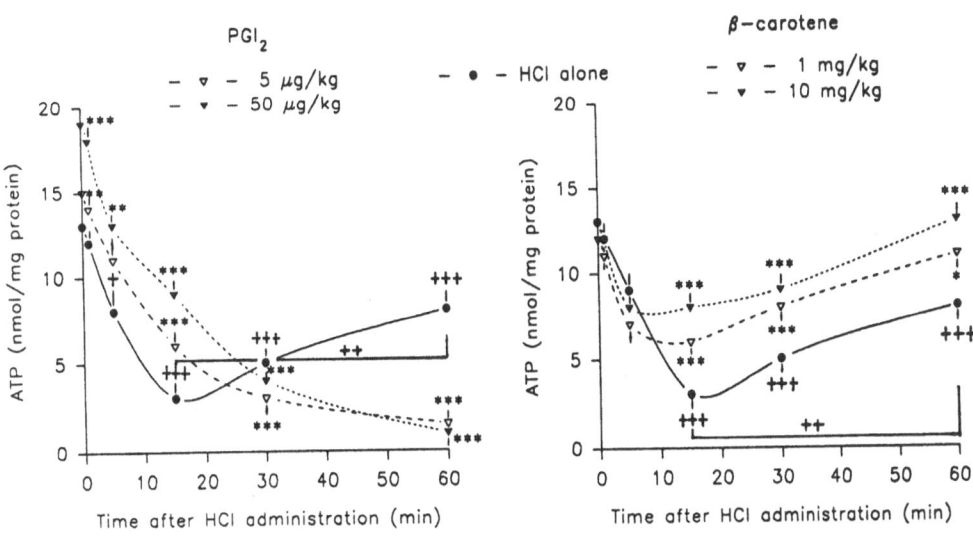

Figure 7. PGI₂-induced (5 and 50 µg/kg ig) and β-carotene-induced (1 and 10 mg/kg ig) changes in the gastric mucosal ATP of HCl-treated rats in relation to dose and time after HCl administration. See Figure 1 for further explanation

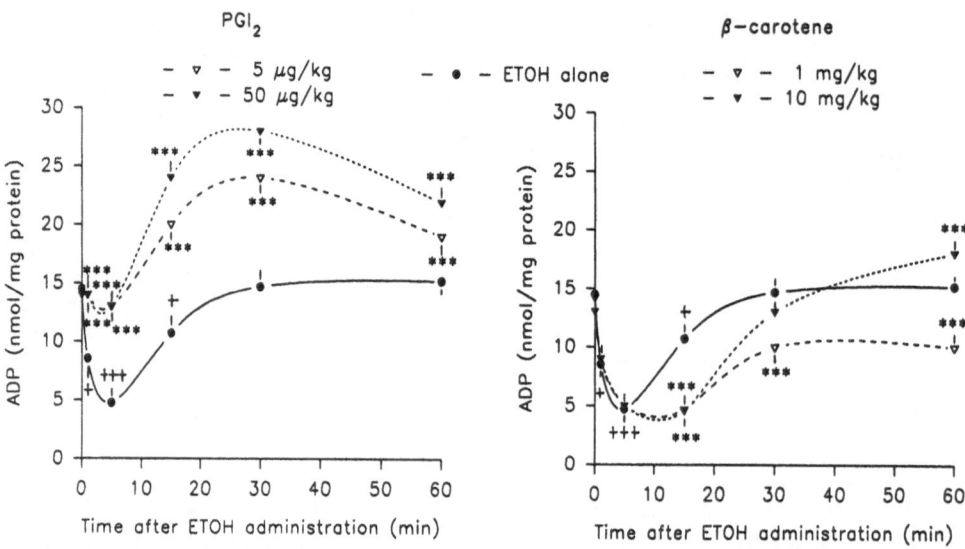

Figure 8. PGI₂-induced (5 and 50 µg/kg ig) and β-carotene-induced (1 and 10 mg/kg ig) changes in the gastric mucosal ADP of EtOH-treated rats in relation to dose and time after EtOH administration. See Figure 1 for further explanation

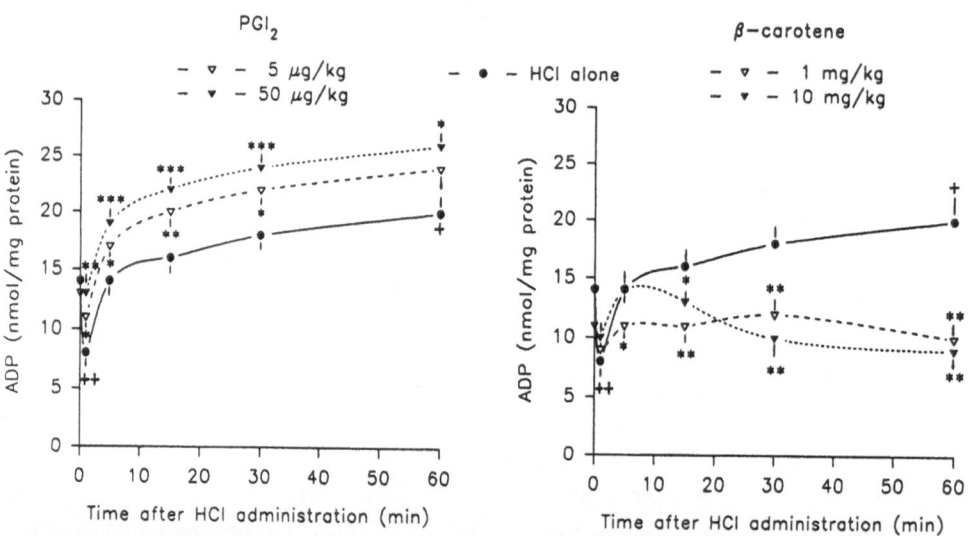

Figure 9. PGI₂-induced (5 and 50 µg/kg ig) and β-carotene-induced (1 and 10 mg/kg ig) changes in the gastric mucosal ADP of HCl-treated rats in relation to dose and time after EtOH administration. See Figure 1 for further explanation

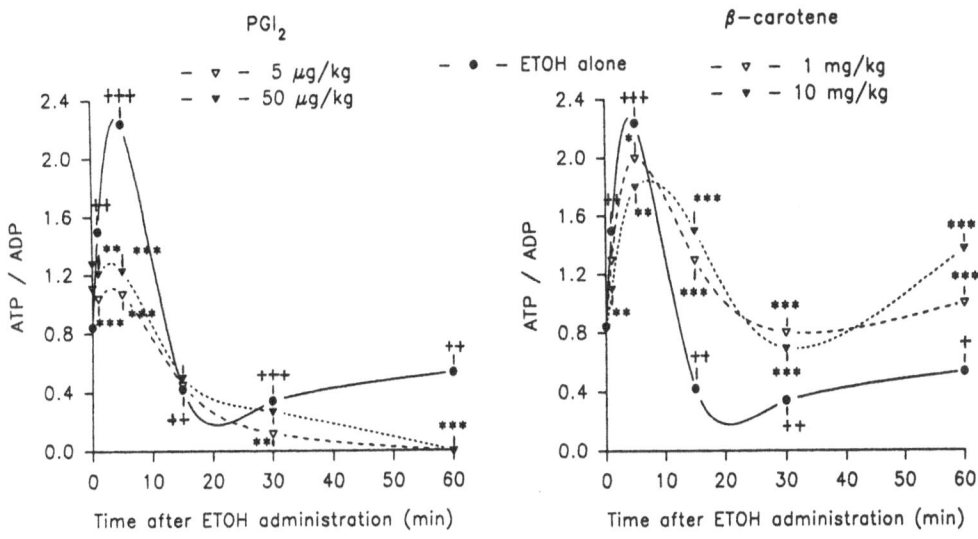

Figure 10. PGI₂-induced (5 and 50 μg/kg ig) and β-carotene-induced (1 and 10 mg/kg ig) changes in the gastric mucosal ATP/ADP of EtOH-treated rats in relation to dose and time after EtOH administration. See Figure 1 for further explanation

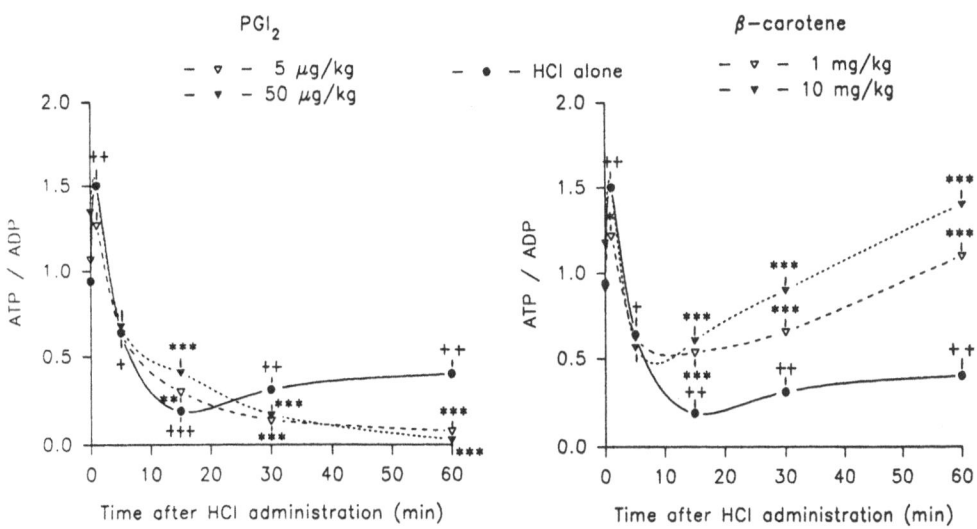

Figure 11. PGI₂-induced (5 and 50 μg/kg ig) and β-carotene-induced (1 and 10 mg/kg ig) changes in the gastric mucosal ATP/ADP of HCl-treated rats in relation to dose and time after HCl administration. See Figure 1 for further explanation

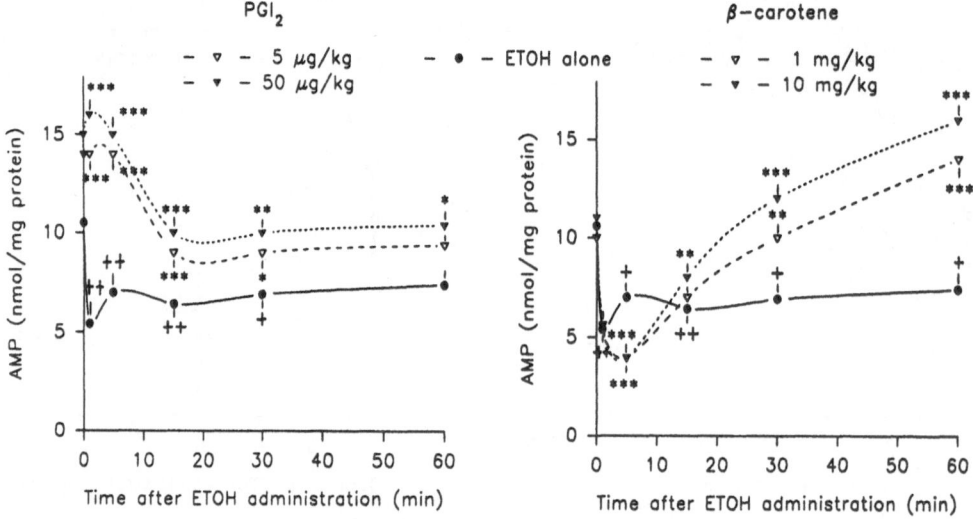

Figure 12. PGI$_2$-induced (5 and 50 µg/kg ig) and β-carotene-induced (1 and 10 mg/kg ig) changes in the gastric mucosal AMP of EtOH-treated rats in relation to dose and time after EtOH administration. See Figure 1 for further explanation

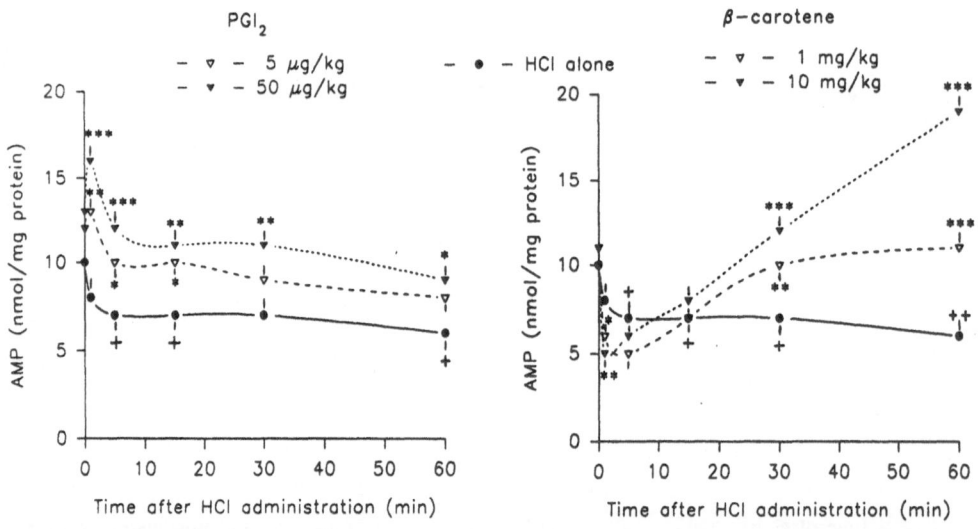

Figure 13. PGI$_2$-induced (5 and 50 µg/kg ig) and β-carotene-induced (1 and 10 mg/kg ig) changes in the gastric mucosal AMP of HCl-treated rats in relation to dose and time after HCl administration. See Figure 1 for further explanation

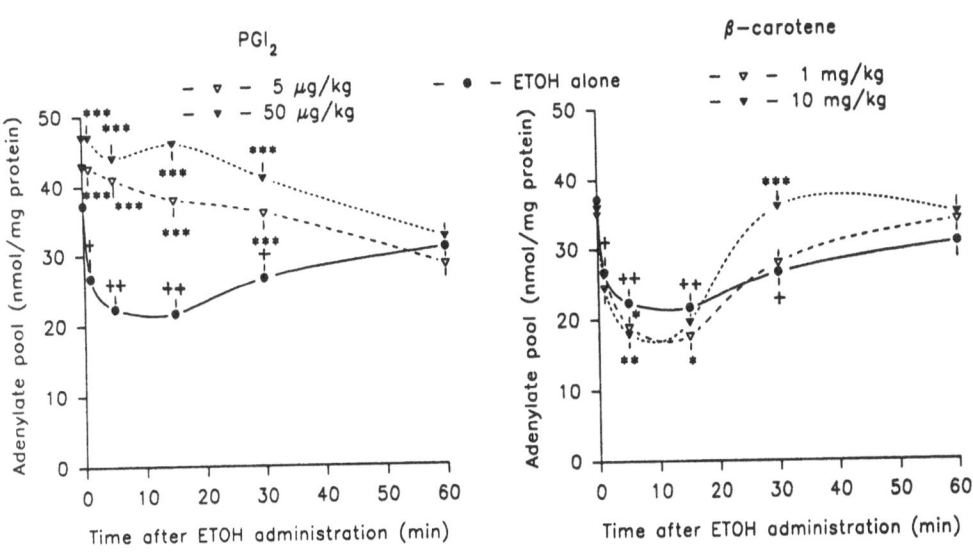

Figure 14. PGI₂-induced (5 and 50 µg/kg ig) and β-carotene-induced (1 and 10 mg/kg ig) changes in the gastric mucosal adenylate pool (ATP+ADP+AMP) of EtOH-treated rats in relation to dose and time after EtOH administration. See Figure 1 for further explanation

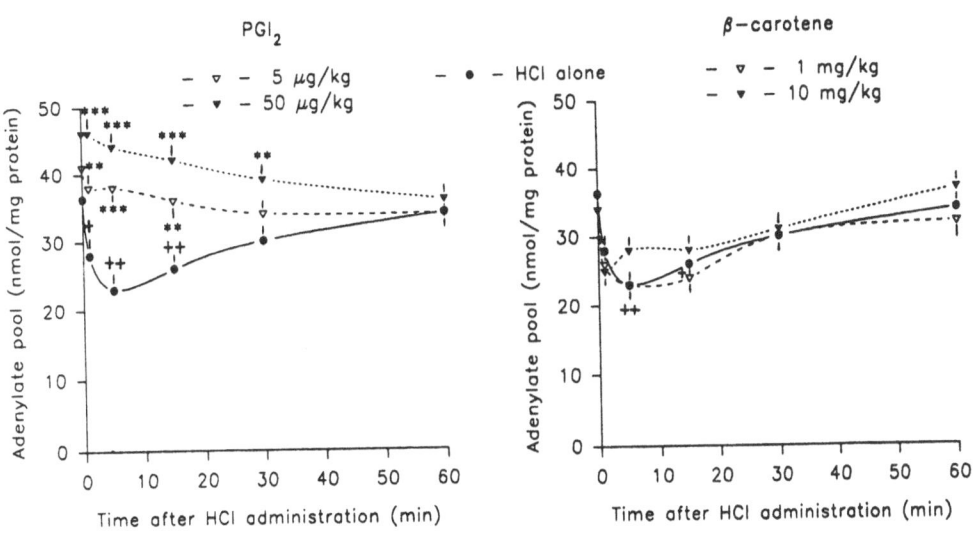

Figure 15. PGI₂-induced (5 and 50 µg/kg ig) and β-carotene-induced (1 and 10 mg/kg ig) changes in the gastric mucosal adenylate pool (ATP+ADP+AMP) of HCl-treated rats in relation to dose and time after HCl administration. See Figure 1 for further explanation

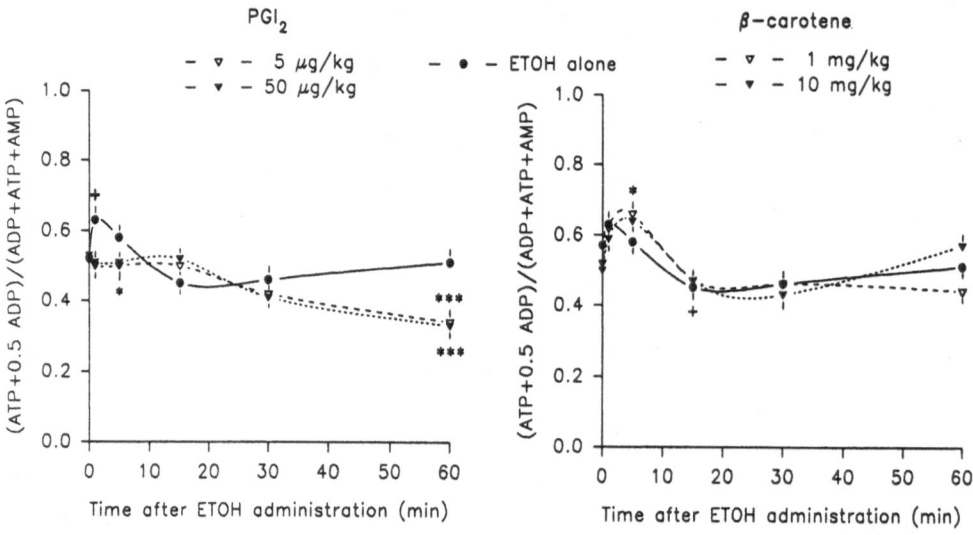

Figure 16. PGI$_2$-induced (5 and 50 µg/kg ig) and β-carotene-induced (1 and 10 mg/kg ig) changes in the 'energy charge' [(ATP+0.5 ADP)/(ATP+ADP+AMP)] in the gastric mucosa of rats treated with EtOH in relation to dose and time after EtOH administration. See Figure 1 for further explanation

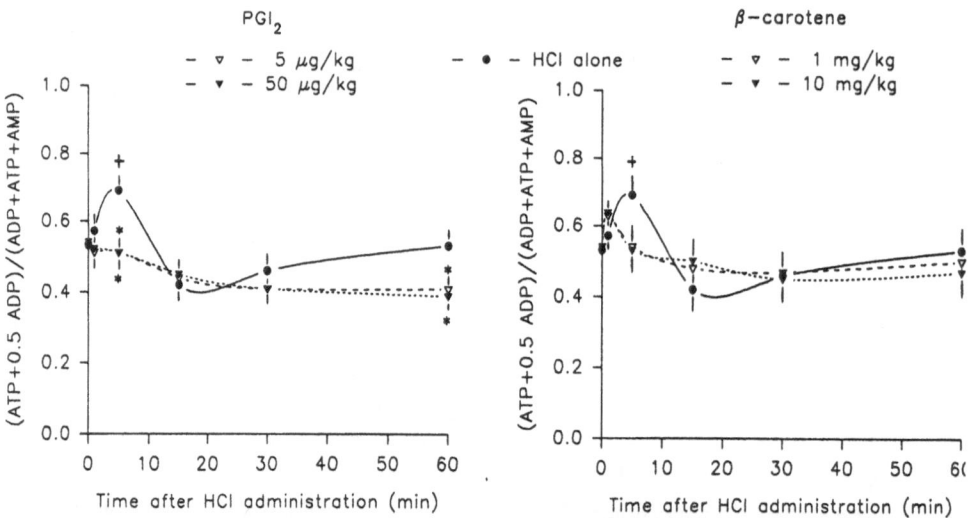

Figure 17. PGI$_2$-induced (5 and 50 µg/kg ig) and β-carotene-induced (1 and 10 mg/kg ig) changes in the 'energy charge' [(ATP+0.5 ADP)/(ATP+ADP+AMP)] in the gastric mucosa of rats treated with HCl in relation to dose and time after HCl administration. See Figure 1 for further explanation

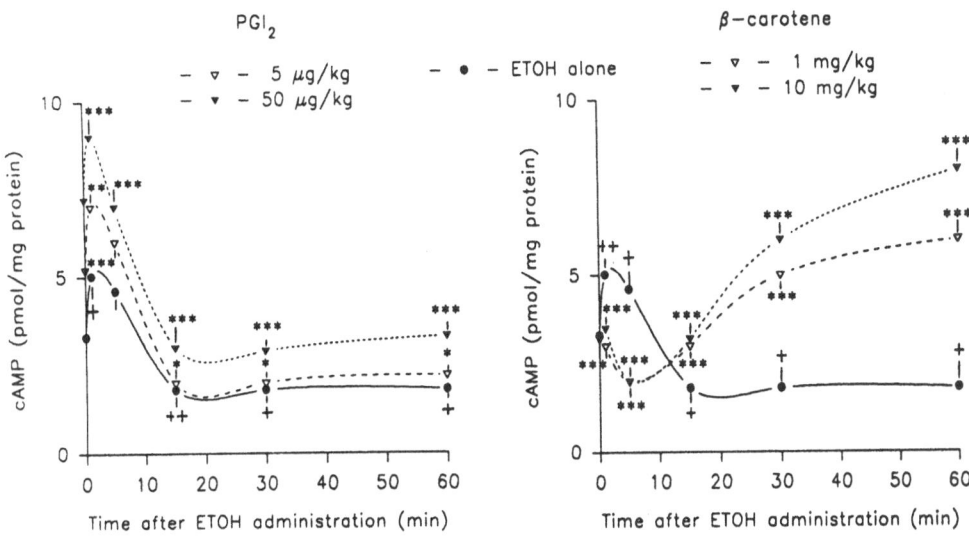

Figure 18. PGI₂-induced (5 and 50 µg/kg ig) and β-carotene-induced (1 and 10 mg/kg ig) changes in the gastric mucosal cAMP of EtOH-treated rats in relation to dose and time after EtOH administration. See Figure 1 for further explanation

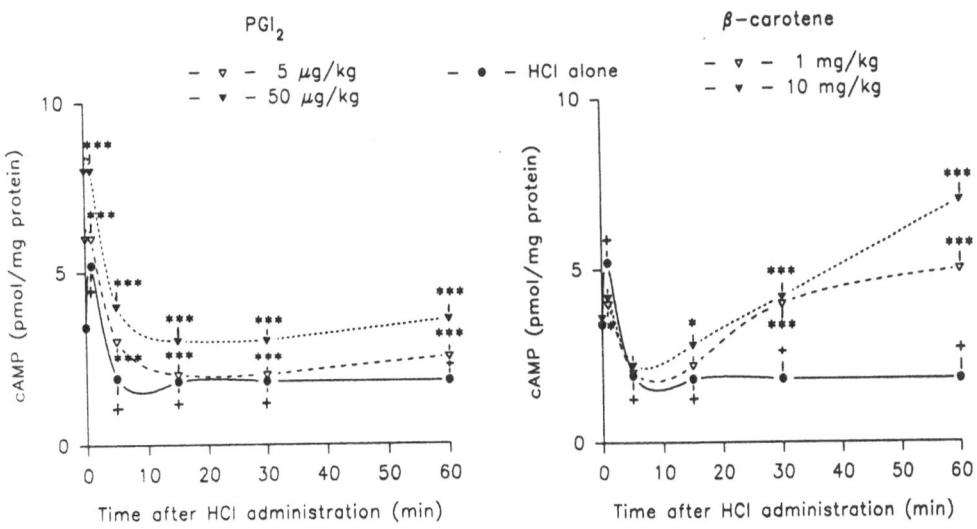

Figure 19. PGI₂-induced (5 and 50 µg/kg ig) and β-carotene-induced (1 and 10 mg/kg ig) changes in the gastric mucosal cAMP of HCl-treated rats in relation to dose and time after HCl administration. See Figure 1 for further explanation

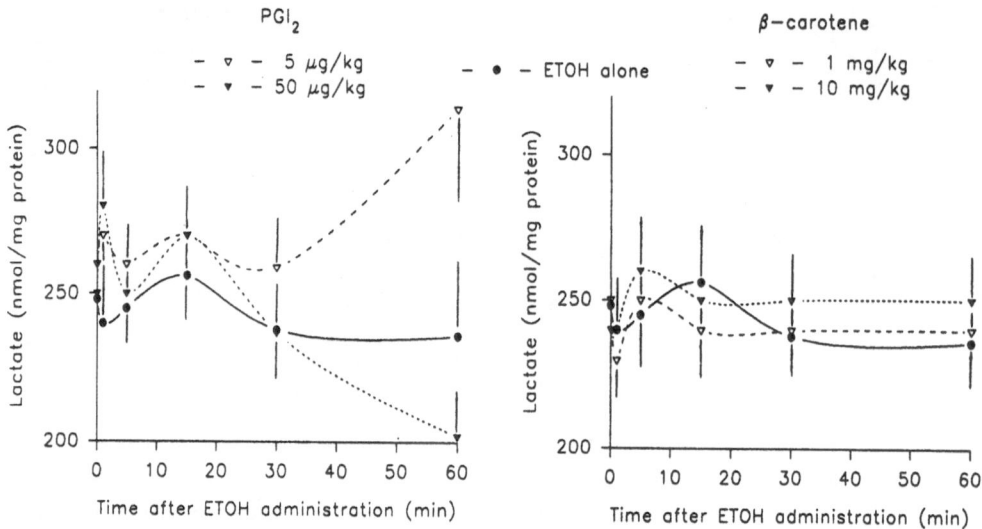

Figure 20. PGI$_2$-induced (5 and 50 µg/kg ig) and β-carotene-induced (1 and 10 mg/kg ig) changes in the gastric mucosal lactate of EtOH-treated rats in relation to dose and time after EtOH administration. See Figure 1 for further explanation

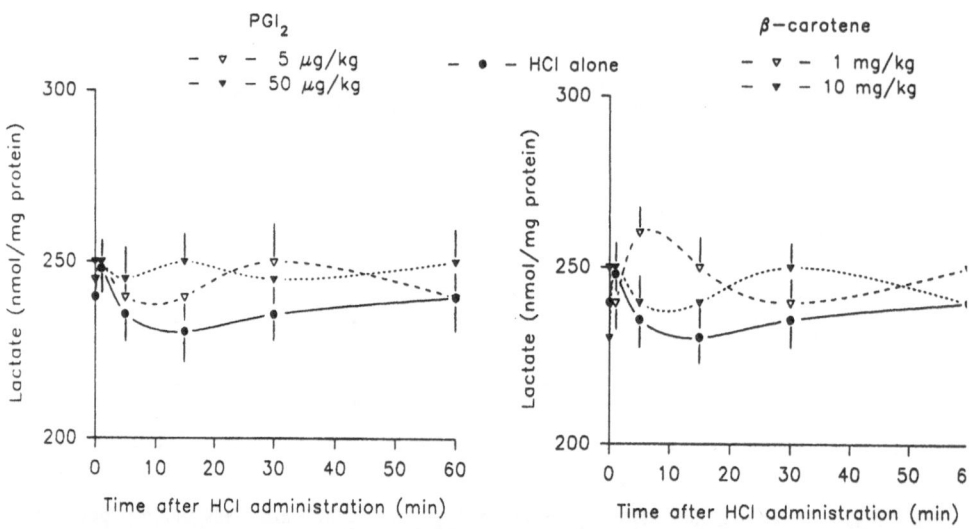

Figure 21. PGI$_2$-induced (5 and 50 µg/kg ig) and β-carotene-induced (1 and 10 mg/kg ig) changes in the gastric mucosal lactate of HCl-treated rats in relation to dose and time after HCl administration. See Figure 1 for further explanation

higher after β-carotene treatment in both models (Figures 10 and 11).

The tissue level of AMP was increased by PGI_2 administration during the entire period, while its level increased in a dose-related manner by β-carotene in both models (Figures 12 and 13).

The adenylate pool (ATP+ADP+AMP) was increased dose-dependently by PGI_2 in both models (Figures 14 and 15) but no significant change was obtained after β-carotene administration.

The values of the 'energy charge' [(ATP+0.5 ADP)/(ATP+ADP+AMP)] were decreased in PGI_2-treated groups (at 60 min after EtOH and HCl administration). However, no significant changes were obtained in β-carotene-treated animals (Figures 16 and 17).

The cAMP was increased in the early phase by PGI_2, and was elevated by β-carotene in the late phase (Figures 18 and 19).

In contrast, no elevation of tissue lactate level was found either in the EtOH- or in the HCl-treated rats with or without application of PGI_2 and β-carotene (Figures 20 and 21).

DISCUSSION

Acid-dependent (HCl) and non-acid-dependent (ethanol) gastric ulcer models were used to study the mucosal protecting effects of PGI_2 and of β-carotene.

The adenine nucleotide metabolism in gastric mucosa offered an excellent opportunity to study the 'cross-section' of mucosal metabolism [9].

Szabó et al. emphasized the pathogenetic role of early vascular reaction in the development of ethanol-induced gastric mucosal damage [17]. In our observations, the changes in gastric mucosal adenine nucleotide metabolism can be divided into an early phase (0–15-min period) and late phase (15–60-min period) after administration of the necrotizing agents, whereas approximately half of the total gastric mucosal damage appears in about 5 min. Furthermore, the mucosal protective effects of PGI_2 and β-carotene, and the changes in adenine nucleotides produced by these agents, can also be identified as early and late reactions (Tables 1–3) supporting our earlier observation (see References 13 and 18).

It is clear that significant changes in the vascular events occur in the early period [17], and impaired oxidative phosphorylation by tissue hypoxia has been suggested by a number of observers based on the changes of gastric mucosal blood flow.

Victor et al. [19] measured the changes in the energy-rich phosphates (ATP, ADP, AMP) from the rat stomach after exposure to different concentrations of ethanol. They found that ATP decreased, while AMP increased after ethanol exposure. However, the authors [19] did not measure the changes in cAMP that we found earlier [9] and have confirmed in the present study. ATP, as a high-energy phosphate, is a common source for both ADP and cAMP [20,21]. Therefore, the decrease in ATP is due to an increased level either of ADP or cAMP. So the decrease in mucosal ATP is not only the result of its breakdown into ADP as suggested by Victor et al. [19], but also due to increased cAMP production [20–22]. Furthermore, the ATP level was unchanged after administration of 50% ethanol [19], and this is in good agreement with our observations (Figures 8 and 9).

The increased level of AMP can be obtained by two ways: increased transformation of ATP→ADP→AMP; and increased transformation of ATP→cAMP→AMP. Consequently, the second pathway mentioned above also offers another explanation for the elevation in mucosal AMP.

Victor et al. [19] reported a slight elevation of mucosal level of lactate, while we did not find any change in the tissue level of lactate (Figures 20 and 21).

We measured tissue ATP in different experimental ulcer conditions and observed that the level increased 60 min after EtOH or HCl administration (compared with the level 15 min after administration of the necrotizing agents).

The elevation of mucosal ATP can be explained in two ways: the complete block of ATP breakdown (which is unlikely); or an increase in the extent of oxidative phosphorylation, which obviously excludes the existence of tissue hypoxia (suggested by the increase in tissue lactate). This second pathway is the likely explanation since the first possibility (block of ATP breakdown) can be easily excluded. In the second pathway, namely increase in oxidative phosphorylation, the exclusion of tissue hypoxia is basically necessary (as in earlier studies we did not find any change in the tissue level of lactate (Figures 20 and 21)). Furthermore, we proved the existence of a very dynamic and complex feedback mechanism between the breakdown of ATP→ADP→AMP (membrane ATPase system) and ATP→cAMP→AMP (adenylate system) and alteration in ATP→cAMP→AMP is needed for the evaluation of changes in ATP, ADP and AMP [20–22].

The changes in the vascular permeability in the gastric mucosa do not affect the development of mucosal damage or its prevention. β-Carotene (acting in the late period) did not change the chemically induced increase in vascular permeability in association with increased repair function of the gastric mucosa [23].

β-Carotene is a representative compound of retinoids. Our results clearly indicate that the beneficial effects of β-carotene only partly depend on its scavenger behaviour (see Figures). Furthermore, an intact vagus nerve [26] and adrenals [25] have been found necessary for the development of β-carotene- [24,25] and PGI_2-induced gastroprotection [27,28]. These are important notes which exclude the possibility that the protective effect of β-carotene in the gastric mucosa is only predominantly due to its scavenging property.

ACKNOWLEDGEMENTS

This study was supported by grants from the Hungarian National Research Fund (OTKA No. T 020098) and Ministry of Health and Welfare (ETT-03 660/93).

REFERENCES

1. Mózsik Gy, Fiegler M, Nagy L, Patty I, Tárnok F. Gastric and small intestinal energy metabolism in mucosal damage. In: Mózsik Gy, Hänninen O, Jávor T, eds. Gastrointestinal Defense Mechanisms. Oxford and Budapest: Pergamon Press and Akademiai Kiadó; 1980:213–76.
2. Robert A, Nezmazis JE, Lanchester C, Hancher AJ. Cytoprotection by prostaglandins in rats. Prevention of gastric mucosal necrosis by alcohol, HCl, NaOH, hypertonic NaCl and thermal injuries. Gastroenterology. 1979;77:433–43.
3. Mózsik Gy, Móron F, Jávor T. Cellular mechanisms of the development of gastric mucosal damage and of gastric cytoprotection induced by prostacyclin in rats. A pharmacological study. Prostagl Leuk Med. 1982;9:71–84.
4. Mózsik Gy, Móron F, Fiegler M et al. Interrelationships between membrane-bound ATP-dependent energy systems, gastric mucosal damage produced by NaOH, hypertonic NaCl, HCl and alcohol, and prostacyclin-induced gastric cytoprotection in rats. Prostagl Leuk Med. 1983;12:423–36.
5. Mózsik Gy, Nagy L, Patty I, Tárnok F. Cellular energy systems and reserpine ulcer. Acta Physiol Hung. 1983;62:107–14.
6. Szabó S, Mózsik Gy, eds. New Pharmacology of Ulcer Disease. New York: Elsevier Science Publishers; 1987.
7. Jávor T, Bata M, Lovász L et al. Gastric cytoprotective effects of vitamin A and other carotenoids. Int J Tiss React. 1983;5:289–93.
8. Mózsik Gy, Móron F, Fiegler M et al. Membrane-bound ATP-dependent energy systems and gastric cytoprotection by prostacyclin, atropine and cimetidine. Int J Tiss React. 1983;5:263.
9. Mózsik Gy, Jávor T. Biochemical and pharmacological approach to the elucidation of ulcer disease. I. A model study of ethanol-induced injury to gastric mucosa in rats. Dig Dis Sci. 1988;33:92–105.
10. Mózsik Gy, Garamszegi M, Jávor T et al. Correlations between the oxygen free radicals, membrane-bound ATP-dependent energy system in relation to development of ethanol- and HCl-induced gastric mucosal damage and of β-carotene-induced gastric cytoprotection. In: Tsuckiya M, Kawai K, Konda M, Yoshikawa T, eds. Free Radicals in Digestive Diseases. Amsterdam: Elsevier Science Publishers; 1988:111–16.
11. Mózsik Gy, Garamszegi M, Fiegler M et al. Mechanisms of gastric injury in the stomach. I. Time sequence analysis of gastric mucosal membrane-bound ATP-dependent energy system, oxygen-free radicals and appearance of gastric mucosal damage. In: Hayaishi O, Niki E, Kondo M, Yoshikawa T, eds. Medical, Biomedical and Chemical Aspects of Free Radicals. Amsterdam: Elsevier Science Publishers; 1989:1427–31.
12. Mózsik Gy, Fiegler M, Garamszegi M et al. Mechanisms of gastric injury in the stomach. I. Time sequence analysis of gastric mucosal membrane-bound ATP-dependent energy sytem, oxygen-free radicals and macroscopic appearance of gastric cytoprotection by PGI$_2$ and β-carotene in HCl-model of rats. In: Hayaishi O, Niki E, Kondo M, Yoshikawa T, eds. Medical, Biomedical and Chemical Aspects of Free Radicals. Amsterdam: Elsevier Science Publishers; 1989:1421–5.
13. Mózsik Gy, Jávor T. Therapy of ulcers with sulfhydryls and non-sulfhydryl antioxidants. In: Swabb EA, Szabó S, eds. Ulcer Disease: Investigation and Basis for Therapy. New York, Basel, Hong Kong: Marcel Dekkel Inc., 1991:321–41.
14. Mózsik Gy, Emerit I, Fehér J, Matkovics B, Vincze A, eds. Oxygen Free Radicals and Scavengers in the Natural Sciences. Budapest: Akadámiai Kiadó; 1993.
15. Lowry OH, Rosenbrough NJ, Farr AL, Randal RJ. Protein measurements with folin phenol reagent. J Biol Chem. 1951;193:265–75.
16. Atkinson DE. The energy charge of the adenylate pool as a regulatory parameter. Interactions with feedback modifiers. Biochemistry. 1968;7:4030–4.
17. Szabó S, Trier JS, Brown A, Schnoor J. Early vascular injury and increased vascular permeability in gastric mucosal injury caused by ethanol in the rat. Gastroenterology. 1985;88:228–36.
18. Sütő G, Garamszegi M, Jávor T, Vincze Á, Mózsik Gy. Similarities and differences in the cytoprotection induced by PGI$_2$ and β-carotene in experimental ulcer. Acta Physiol Hung. 1989;73:155–8.
19. Victor BE, Taegtmeyer H, Miller TA. Gastric mucosal high-energy phosphate metabolism. Influence of ethanol and PGI$_2$. Dig Dis Sci. 1995;40:120–7.
20. Mózsik Gy. Some feedback mechanisms by drugs in the interrelationships between the active transport system and adenylate system localized in the cell membrane. Eur J Pharmacol. 1969;7:318–27.
21. Mózsik Gy. Direct inhibitory effect of adenosine monophosphate on Na$^+$–K$^+$-dependent ATP-ase prepared from human gastric mucosa. Eur J Pharmacol. 1970;9:207–10.

22. Mózsik Gy, Király Á, Sütő G, Vincze Á. ATP breakdown and resynthesis in the development of gastrointestinal mucosal damage and its prevention in animals and human. An overview of 25 years ulcer research studies. In: Mózsik Gy, Pár A, Csomós G et al., eds. Cell Injury and Protection in the Gastrointestinal Tract: From Basic Sciences to Clinical Perspectives. Budapest: Akademiai Kiadó; 1993:39–80.

23. Mózsik Gy, Király Á, Garamszegi M et al. Failure of prostacyclin, β-carotene, atropine, and cimetidine to produce gastric cyto- and general mucosal protection in surgically vagotomized rats. Life Sci. 1991;49:1383–9.

24. Vincze Á, Garamszegi M, Jávor T , Sütő G, Mózsik Gy. The prevention of increased vascular permeability is not involved in gastric cytoprotective effect of β-carotene. Dig Dis Sci. 1990;35:1033–7.

25. Mózsik Gy, Bódis B, Garamszegi M et al. Role of the vagal nerve in the development of gastric mucosal injury and its prevention by atropine, cimetidine, β-carotene and prostacyclin in rats. In: Szabó S, Taché Y, eds. Neuroendocrinology of Gastrointestinal Ulceration. New York: Plenum Press; 1995:175–90.

26. Mózsik Gy, Király Á, Garamszegi M et al. Mechanisms of vagal nerve in the gastric mucosal defences: unchanged gastric emptying and increased vascular permeability. J Clin Gastroenterol. 1992;14(suppl 1):S140–4.

27. Bódis B, Balaskó M, Csontos Zs et al. Changes of gastric mucosal prostaglandin contents in intact and vagotomized rats, without and with β-carotene treatment. Dig Dis Sci. 1990;35:1015–18.

28. Mózsik Gy, Király Á, Garamszegi M et al. Gastric cytoprotection mediating in SH groups is failured by surgical vagotomy. Acta Physiol Hung. 1990;75(suppl):219–25.

G Mózsik et al. Cell Injury and Cytoprotection in the GI Tract. 51–61.
© 1997 Kluwer Academic Publishers.

REDUCTION IN GASTRIC BICARBONATE SECRETORY RESPONSE INDUCED BY N^G-NITRO-L-ARGININE METHYL ESTER FOLLOWING REPEATED ADMINISTRATION IN RATS

K. TAKEUCHI*, S. KATO, K. TAKEHARA AND T. YASUHIRO

Department of Pharmacology and Experimental Therapeutics, Kyoto Pharmaceutical University, Misasagi, Yamashina, Kyoto 607, Japan
*Correspondence

ABSTRACT

Gastric HCO_3^- secretory response induced by the nitric oxide (NO) synthase inhibitor, N^G-nitro-L-arginine methyl ester (L-NAME), was examined in rats before and after the repeated administration of this agent. HCO_3^- secretion was determined in ex-vivo chambered stomachs of anaesthetized rats. Intravenous administration of L-NAME (5 mg/kg) increased gastric HCO_3^- secretion with a con-comitant rise in arterial blood pressure (BP). The HCO_3^- stimulatory action of iv L-NAME diminished when they were pretreated with L-NAME (20 mg/kg × 2, po) for 1 or 3 days, and an inverse relationship was found between the degree of stimulation and the period of treatment. The increased BP response to iv L-NAME was also significantly lessened following repeated administration; the basal BP showed a step-wise increase during treatment and did not change at all in response to iv L-NAME after 3 days treatment. When ΔHCO_3^- output induced by iv L-NAME was plotted against ΔBP change during repeated treatment with L-NAME po, a significant relationship was found between these two factors. The reduction of HCO_3^- response to iv L-NAME was significantly restored when the animals were given L-arginine (500 mg/kg × 2 ip) simultaneously with po L-NAME. However, prostaglandin E_2 (300 µg/kg iv) caused a gastric HCO_3^- response similar in degree regardless of whether the animals were pretreated with L-NAME po or not. These results suggest that: (1) the repeated po treatment with L-NAME diminishes the HCO_3^- stimulatory action of iv L-NAME; (2) this phenomenon may be explained by the lack of further elevation of blood pressure to iv L-NAME following the repeated treatment; and (3) the stimulation of HCO_3^- secretion by iv L-NAME may be causally related to the increased blood pressure response to this agent.

Keywords: gastric bicarbonate secretion, nitric oxide, NO synthase inhibitor, L-NAME

INTRODUCTION

It has been demonstrated that the nitric oxide (NO) synthase inhibitor N^G-nitro-L-arginine methyl ester (L-NAME) causes stimulation of HCO_3^- secretion in the gastroduodenal mucosa of rats [1–3]. Since the HCO_3^- stimulatory effect of L-NAME is mimicked by another NO synthase inhibitor, N^G-monomethyl L-arginine and is antagonized by the simultaneous administration of L-arginine, this action may be associated with the inhibition of endogenous NO production.

NO is constitutively formed in the vascular endothelium and plays an important role in the regulation of blood pressure by dilating the vascular smooth muscle [4–6].

This paper was presented at the Symposium on 'Cell injury and protection in the gastrointestinal tract: from basic science to clinical perspectives', October 8–11, 1995, Pécs, Hungary.

Indeed, the administration of L-NAME causes a marked elevation of arterial blood pressure at the doses that stimulate HCO_3^- secretion in the gastroduodenal mucosa [3]. Since the marked elevation of blood pressure is followed by a neuronal reflex, it might be possible to speculate that the HCO_3^- stimulatory action of L-NAME is related to changes in such neuronal activity resulting from elevation of blood pressure [7]. We also found that the increased blood pressure response to L-NAME was less marked in rats when they were treated repeatedly with L-NAME. If the HCO_3^- stimulatory effect of L-NAME is related to the neuronal reflex resulting from the pressor response, this action would also become less pronounced following the repeated administration of L-NAME.

In the present study, we thus examined the effect of iv administration of L-NAME on gastric HCO_3^- secretion and systemic blood pressure in the rat before and after repeated treatment with po L-NAME, and investigated the relationship of HCO_3^- response to blood pressure changes induced by iv L-NAME under the inhibition of endogenous NO production.

MATERIALS AND METHODS

Animals

Male Sprague–Dawley rats, weighing 230–250 g (Charles River, Shizuoka, Japan) were used. All studies were carried out using 4–6 animals per group.

General procedures

The animals were administered L-NAME (20 mg/kg) po twice daily (9.00 am and 6.00 pm) for 1 or 3 days. These animals were then kept in individual cages and deprived of food but allowed free access to tap water for 18 h. In these animals, both gastric HCO_3^- secretory and blood pressure responses to a single iv administration of L-NAME (5 mg/kg) were measured under anaesthetized conditions induced by urethane (1.25 g/kg ip). Some of the animals treated with L-NAME po for 3 days were fed normally for another 3 days, and were used in the measurement of HCO_3^- secretion and blood pressure. In some experiments, the animals were simultaneously administered with L- or D-arginine (500 mg/kg ip) together with L-NAME po for 1 or 3 days, and they were subjected to similar experiments. In addition, the effect of prostaglandin E_2 (PGE_2) on gastric HCO_3^- secretion was also determined in the animals treated with L-NAME po for 1 or 3 days.

Determination of gastric HCO_3^- secretion and blood pressure

HCO_3^- secretion was measured in a chambered stomach according to the previously published papers [3,8]. The stomach, mounted on an ex-vivo chamber, was perfused with saline that was gassed with 100% O$_2$, heated at 37°C and kept in a reservoir. Gastric HCO$_3^-$ secretion was measured at pH 7.0 using a pH-stat method (Hiranuma Comtite-7, Mito, Japan) and by adding 10 mmol/L HCl to the reservoir. For unmasking HCO$_3^-$ in the stomach, acid secretion was inhibited by omeprazole (60 mg/kg ip). After basal HCO$_3^-$ secretion had stabilized, L-NAME (5 mg/kg) or PGE$_2$ (300 µg/kg) was administered iv as a single injection. The femoral artery was cannulated, and both arterial blood pressure and heart rate was monitored using a pressure transducer and polygraph device (Sanei, CASE-7903, Tokyo, Japan).

Preparation of drugs

Drugs used were urethane (Tokyo Kasei, Tokyo, Japan), N^G-nitro-L-arginine methyl ester, L-arginine, D-arginine (Sigma Chemicals, St. Louis, MO, USA), prostaglandin E$_2$ (Funakoshi, Tokyo, Japan) and omeprazole (Hessle, Mondale, Sweden). Urethane, L-NAME, L- and D-arginine were dissolved in saline. PGE$_2$ was first dissolved in 100% ethanol and diluted with saline to the desired concentration. Each agent was prepared immediately before use and was given in a volume of 0.1 ml per 100 g body weight in the case of iv administration or in a volume of 0.5 ml per 100 g body weight in cases of ip and po administration. Control animals received saline as the vehicle.

Statistics

Data are presented as the mean $\pm$ SE of 4–6 rats per group. Statistical analyses were performed using a two-tailed Dunnett's multiple comparison test [9], and values of $p < 0.05$ were regarded as significant. Correlation between gastric HCO$_3^-$ secretion and blood pressure responses was assessed by linear-regression analysis.

RESULTS

Effects of repeated treatment with L-NAME on gastric HCO$_3^-$ secretion

Under our experimental conditions, the gastric mucosa secreted HCO$_3^-$ spontaneously at steady rates of 0.2$\pm$0.4 µEq/5 min in the absence of acid secretion. Intravenous administration of L-NAME (5 mg/kg) caused an increase of gastric HCO$_3^-$ secretion to reach a maximal level of 2.5 times greater than basal values; ΔHCO$_3^-$ output was 4.6$\pm$0.3 µEq/h (Figure 1). The HCO$_3^-$ stimulatory action of iv L-NAME became diminished when the animals were pretreated with L-NAME (20 mg/kg $\times$, po). In the animals subjected to 1 day of treatment with po L-NAME, the subsequent iv administration of L-NAME did stimulate HCO$_3^-$ secretion in the stomach, but the degree of stimulation was significantly weak compared with that observed in intact animals. Following 3 days treatment with po L-NAME, the stimulatory effect of iv L-NAME on HCO$_3^-$ secretion almost totally disappeared, ΔHCO$_3^-$ output being 0.4$\pm$0.3

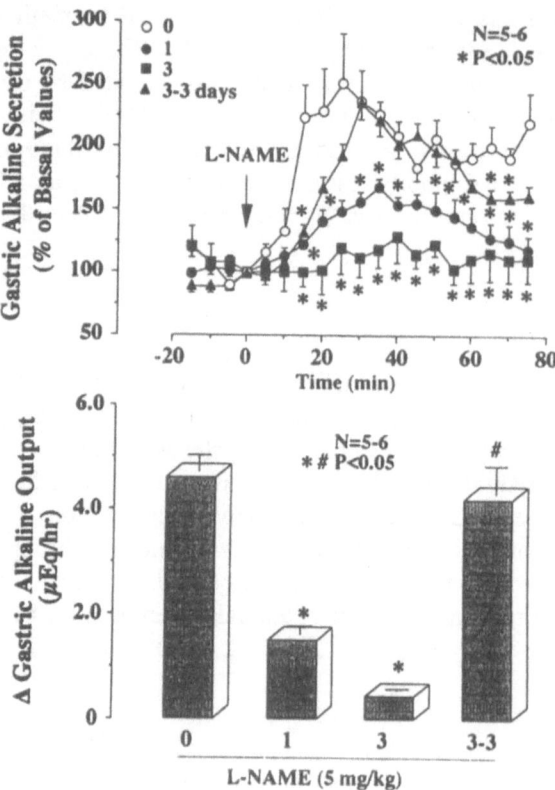

Figure 1. Effect of L-NAME on gastric HCO$_3^-$ secretion in anaesthetized rats after repeated treatment with L-NAME. The animals were given L-NAME orally (20 mg/kg × 2) for 1 or 3 days, and half the latter group remained for 3 days after the final treatment. On the day of the experiment, L-NAME was given iv in a dose of 5 mg/kg as a single injection. Data are expressed as % of basal values and represent the mean ± SE of values determined every 5 min from 5–6 rats. *Statistically significant differences from control (day 0) at $p < 0.05$. The lower panel shows ΔHCO$_3^-$ output induced by L-NAME after repeated treatment with L-NAME. Values are presented as ΔHCO$_3^-$ output for 1 h after administration of L-NAME (5 mg/kg), and represent the mean ± SE from 5–6 rats. Statistically significant difference at $p < 0.05$; *from day 0; #from day 3

μEq/h, which is only 10% of that obtained in control animals. However, when the rats were fed normally for another 3 days after 3 days treatment with po L-NAME, they again responded to iv L-NAME by a marked increase in gastric HCO$_3^-$ secretion similar to control rats without pretreatment with po L-NAME; ΔHCO$_3^-$ output was 4.2 ± 0.5 μEq/h, which is not significantly different from that observed in control animals.

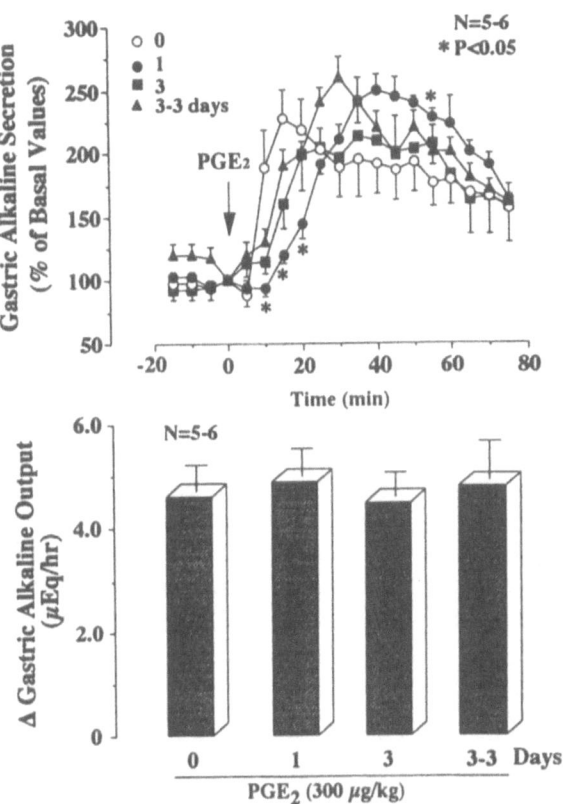

Figure 2. Effect of PGE_2 on gastric HCO_3^- secretion in anaesthetized rats after repeated treatment with L-NAME. The animals were given L-NAME orally (20 mg/kg × 2) for 1 or 3 days, and half the latter group remained for 3 days after the final treatment. On the day of the experiment, PGE_2 was given in a dose of 300 μg/kg as a single iv injection. Data are expressed as % of basal values and represent the mean ± SE of values determined every 5 min from 5–6 rats. *Statistically significant differences from control (day 0) at $p < 0.05$. The lower panel shows ΔHCO_3^- output induced by PGE_2 after repeated treatment with L-NAME. Values are presented as ΔHCO_3^- output for 1 h after administration of PGE_2 (300 μg/kg), and represent the mean ± SE from 5–6 rats. Statistically significant difference at $p < 0.05$; *from day 0

On the other hand, gastric HCO_3^- secretion was significantly increased in response to iv administration of PGE_2 (300 μg/kg), and the ΔHCO_3^- output (4.6 ± 0.5 μEq/h) was equivalent to that induced by L-NAME (5 mg/kg, iv) (Figure 2). However, this effect of PGE_2 on HCO_3^- secretion was similarly observed in the rats, irrespective of whether they were pretreated with po L-NAME for 1 or 3 days, or fed for another 3 days following the 3 days treatment; the ΔHCO_3^- output was 4.9 ± 0.5 μEq/h, 4.5 ± 0.5 μEq/ h or 4.8 ± 0.7 μEq/h, respectively.

Effect of repeated treatment with L-NAME on blood pressure response

Intravenous administration of L-NAME caused a marked elevation of arterial blood pressure at the dose (5 mg/kg) which stimulates HCO_3^- secretion in the stomach; the mean blood pressure rose from 90.6 ± 6.0 mmHg to 147.8 ± 13.5 mmHg and the heart rate decreased from 392.4 ± 11.5 beats/min to 321.6 ± 18.1 beats/min within 5 min. On the other hand, repeated po treatment with L-NAME (20 mg/kg $\times 2$) increased basal blood pressure to 117.3 ± 3.2 mmHg and 123.3 ± 3.5 mmHg after 1 and 3 days treatment, respectively (Table 1). In these animals, however, acute iv administration of L-NAME (5 mg/kg) caused less significant elevation of blood pressure; Δ increase in blood pressure was $19.9 \pm 5.1\%$ and $7.9 \pm 6.0\%$ in animals treated with L-NAME for 1 and 3 days, respectively, which is significantly lower than that ($75.0 \pm 9.6\%$) in control rats. When the animals were treated with po L-NAME for 3 days and fed for another 3 days without any treatment, the blood pressure reverted to control levels (83.0 ± 4.9 mmHg) and again responded to subsequent iv administration of L-NAME by a marked increase of blood pressure ($97.9 \pm 18.1\%$). When ΔHCO_3^- output induced by iv administration of L-NAME in the animals treated with po L-NAME was plotted against changes in blood pressure (Δ increase in blood pressure from basal values) observed in these rats, a significant relationship was obtained between these two parameters; the correlation coefficient (r) being 0.951 ($p < 0.05$) (Figure 3).

TABLE 1

Changes in blood pressure responses to iv L-NAME in anaesthetized rats before and after the repeated po administration of L-NAME

Group	Number of rats	Basal BP (mmHg)	Δ to iv L-NAME (%)
Control	6	90.6 ± 6.0	75.0 ± 9.6
L-NAME treatment			
1 day	5	117.3 ± 3.2[a]	19.9 ± 5.1[a]
3 days	5	121.3 ± 3.5[a]	7.9 ± 6.0[a]
+L-arginine	4	97.3 ± 8.1[b]	38.9 ± 10.4[b]
+D-arginine	4	128.5 ± 5.1[a]	5.2 ± 4.8[a]
3 days treatment and 3 days off	5	83.0 ± 4.9[b]	97.9 ± 18.1[b]

Values are presented as the mean $\pm$ SE of 4–6 rats per group. The animals were given L-NAME po (20 mg/ kg $\times 2$) for 1 or 3 days, and some of the animals remained without treatment for 3 days after the final administration. Then, L-NAME was given iv as a single injection 18 h (1- and 3-days treatment) or 90 h (3 days treatment and 3 days off) after the final administration of po L-NAME. L-arginine or D-arginine (500 mg/kg $\times 2$, ip) was administered for 3 days simultaneously with L-NAME. Data indicate both basal blood pressure (mmHg) and % increase in blood pressure from basal values. Statistically significant difference at $p < 0.05$: [a]from contro; [b]from the values in the group treated for 3 days with L-NAME alone

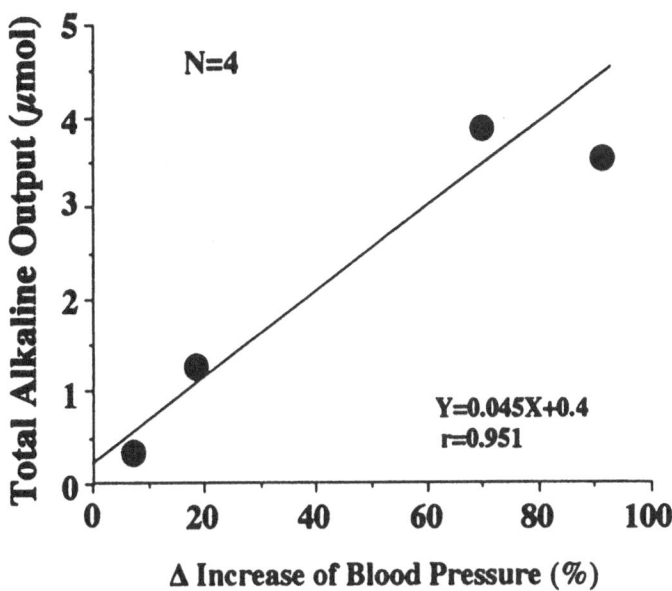

Figure 3. The relationship between HCO$_3^-$ secretion (ΔHCO$_3^-$ output) and Δblood pressure changes induced by L-NAME in anaesthetized rats. The animals were given L-NAME orally (20 mg/kg × 2) for 1 or 3 days, and half the latter group were untreated for 3 days after the final treatment. L-NAME was given in a dose of 5 mg/kg as a single iv injection

Effect of simultaneous treatment with L-NAME plus L-arginine on gastric HCO$_3^-$ and blood pressure responses

The repeated po treatment of animals with L-NAME (20 mg/kg × 2) significantly reduced the magnitude of gastric HCO$_3^-$ secretion and blood pressure changes in response to iv administration of L-NAME (5 mg/kg). These effects of repeated po treatment with L-NAME were significantly antagonized by the co-administration of L-arginine (500 mg/kg × 2 ip) together with L-NAME. As shown in Figure 4, a single iv administration of L-NAME (5 mg/kg) increased gastric HCO$_3^-$ secretion by about 60% over basal values in the animals treated with L-NAME plus L-arginine for 3 days, and the degree of HCO$_3^-$ stimulation in these rats was significantly greater when compared with control animals treated with po L-NAME alone (20%). The ΔHCO$_3^-$ output induced by iv L-NAME in these rats following 1 and 3 days pretreatment with po L-NAME plus L-arginine was 4.1±0.6 µEq/h and 3.2±0.2 µEq/h, which are significantly greater than those (1.5±0.2 µEq/h and 0.4±0.03 µEq/h) obtained in animals pretreated with po L-NAME alone. The simultaneous administration of D-arginine with po L-NAME did not affect the reduced HCO$_3^-$ response to iv administration of L-NAME, and the values were equivalent to those observed in rats after the repeated po treatment with L-NAME for 1 or 3 days.

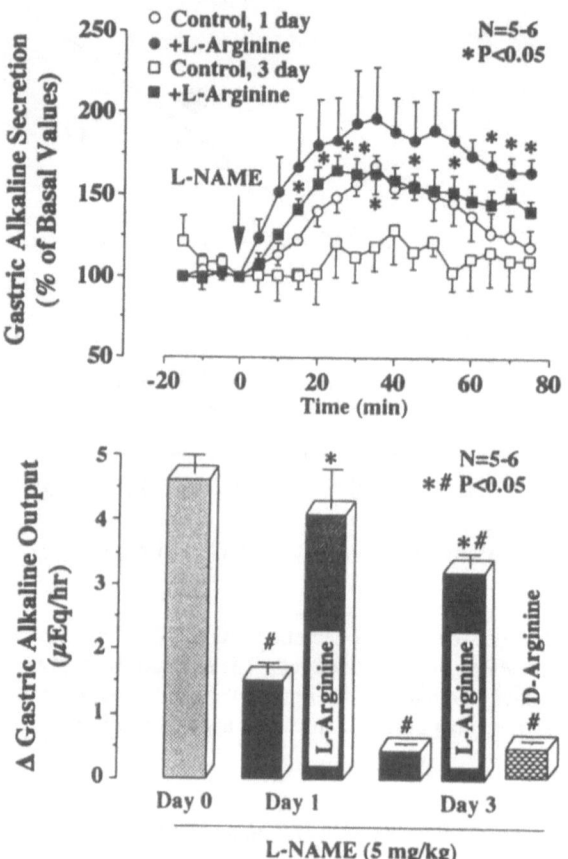

Figure 4. Effect of co-administration of L- or D-arginine on changes in gastric HCO₃⁻ response to L-NAME in anaesthetized rats after repeated treatment with L-NAME. The animals were given L-NAME (20 mg/kg × 2, po) plus L- or D-arginine (500 mg/kg × 2, ip) for 1 or 3 days. In each rat, L-NAME was given iv in a dose of 5 mg/kg as a single injection. Data in the upper panel are expresssed as % of basal values and represent the mean ± SE of values determined from 5 rats. *Statistically significant differences from animals without L-arginine, at $p < 0.05$. Values in the lower panel indicate the total HCO₃⁻ output for 1 h (ΔHCO₃⁻ output) induced by L-NAME (iv) and are presented as the mean ± SE of 5–6 rats. Statistically significant difference at $p < 0.05$; *from L-NAME alone; #from day 0

Similar results were obtained in the blood pressure response to iv administration of L-NAME when the animals were pretreated with L-arginine together with po L-NAME (Table 1). Co-treatment with L-arginine but not D-arginine (500 mg/kg × 2, ip) partially but significantly restored the increased blood pressure response to iv administration of L-NAME in the animals pretreated with po L-NAME for 3 days.

Repeated po treatment with L-NAME alone for 3 days increased basal blood pressure from 90.6 ± 6.0 mmHg to 123.5 ± 4.1 mmHg and almost totally abolished the pressor response to iv L-NAME. However, in the animals given L-arginine simultaneously with po L-NAME for 3 days, the basal blood pressure significantly decreased to 97.3 ± 8.1 mmHg, and the subsequent iv administration of L-NAME again caused a significant elevation in blood pressure to 134.2 ± 7.8 mmHg (Δ increase: $38.0 \pm 8.2\%$).

DISCUSSION

We confirmed our previous finding that iv administration of L-NAME caused an increase of HCO_3^- secretion in the rat stomach with concomitant rise in arterial blood pressure [1–3,8]. Since this HCO_3^- response was significantly antagonized by prior administration of L-arginine but not D-arginine, it is considered that the HCO_3^- stimulatory action of L-NAME is associated with the inhibition of endogenous NO production [2,3]. In the present study, we demonstrated that both the increased HCO_3^- and blood pressure responses to L-NAME become less pronounced after repeated po treatment with L-NAME and suggest a close relationship between these two responses induced by iv L-NAME.

In previous papers [3,7], we have reported that the stimulatory effect of iv L-NAME on HCO_3^- secretion is significantly attenuated by vagotomy and pretreatment with atropine or indomethacin, suggesting that the mechanism of HCO_3^- secretion in response to L-NAME involves vagal–cholinergic pathways and is partly mediated by endogenous PGs. Vagal excitation stimulates HCO_3^- as well as acid secretions and increases the release and/or biosynthesis of endogenous PGs in the stomach of various species of animals [10,11]. We also observed that L-NAME caused a marked increase of blood pressure and a decrease in heart rate at the dose that stimulates HCO_3^- secretion [12]. It was further reported that the HCO_3^- response caused by L-NAME was significantly mitigated by prior administration of α-adrenoceptor antagonists, such as prazosin or yohimbine [7]. These agents alone caused a profound decrease in blood pressure and significantly reduced the pressor response to L-NAME, leading to attenuation of the bradycardic response caused by the NO synthase inhibitor. Based on these findings, we hypothesized that iv administration of L-NAME stimulates HCO_3^- secretion, at least partly, mediated by a neural reflex through vagal efferent nerves, resulting from the marked increase in blood pressure. A decrease in heart rate following the increase in blood pressure caused by L-NAME supports a reflex activation of the vagus nerves. Indeed, vagotomy mitigated both HCO_3^- and heart rate responses induced by L-NAME without affecting the increase in blood pressure.

Of most interest is the finding that the increased HCO_3^- and blood pressure responses caused by iv administration of L-NAME diminished by pretreatment of animals with L-NAME po repeatedly for 1–3 days, and the magnitude of such changes became greater depending upon the period of L-NAME treatment. After 3 days treatment with po L-NAME, the blood pressure remained elevated and did not respond further to iv administration of L-NAME. In such animals, iv L-NAME also failed to stimulate gastric HCO_3^- secretion. Of interest, when the rats were first treated with po L-NAME for 3 days, then L-NAME administered iv to these animals, 3 days after such treatment, the increased HCO_3^- and blood pressure responses to iv L-NAME were observed again, similar to those in intact animals without any pretreatment. These findings strongly suggest that the elevated blood pressure response is a prerequisite for the increase of HCO_3^- secretion seen after iv administration of L-NAME. This contention is also supported by the close relationship between the degree of HCO_3^- secretion and pressor response induced by iv L-NAME. Since iv administration of PGE_2 stimulated gastric HCO_3^- secretion to a similar degree in rats, irrespective of whether or not they were pretreated with po L-NAME for 1–3 days, it is unlikely that repeated po treatment with L-NAME impairs the HCO_3^- secretory ability of the surface epithelial cells in the stomach.

NO formed in the vascular endothelium plays an important role in regulation of blood pressure [4,5]. Since L-NAME increases blood pressure by inhibiting the NO synthase, this action is antagonized by co-administration of L-arginine, the precursor amino acid in the NO biosynthesis. We previously showed that the stimulatory effect of L-NAME on gastric HCO_3^- secretion is also antagonized by the simultaneous administration of L-arginine but not that of D-arginine, strongly suggesting that this phenomenon is associated with the inhibition of endogenous NO production [2,3]. In the present study, the simultaneous administration of L-arginine significantly antagonized the increase in basal blood pressure following repeated treatment with po L-NAME and recovered the increased blood pressure response caused by iv L-NAME. Such treatment with L-arginine also restored gastric HCO_3^- response to iv L-NAME, again indicating a cause–effect relationship between HCO_3^- and blood pressure responses. These results also suggest that the phenomena observed in this study are attributable to NO synthase inhibition but not to non-specific actions of the repeated po treatment with L-NAME.

Previously, Hallgren et al. [13,14] found that the NO synthase inhibitors, such as L-NAME, caused an increase of both luminal alkalinization and luminal pressure in the rat duodenum and postulated that the HCO_3^- stimulatory action of L-NAME may be due to the neural reflex resulting from the rise in luminal pressure through mechano-receptors. In the present study, the experiments were performed using ex-vivo stomachs that were mounted on a chamber and superfused at a constant flow rate with saline. Under these conditions, the pressure of the stomach lumen was relatively constant, yet L-NAME caused a marked increase of luminal alkalinization. Thus, it seems likely that stimulation by L-NAME of HCO_3^- secretion is not simply brought about by an increase of the luminal pressure in these tissues. Certainly, further studies are required to clarify this point.

In conclusion, the present study showed that repeated po treatment with L-NAME diminishes the stimulatory effect of iv L-NAME on HCO_3^- secretion, and this phenomenon may be due to the lack of further elevation of blood pressure in response to iv L-NAME. These results also support the hypothesis that the HCO_3^- stimulatory action of iv L-NAME is mediated by a neural reflex through vagal efferent nerves, resulting from the marked pressor response [7]. Certainly, since we have reported that the exogenous NO donor, nitroprusside, not only antagonizes the stimulatory effect of L-NAME on HCO_3^- secretion but also causes a dose-dependent reduction in the HCO_3^-

response induced by 16,16-dimethyl PGE_2 [3,15], it is possible that the HCO_3^- stimulatory effect of L-NAME may be partly accounted for by removal of the negative influence of endogenous NO on this secretion. Although NO is a stimulator of soluble guanylate cyclase, leading to accumulation of cyclic GMP [5], it remains unknown at present whether L-NAME affects HCO_3^- secretion directly through changes in the guanylate cyclase/cyclic GMP system.

REFERENCES

1. Takeuchi K, Ohuchi T, Miyake H, Sugawara H, Okabe S. Effects of nitric oxide synthase inhibitors on gastric alkaline secretion in rats. Jpn J Pharmacol. 1992;60:303–5.
2. Takeuchi K, Ohuchi T, Miyake H, Niki S, Okabe S. Effects of nitric oxide synthase inhibitors on duodenal alkaline secretion in anesthetized rats. Eur J Pharmacol. 1993;231:135–8.
3. Takeuchi K, Ohuchi T, Miyake H, Okabe S. Stimulation by nitric oxide synthase inhibitors of gastric and duodenal HCO_3^- secretion in rats. J Pharmacol Exp Ther. 1993;266:1512–19.
4. Furchgott RF. The role of endothelium in the response of vascular smooth muscle to drugs. Ann Rev Pharmacol Toxicol. 1984;24:175–97.
5. Moncada S, Palmer RMJ, Higgs EA. Nitric oxide: Physiology, pathophysiology and pharmacology. Pharmacol Rev. 1991;43:109–42.
6. Whittle BJR, Lopes-Bermonte J, Moncada S. Regulation of gastric mucosal integrity by endogenous nitric oxide: Interactions with prostanoids and sensory neuropeptides in the rat. Br J Pharmacol. 1990;99:607–11.
7. Takeuchi K, Takehara K, Okabe S. Mechanisms underlying stimulation of gastroduodenal HCO_3^- secretion by N^G-nitro-L-arginine methyl ester, an inhibitor of nitric oxide synthase, in rats. Jpn J Pharmacol. 1994;66:295–302.
8. Takeuchi K, Ueshima K, Matsumoto J, Okabe S. Role of capsaicin-sensitive sensory nerves in acid-induced bicarbonate secretion in rat stomach. Dig Dis Sci. 1992;37:737–43.
9. Dunnett CW. A multiple comparison procedure for comparing several treatments with a control. Am J Stat Assoc. 1955;50:1096–121.
10. Cocearni F, Pace-Asciak C, Volta F, Wolff LS. Effect of nerve stimulation on prostaglandin formation and release from the rat stomach. Am J Physiol. 1967;213:1056–67.
11. Jonson C, Nylander O, Flemstrom G, Fandriks L. Vagal stimulation of duodenal HCO_3^- secretion in anesthetized rats. Acta Physiol Scand. 1986;128:65–70.
12. Takeuchi K, Ohuchi T, Tachibana M, Okabe S. Mechanisms underlying stimulation of gastric HCO_3^- secretion by N^G-nitro-L-arginine methyl ester, an inhibitor of nitric oxide synthase, in rats. J Gastroenterol Hepatol. 1994;9:S50–4.
13. Hallgren G, Flemstrom G, Nylander O. Effects of nitric oxide synthase inhibitors on bicarbonate secretion, net fluid transport, mucosal permeability, blood flow and motility in rat duodenum. Gastroenterology (Abstract). 1993;105:A-1531.
14. Hallgren A, Nylander O. The acid-induced increase in duodenal mucosal permeability is augmented by nitric oxide synthase inhibitor or vasopressin. Gastroenterology (Abstract). 1994;106:A-2450.
15. Takeuchi K, Takehara K, Okabe S. Effects of endogenous and exogenous nitric oxide on gastric alkaline secretion in anesthetized rats. Asia Paci J Pharmacol. 1994;9:259–65.

G Mózsik et al. Cell Injury and Cytoprotection in the GI Tract. 63–70.
© 1997 Kluwer Academic Publishers.

ROLE OF BASIC FIBROBLAST GROWTH FACTOR (bFGF) AND PLATELET-DERIVED GROWTH FACTOR (PDGF) IN ULCER HEALING

S. SZABO[1,2*], Á. VINCZE[1,2], Zs. SANDOR[1,2], S. KUSSTATSCHER[1], G. SAKOULAS[1] AND H. SATOH[3]

[1]Department of Pathology, Brigham and Women's Hospital, Harvard Medical School, Boston, MA; [2]Departments of Pathology and Pharmacology, University of California, Irvine, VA Medical Center, Long Beach, CA, USA; [3]Pharmaceutical Research Division, Takeda Chemical Industries, Ltd., Osaka, Japan
*Correspondence

ABSTRACT

Growth factors stimulate virtually all the cellular determinants of ulcer healing (e.g. angiogenesis, granulation tissue production, re-epithelialization). Oral treatment of rats with the natural bFGF-wild, acid-resistant mutein bFGF-CS23 or PDGF-BB accelerated the healing of cysteamine-induced chronic duodenal ulcers. Parallel treatment with marginally effective doses of bFGF + cimetidine or lansoprazole or sucralfate resulted in additive/synergistic ulcer healing. In the ethanol model of acute gastric haemorrhagic erosions, PDGF offered partial gastroprotection, while bFGF was not effective. To investigate the role of endogenous bFGF in the natural history of gastroduodenal ulceration, the heparin-binding fraction of protein extract from duodenal mucosa was analysed by Western blot. A transient 2–3 fold increase in the high-molecular-weight (HMW) nuclear forms of bFGF (21–25 kDa) was seen at 12 h along with the simultaneous decrease (about 50%) in the cytoplasmic 18-kDa bFGF. At 24 and 48 h, the levels of the HMW forms declined and the 18-kDa form increased when compared with 12 h samples. Thus, bFGF and PDGF may be new pharmacological and pathophysiological mediators of ulcer healing.

Keywords: ulcer healing, duodenal ulcer, basic fibroblast growth factor (bFGF), platelet-derived growth factor (PDGF), cysteamine, ethanol, gastroprotection

INTRODUCTION

Gastroduodenal ulceration has been investigated mainly from the point of view of aggressive factors, such as acid and pepsin secretion, *Helicobacter pylori*, and, less intensively, from the aspect of defensive mechanisms, mucus and bicarbonate secretion, and healing processes [1–3]. Therapeutic interventions were thus designed to counter aggressive factors, e.g. antacids, H_2-receptor blockers, proton pump inhibitors. With all these interventions, the ulcer is then left to heal by itself and only a few currently available drugs are able to influence the defensive factors, e.g. sucralfate, bismuth-containing compounds.

This paper was presented at the Symposium on 'Cell injury and protection in the gastrointestinal tract: from basic science to clinical perspectives', October 8–11, 1995, Pécs, Hungary.

8The observation that the spontaneously healed duodenal ulcer contains 2–3 times fewer microvessels than the surrounding intact tissue suggests that healing is far from optimal and indicates new ways to directly enhance the healing processes in ulcer disease, gastritis and colitis [4–6]. Namely, stimulation of ulcer healing is possible by enhancing angiogenesis, granulation tissue formation and re-epithelialization. One of the best candidates might be growth factors which act locally via autocrine and paracrine pathways. Epidermal growth factor (EGF) which inhibits acid secretion was first found to exert antiulcer activity [7,8]. Subsequently, basic fibroblast growth factor (bFGF) was found to be about 7 million times more potent on a molar basis than the antiulcerogenic effect of cimetidine in the healing of cysteamine-induced chronic duodenal ulcers in rats [4,5]. The mechanisms of action of bFGF and EGF are nevertheless different since the ulcer healing properties of bFGF were not associated with decreased acid or pepsin secretion, implying that the ulcer healing action of bFGF is direct, and involves the upper and lower gastrointestinal (GI) tract [4–6,9]. More recently, platelet-derived growth factor (PDGF) was also shown to exert a strong healing effect in experimental chronic duodenal ulcers, chronic gastritis and ulcerative colitis [10–13].

The therapeutic success of these growth factors suggests that many mechanisms and regulators are involved in ulcer healing. These include angiogenesis, the proliferation and migration of epithelial cells, the production of granulation tissue (i.e. deposition of collagen, proliferation of fibroblasts and neovascularization). Some of these cytokines may also become new 'endogenous drugs' for ulcer healing [14].

Since our laboratory was first to use bFGF and PDGF in animal models of ulcerative and inflammatory lesions of the GI tract [4–6,9], this minireview is focused mainly on our recent data on the role of these two growth factors in ulcer healing.

FIBROBLAST GROWTH FACTOR

Fibroblast growth factors exist in multiple forms, e.g. acidic (aFGF) and basic (bFGF) derivatives, and are expressed in most cells of the body, especially in endothelial cells, fibroblasts and macrophages [15,16]. These molecules are stored within the basal membrane or extracellular matrix and are released in an active form to stimulate tissue repair and healing [17]. The bFGF isoform is one of the most potent endothelial mitogens, and it also stimulates the proliferation of fibroblasts, smooth muscle and neural cells [18,19] (Table 1).

Basic FGF influences the restoration of virtually all the elements needed to replace the lost tissue in GI ulcers. Since angiogenesis or neovascularization is one of the most important processes in ulcer healing, and bFGF is one of the most potent angiogenic peptides so far isolated, we hypothesized that bFGF might exert potent ulcer-healing properties.

The initial studies in our laboratory demonstrated that oral treatment of rats with either the naturally occurring bFGF or its acid-resistant mutein, in which the second and third cysteines are replaced with site-specific mutagenesis by serines [20], bFGF-CS23 (100 ng/100 g, twice a day) accelerated the healing of chronic cysteamine-

TABLE 1

The actions of bFGF and PDGF in ulcer pathogenesis, prevention and healing

	bFGF	PDGF
Gastric acid secretion	No change or stimulation	No change
Duodenal alkaline secretion	No	No
Angiogenesis stimulation	Potent	Mild or minimal
Fibroblast proliferation	Yes	Yes
Epithelial restitution	Yes	?
Epithelial proliferation	Yes	?
Smooth muscle regeneration	Yes	Yes
Neuronal regeneration	Yes	?
Acute gastroprotection	No	Mild
Chronic ulcer healing	Potent	Potent

Updated from Reference 34

induced duodenal ulcers [4,5]. This effect was equal to or more potent than the oral administration of cimetidine (10 mg/100 g, twice a day for 3 weeks); however, only treatment with the acid-resistant mutein, bFGF-CS23 (100 ng/100 g, twice a day for 3 weeks) decreased significantly both the size ($p < 0.01$ vs control) and the incidence ($p < 0.05$ vs control) of experimental chronic duodenal ulcers. Secretory studies showed that a single dose of bFGF had no effect on gastric output of acid and pepsin, whereas daily treatment for 2 or 3 weeks resulted in enhanced output of both products [5,21]. On a molar basis, the antiulcer effect of bFGF-CS23 (100 ng/100 g) was about 7 million times more potent than that of cimetidine (10 mg/100 g).

Our next series of pharmacological experiments were related to the possibility of combination therapy involving both direct and indirect treatment of duodenal ulcers. Namely, we found that since the natural form of bFGF (bFGF-w) is sensitive to acid–peptic degradation, treatment of rats with antisecretory drugs like cimetidine increased the concentration of bFGF in the stomach [22] (Figure 1). Sucralfate, because of its similarity to heparin, also binds bFGF-w and increases the local bioavailability of bFGF in the rat stomach [22]. We thus tested the hypothesis that exogenous bFGF and cimetidine or lansoprazole might exert an additive or potentiating interaction in the healing of experimental ulcers. The duodenal ulcer size in the cimetidine (10 mg/100 g) plus bFGF (50 ng/100 g) treated group was significantly lower (2.0 ± 0.6 mm^2, $p < 0.05$) than in the group given only cimetidine (10 mg/100 g) (7.5 ± 2.1 mm^2), while, in the combination therapy with the smaller dose of bFGF (10 ng/100 g), the difference was at the border of statistical significance (2.5 ± 0.6 mm^2, $p = 0.06$). Lansoprazole alone (1 mg/100 g) reduced the ulcer size to 3.0 ± 1.6 mm^2 ($p < 0.05$). The combination of lansoprazole (1 mg/100 g) and bFGF-CS23 (2 and 50 ng/100 g) resulted in smaller ulcer sizes (2.5 ± 0.8 and 2.0 ± 0.9 mm^2, respectively). Histological evaluation revealed that the combination treatment reduced the extent of necrosis and inflammation in the ulcer crater [23,24].

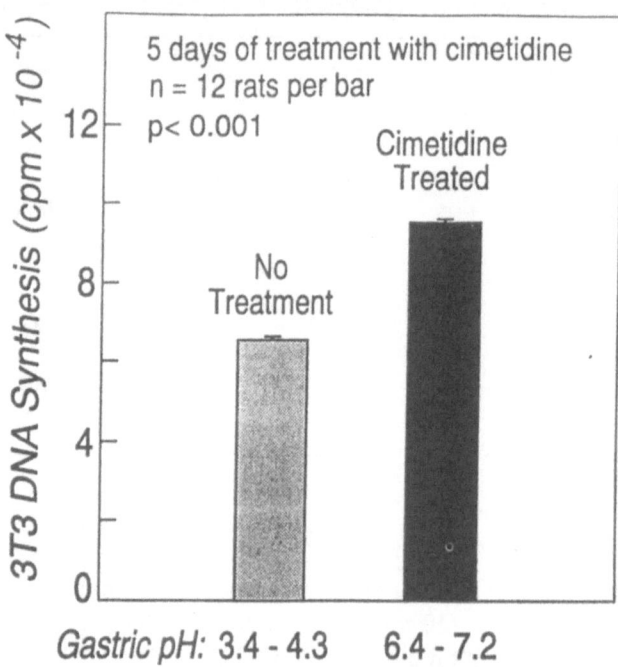

Figure 1. Effect of treatment with cimetidine on the concentration of endogenous bFGF in the rat stomach. Twenty-four rats with chronic duodenal ulcers induced by cysteamine were divided randomly into two groups of 12 rats each. The first group received no treatment except for gavage with vehicle (water) twice daily. The second group received cimetidine, 20 mg/100 g by intragastric gavage twice daily for 5 days. All animals were killed on day 6, and the pH of the gastric juice was measured. The untreated animals had a pH range of 3.4–4.3; the cimetidine-treated animals had a pH of 6.4–7.2. The ulcer beds were excised and the bFGF in the ulcer bed was analysed for DNA synthesis activity on the 3T3 fibroblasts. Cimetidine-treated animals had significantly higher levels of biologically active bFGF in the ulcer bed than the untreated animals ($p < 0.001$). (Reprinted with permission from Folkman et al., Ann Surg. 1991;214:414–27, Reference 22)

The efficacy of bFGF was also shown in preliminary human studies. Namely, previously therapy-resistant duodenal and antral ulcers were found to heal rapidly after oral treatment with bFGF-CS23 for four weeks, without any adverse effect on systemic absorption of the compound [25].

Subsequently, we investigated the effects of mucosal bFGF on the natural history of ulcer disease [26]. We postulated that endogenous bFGF, presumably occurring in the ulcer bed in the gut mucosa, might be critical to ulcer healing because of its angiogenic and other mitogenic properties. To test this hypothesis, rats were treated with the duodenal ulcerogen cysteamine three times at 4-h intervals and were killed 12, 24 and 48 h after the first dose of cysteamine. Mucosal scrapings from proximal duodenum

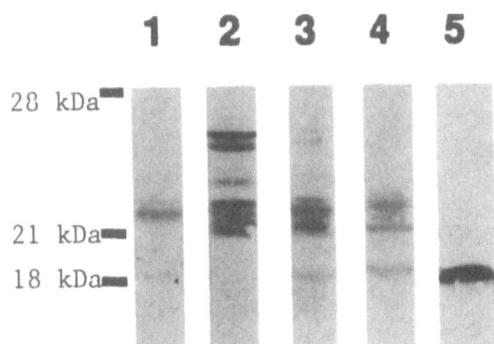

Figure 2. To assess the changes in molecular forms of basic fibroblast growth factor (bFGF) during duodenal ulceration, heparin-binding proteins from rat duodenal mucosa were extracted, separated on a 15% polyacrylamide gel and analysed for bFGF expression by Western blot. Lanes: 1, control rat; 2, 12 h after the first of three cysteamine injections; 3, 24 h after cysteamine; 4, 48 h after cysteamine; 5, low-molecular-weight (18-kDa) bFGF control. (Reprinted with permission from Szabo et al., Eur J Gastroenterol Hepatol. 1993;5(Suppl. 3):S53–7, Reference 26)

were homogenized in 2 mol/L sodium chloride buffered at pH 7.4. The high salt concentration was necessary to ensure the complete removal of bFGF from cationic factors in the extracellular matrix [27]. The extract was then diluted 10-fold and the heparin-binding fraction was isolated on heparin-sepharose beads, since sulphated saccharides, such as heparin, have high affinity for fibroblast growth factors [22,27], followed by Western blotting. The primary antibody was monoclonal anti-bFGF antibody (MAb 77R, Takeda Chemicals, Japan). After 12 h, a reduction in the low-molecular-weight (LMW, 18-kDa) form of bFGF (localized to the cytoplasm and extracellular space) was found, with a simultaneous increase in the high-molecular-weight (HMW, 20-, 21- and 25-kDa) forms (localized to the nuclei of cells), compared with the controls (Figure 2). After 24 h, the HMW forms decreased, with an increase in the LMW, compared with the 12-h samples. The 48-h samples showed a continuation of this trend towards the pattern seen in the controls [26].

Our more recent studies combining Western blot and ELISA analysis of bFGF and PDGF are summarized in another paper in this issue [28].

PLATELET-DERIVED GROWTH FACTOR

PDGF, unlike bFGF, is acid resistant in its natural form and is a potent mitogen for fibroblasts, epithelial and endothelial cells. It has a chemoattractant property for monocytes, neutrophils, fibroblasts and some smooth muscle cells (Table 2). It stimulates the production of collagen by fibroblasts in culture which is essential for

TABLE 2

Comparative effects and doses of bFGF and PDGF in ulcer healing and prevention

	bFGF-w	bFGF-CS23	PDGF-BB
Chronic duodenal ulcer (cysteamine–HCl)	100 ng/100 g	10, 50, 100 ng/100 g	100, 500 ng/100 g
Chronic erosive gastritis (iodoacetamide)	25 ng/100 g	25, 100 ng/100 g	500, 2500 ng/100 g
Gastric secretion (pylorus ligation)	NE or ↑	NE or ↑	NE
Acute gastroprotection (ethanol model)	No	No	2.5 µg/100 g
Endogenous peptides involved	Yes	–	Yes

NE, no effect

tissue repair [29,30]. PDGF consists of A and B peptides, and exists in three isoforms: AA, BB and AB [31]. The molecular forms of PDGF which contain the A chain can activate only the α or A receptor of PDGF, while PDGF-BB can act on both α and β receptors [31,32]. The gene encoding PDGF-A is on human chromosome 7, while PDGF-B is encoded by human chromosome 22 [32].

Since PDGF-BB may activate both α and β receptors, we used this homodimer in acute gastroprotection and chronic ulcer healing studies. In the acute series of experiments, gastric haemorrhagic erosions were produced by 1 ml 75% ethanol in fasting rats, while PDGF-BB (2.5 µg/100 g, sc or ig) and, for comparison, bFGF (1 µg/ 100 g sc) were given 30 min before ethanol. The rats were killed 1 h after the administration of damaging agent, and the area of acute haemorrhagic mucosal lesions was measured by computerized stereomicroscopic planimetry. bFGF and the sc administration of PDGF did not reduce the area of mucosal lesions (8.5 ± 2.0 and 7.0 ± 1.3 vs $10.3 \pm 1.5\%$ of glandular stomach in the control animals, respectively), while the intragastric administration of PDGF was slightly effective (6.3 ± 1.7, $p = 0.09$ with Mann–Whitney U test). Thus, while EGF exerts strong gastroprotection in small doses which do not influence gastric acid secretion [8], PDGF had only mild, and bFGF did not exert, acute gastroprotective effects.

In chronic healing studies, oral administration of PDGF-BB (100 and 500 ng/100 g, twice daily for 3 weeks) significantly accelerated the healing of chronic duodenal ulcer induced by cysteamine (the ulcer sizes were 2.5 ± 1.1 mm^2 [$p = 0.051$] and 2.0 ± 1.4 mm^2 [$p = 0.048$], respectively, vs 16.9 ± 6.8 mm^2 in controls). Mechanistically, it is important that gastric acid secretion was not influenced by these doses of PDGF-BB [10].

Oral treatment with PDGF-BB (0.5 and 2.5 µg/100 g, twice a day), like bFGF, also dose-dependently decreased the severity of chronic gastritis induced by the sulphydryl alkylator iodoacetamide (0.1% in drinking water) in rats [6,11]. More recently, we also found that intracolonic administration of PDGF-BB, like bFGF [9], accelerated the healing of experimental ulcerative colitis [12,13].

Our preliminary results with ELISA and Western blotting on the role of endogenous PDGF in ulcer healing are also summarized in a recent paper [28]. Nakamura et al. recently reported an 'increased effector site' of PDGF and bFGF during acetic acid-induced gastric ulcer healing in rats [33].

Thus, in addition to bFGF, PDGF is also a very potent and naturally occurring antiulcer agent which may be active both in the upper and lower GI tract.

REFERENCES

1. Allen A, Flemström G, Garner A, Kivilaakso E. Gastroduodenal mucosal protection. Physiol Rev. 1993;73:823.
2. Hunt RH, Tytgat GNJ, eds. Helicobacter pylori. Basic Mechanisms to Clinical Cure. Dordrecht, Boston, London: Kluwer Academic Press; 1994.
3. Szabo S, Mózsik Gy, eds. New Pharmacology of Ulcer Disease: Experimental and New Therapeutic Approaches. New York: Elsevier; 1987.
4. Szabo S, Folkman J, Vattay P et al. Duodenal ulcerogens: The effect of FGF on cysteamine-induced duodenal ulcer. In: Halter F, Garner A, Tytgat GNJ, eds. Mechanisms of Peptic Ulcer Healing. Dordrecht, Boston, London: Kluwer Academic Publishers; 1991:139–50.
5. Szabo S, Folkman J, Vattay P, Morales RE, Pinkus GE, Kato K. Accelerated healing of duodenal ulcers by oral administration of a mutein of fibroblast growth factor in rats. Gastroenterology. 1994;106:1106–11.
6. Szabo S, Kusstatscher S, Stovroff M. Role of bFGF and angiogenesis in ulcer healing and the treatment of gastritis. In: Domschke W, Konturek SJ, eds. The Stomach. Berlin, Heidelberg: Springer-Verlag; 1993:193–7.
7. Poulsen SS, Olsen PS, Kirkegaard P. Healing of cysteamine-induced duodenal ulcers in the rat. Dig Dis Sci. 1985;30:161–7.
8. Konturek SJ, Brzozowski T, Dembinski A et al. Gastric protective and ulcer-healing action of epidermal growth factor. In: Garner A, Whittle BJR, eds. Advances in Drug Therapy of Gastrointestinal Ulceration. New York: John Wiley and Sons; 1989:261–73.
9. Satoh H, Takami K, Kato K et al. Effect of bFGF and its mutein on healing of colonic ulcers induced by N-ethyl-maleimide in rats. Gastroenterology. 1990;98:A203.
10. Vattay P, Gyömbér E, Morales RE et al. Effect of orally administered platelet-derived growth factor (PDGF) on healing of chronic duodenal ulcers and gastric secretion in rats. Gastroenterology. 1991;100:A183.
11. Kusstatscher S, Szabo S. Effect of platelet-derived growth factor (PDGF) on the healing of chronic gastritis in rats. Gastroenterology. 1993;104:A125.
12. Sandor Z, Szeli D, Charette M et al. Platelet-derived growth factor (PDGF) accelerates the healing of experimental ulcerative colitis in rats. Gastroenterology. 1995;108:A208.
13. Sandor Z, Kusstatscher S, Szeli D, Szabo S. The effect of platelet-derived growth factor (PDGF) on experimental inflammatory bowel disease. Orvosi Hetilap. 1995;136:24–6.
14. Szabo S, Kusstatscher S, Sakoulas G, Sandor Z, Vincze Á, Jadus M. Growth factors: New 'endogenous drugs' for ulcer healing. Scand J Gastroenterol. 1995;30(Suppl.210):15–18.
15. Gospodarowicz D, Neufeld G, Schweigerer L. Fibroblast growth factor. Mol Cell Endocrinol. 1986;46:187–206.
16. Gospodarowicz D, Ferrara N, Schweigerer L, Neufeld G. Structural characterization and biological functions of fibroblast growth factors. Endocr Rev. 1987;8:95–114.

17. Folkman J, Klagsbrum M, Sasse I, Wadzinski M, Ingberg D, Vlodavsky I. A heparin binding angiogenic protein – basic fibroblast growth factor – is stored within basement membrane. Am J Pathol. 1988;130:393–400.
18. Folkman J, Klagsbrum M. Angiogenic factors. Science. 1987;235:442–7.
19. Gospodarowicz D. Fibroblast growth factors. In: Aggarwal BB, Gutterman JU, eds. Human Cytokines: Hand book for Basic and Clinical Research. Boston: Blackwell Scientific Publications; 1992:330–51.
20. Seno K, Sasada R, Iwane K et al. Stabilizing basic fibroblast growth factor using protein engineering. Biochem Biophys Res Commun. 1988;151:701–8.
21. Konturek SJ, Brzozowski T, Majka J et al. Fibroblast growth factor in gastroprotection and ulcer healing: interaction with sucralfate. Gut. 1993;34:881–7.
22. Folkman J, Szabo S, Stovroff M, McNeil P, Li W, Shing Y. Duodenal ulcer: Discovery of a new mechanism and development of angiogenic therapy that accelerates healing. Ann Surg. 1991;214:414–27.
23. Kusstatscher S, Nagy L, Morales RE et al. Additive effect of basic fibroblast growth factor (bFGF) and cimetidine on chronic duodenal ulcer healing in rats. Gastroenterology. 1992;102:A104.
24. Vincze Á, Kusstatscher S, Satoh H et al. Additive effect of basic fibroblast growth factor (bFGF) and lansoprazole on chronic duodenal ulcer healing in rats. Gastroenterology. 1995;108:A762.
25. Wolfe MM, Bynum TE, Parsons WG et al. Safety and efficacy of an angiogenic peptide, basic fibroblast growth factor (bFGF), in the treatment of gastroduodenal ulcers: A preliminary report. Gastroenterology. 1994;106:A212.
26. Szabo S, Sakoulas G, Kusstatscher S, Sandor Z. Effects of endogenous and exogenous basic fibroblast growth factor in ulcer healing. Eur J Gastroenterol Hepatol. 1993;5(Suppl. 3):S52–7.
27. Klagsbrun M, Shing Y. Heparin affinity of anionic and cationic capillary endothelial cell growth factors: analysis of hypothalamus-derived growth factor and fibroblast growth factor. Proc Soc Exp Biol Med. 1985;82:805–9.
28. Vincze Á, Nagata M, Sandor Z, Szabo S. ELISA and Western blot studies with basic fibroblast growth factor (bFGF) and platelet-derived growth factor (PDGF) in experimental duodenal ulceration and healing. Inflammopharmacology. 1996;4(3):261–5.
29. Ross R. Platelet-derived growth factor. Annu Rev Med. 1987;38:71.
30. Deuel TF, Kawahara RS. Platelet-derived growth factor. In: Aggarwal BB, Gutterman JU, eds. Human Cytokines: Handbook for Basic and Clinical Research. Boston: Blackwell Scientific Publications; 1992:301–27.
31. Heldin C-H, Westermark B. Platelet-derived growth factor: three isoforms and two receptor types. Trends Genet. 1989;5:108.
32. Pimentel E, ed. Handbook of Growth Factors. Vol. III: Hematopoietic Growth Factors and Cytokines. Boca Raton: CRC Press; 1994.
33. Nakamura M, Akiba Y, Oda M et al. Increased effector site of platelet-derived growth factor-AA, BB and basic fibroblast growth factor during acetic acid-induced gastric ulcer healing. Gastroenterology. 1995;108:A175.
34. Szabo S, Folkman J, Kusstatscher S, Sandor Zs, Wolfe MM. The effect of bFGF and PDGF on acute gastric mucosal lesions, chronic gastritis and chronic duodenal ulcer. In: Szabo S, Taché Y, Glavin GB, eds. Neuroendocrinology of Gastrointestinal Ulceration. New York: Plenum Press; 1995:61–71.

G Mózsik et al. Cell Injury and Cytoprotection in the GI Tract. 71–81.

THE RESPONSE OF ODONTOBLASTS TO INJURY TO EPITHELIAL INTEGRITY: REVIEW

J. SZABÓ* AND G. VARBIRÓ

School of Dentistry, Medical University of Pécs, Pécs, Hungary
*Correspondence

ABSTRACT

The odontoblast cells can be exposed to the irritating effect of various noxious agents under carious lesions or abrasion of enamel and under the damaged cells of the epithelial sulcus. The odontoblasts have the potential for recovery and repair which can be detected at the light and electron-microscopical levels. The corresponding dentine reactions represent a continuum of dentineal reactions. Bacterial invasion into the dentine in relation to the activity of underlying odontoblasts has been examined by several authors. Two different types of reaction may occur: secondary dentine formation at the pulp-dentine border and the dentinal tubules may become obturated by growth of the peritubular dentine or by precipitation of materials within the tubules. Precipitation of materials is considered to be a passive physical–chemical process but the growth of peritubular dentine and secondary dentine formation is a typical vital response, requiring odontoblast activity. Lesions restricted to the outer third of the dentine have a positive effect on the metabolism of injured odontoblasts, which appears as an increased rate of synthesis observed by measurement of enzyme activities. The effect of growth factors, peptide hormones and brain–gut peptides on odontoblast response requires further studies.

Keywords: odontoblast injury, active cellular reactions, passive dentine sclerosis

EPITHELIAL INTEGRITY

The epithelial integrity of the oral cavity, the first part of the respiratory and alimentary tracts, involves teeth being covered by intact enamel, healthy sulcus epithelial cells adhering to the enamel and oral mucosa cells without any alteration. The various diseases of the masticatory, specialized and lining oral mucosa and the different enamel lesions are collectively termed as the loss of epithelial integrity.

THE ORAL CAVITY AS PART OF THE ALIMENTARY AND RESPIRATORY TRACTS

Gastrointestinal diseases, like coeliac disease or tropical sprue, Crohn's disease or ulcerative colitis, are usually connected with oral cavity symptoms. Interestingly enough, the sprue was derived from a Dutch word for aphthosus ulcer, indicating the high proportion of sufferers with oral ulcerations [1]. Although the passage of food and fluids through the oral cavity is rapid compared with the lower intestinal tract, the

This paper was presented at the Symposium on 'Cell injury and protection in the gastrointestinal tract: from basic science to clinical perspectives', October 8–11, 1995, Pécs, Hungary.

mastication and the start of digestion by saliva enzymes [2] have an effect on the function of the gastrointestinal tract. Contrary to swallowing, mastication is a learned reflex mechanism and a very individual one though it has a major effect on enzymatic digestion. The upper portion of the alimentary tract has some morphological and functional features. A unique and special organ is the tooth, being the only hard tissue intraluminally in the alimentary tract.

The oral cavity as the first part of the respiratory tract, as well, shows a different gas content [3] from the lower intestinal and respiratory tracts. It has to be emphasized that the average oxygen concentration in the mandibular and buccal fold is about 0.3–0.4%; cf. the dorsal surface of the tongue where it is 12–16%. This allows a wide variety of intraoral micro-organisms, such as various Treponema species and Bacteroides species, to be present primarily in the gingiva crevice area and these cannot be recovered from the surface of the tongue. Moreover, these low oxygen concentrations are consistent with the relatively low redox potential (Eh) levels found in the gingival sulcus. A low Eh is an essential component of an ecosystem supporting the growth and survival of subgingival anaerobic bacteria. Injury to the gingival sulcus epithelial cells in connection with low Eh is an intensively studied field of cell injuries in the oral cavity [4–8] because the periodontal chronic inflammation is associated with the loss of teeth in the adult population and is found in all people, in all nations. On the enamel surface of the teeth, the adhesion of micro-organisms causing caries of the enamel is governed together with other factors by a thin layer of saliva macromolecules called the acquired pellicle [9–11].

MESENCHYMAL STRUCTURES UNDERLYING THE ENAMEL

The dentine, as a mineralized tissue forms the bulk of teeth. It is covered by enamel, a cell-free and non-regenerating epithelial structure. The dentine-forming cells are layered in the pulp near to the predentine. In contrast to tooth enamel, which developmentally is an ectodermal product, dentine is mesodermally derived [12,13]. In this sense, dentine is related to bone and dental cement. The similarities prevail but the epithelial-like configuration of tightly connecting odontoblast cells and the definite differences in chemistry and mode of formation may be used for comparative purposes to elucidate cell injury mechanisms [14–17].

Primary dentine is the dentine formed at a relatively high rate during formation of the tooth. After root formation of the tooth is complete, the odontoblasts continue to form dentine on the pulpal aspect of the primary dentine, although at a much reduced rate [18].

The odontoblast cell process [19–21], which is called Tomes fibre, can be found in the dentinal tubules running to the periphery of dentine. Circumpulpal dentine may be divided into peritubular and intertubular dentine. Beside the Tomes fibre, the axons and nerve endings of the trigeminal nerve are present in the dentinal tubules [22]. No cell organelles can be found in healthy dentine. Ribosomes are present only in the cell body of nerve cells and odontoblast so no protein synthesis occurs in the axons and Tomes fibres [23–25].

It is generally believed that initiation of each mineral crystal is facilitated by some kind of nucleation. This term refers to a specific stereochemical arrangement of reactive groups with electrical charge or other properties that lower the energy barrier, so that some solid phase of calcium phosphate is formed from an otherwise stable solution [26]. This is why dentinogenesis is a convenient experimental system for the study of biomineralization mechanisms. Non-collagenous proteins, NCPs, are extensively studied for their role in tissue mineralization. Proteoglycans, PGs, are inhibitory to mineralization, whereas highly phosphorylated phosphoproteins, PP-H, are reported to be directly transported to the dentine mineralization front [27–29].

CELL INJURY

Cell injury, which may be induced by external noxious stimuli or by the activation of various endogenous systems and mediators, provokes inflammation or disturbed cell growth and transformation. Diseases with altered or overgrowth of the oral mucus membrane cells could be used as models for studying the roles of different mediators and immune responses, e.g. reduced natural killer cell activity was observed in patients with oral leukoplakia [30]. Natural killer cell activity is an important effector in immunosurveillance against tumours and can be stimulated by interferon. The oral cavity lesions can be used for detection of natural killer cell effectiveness. Similarly, soft-tissue oral lesions can be used as models for immunological pathogenesis of injured cells [31].

Under the epithelial lesions, injury to the subjacent mesenchymal cells could influence the pathomechanism and the reparation of the lesions alongside the gastrointestinal tract. Therefore, the odontoblast layer could be used as a model for studying the pathogenesis and pathomechanism of injured mesenchymal cells in the alimentary tract. Some details of odontoblast response to enamel injury are well known and understood [32–34].

Response of odontoblasts to the injury

As a response to external stimuli, such as chemical irritants, caries, attrition or other trauma, tertiary dentine may form. This is often referred to as *reparative* or *irritation* dentine. The site of formation of reparative dentine is at the pulpal end of the injured odontoblasts and this tertiary dentine is produced by differentiated fibroblasts of the pulp [35,36].

Studying the pathomechanism of dentine caries could result in understanding of calcium transport and deposition governed by active cell function or by passive physicochemical mechanisms [37,38].

The earliest possible stage of dental development when a carious process may attack the dental tissues is when primary dentine formation has already ceased in the coronal areas. Then odontoblasts, after the active period of synthesis and secretion, enter a new stage of their life cycle, i.e. the stage of slow metabolism [39].

There are no reports so far about alteration of the cell process due to ageing. However, ageing appears as a slightly reduced height of cells accompanied by a reduced number of intracellular organelles. Moreover, a specific age-related relocation of the intracellular synthetic machinery has been reported. Frequently, large lipid-filled vacuoles have been demonstrated in aged odontoblasts. All these alterations result in reduced protein synthesis and increased autolytic activity. The remaining organelles are sufficient for slow but continuous dentine formation and for a limited reactivation if needed [40].

The alterations in ultrastructure are in accordance with those demonstrated in the secretory rate of the aged odontoblasts: the formation of dentine matrix by rat incisor odontoblasts is approximately four times faster than that displayed by the fully formed rat molar odontoblast. Also, in humans it is estimated that the formative rate of aged odontoblasts decreases to one quarter of the value displayed by the actively functioning cells. The amount of ATP, and the activity of ATPase enzymes, may partly reflect the level of energy consumption in cells. The peripulpal dentine of developing teeth, representing active secretory odontoblasts, has been shown to contain amounts of ATP and ATPase activity levels approximately equal to those of odontoblasts which are in the stage of secondary dentine formation. It may be concluded that the formation of secondary dentine requires amounts of ATP-related energy approximately equal to those required for the formation of primary dentine [41].

Caries-induced injury represents a chronic type of cell damage, whereas the treatment for the disease is a sudden acute type of injury. In studies, alterations related to chronic sublethal cell injuries have been described: these include lipid accumulation; formation of autophagic lysosomes and pigmented residual bodies; formation of several kinds of watery vacuolation; dilation of the endoplasmatic reticulum or of the phagolysosomal system; modification in the microtubules; formation of cytoplasmic or nuclear inclusions; atrophy or reduction in the size of the nuclei have been demonstrated.

In a series of studies using biochemical methods, the metabolic activity of odontoblasts [35] was determined by measuring the levels of various enzyme activities as a function of the propagation of caries. The enzymes were selected to reflect the rate of mineralization (ALP, phosphoserine phosphatase), the levels of energy requirement (ATPase), the pattern of metabolism whether aerobic or anaerobic (lactate and malate dehydrogenase activity), the possible activation of the inflammatory process (arginin aminopeptidase activity) and the activation of the autophagic system (acid phosphatase). The biochemical findings suggest that the aged odontoblasts of fully matured teeth, if mildly injured, are capable of a limited reactivation of both the rate of mineralization and collagenous matrix formation. If no intervention occurs and the process is allowed to proceed, several enzyme activities decrease below the level displayed by aged healthy odontoblasts. Judging from the activation of autophagic lysosomal enzymes, the odontoblasts are no longer capable of maintaining a steady homeostasis.

Lesions extending no further than the peripheral third of the dentine caused a moderate reactivation of the aged odontoblasts which could be measured biochemically as increased rates of matrix formation and mineralization. Histologically,

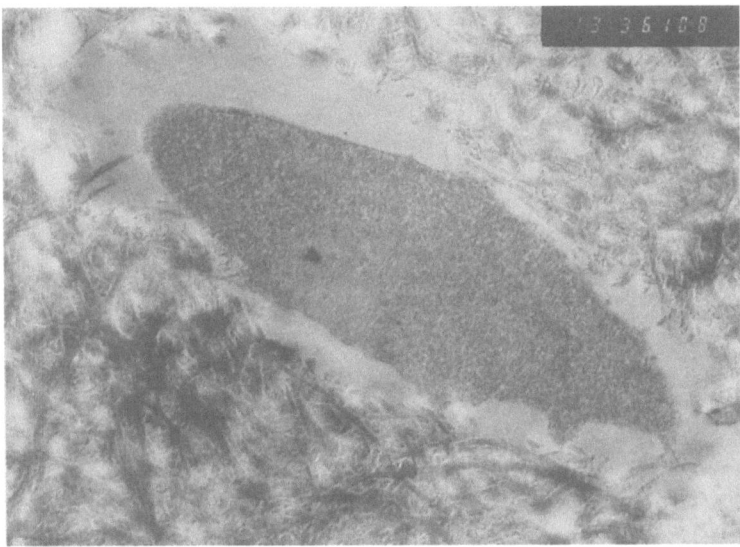

Figure 1. Transmission electron microscopic view of an obliquely sectioned dentineal tubule in the inner third of the carious dentine. Note the preserved structure of collagen fibres and the small number of secretory granules. (Original magnification × 36 000)

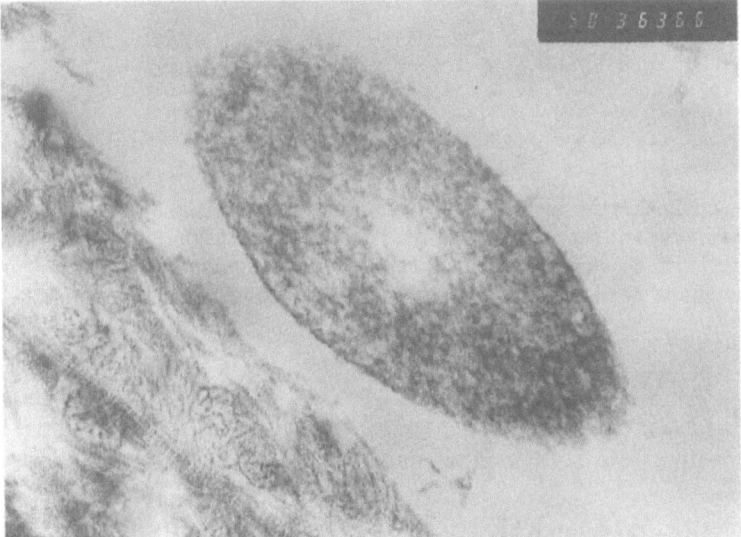

Figure 2. Transmission electron microscopic view of an obliquely sectioned dentineal tubule in the middle third of the carious dentine. Note the preserved structure of collagen fibres and the central degeneration of the odontoblast process. (Original magnification × 36 000)

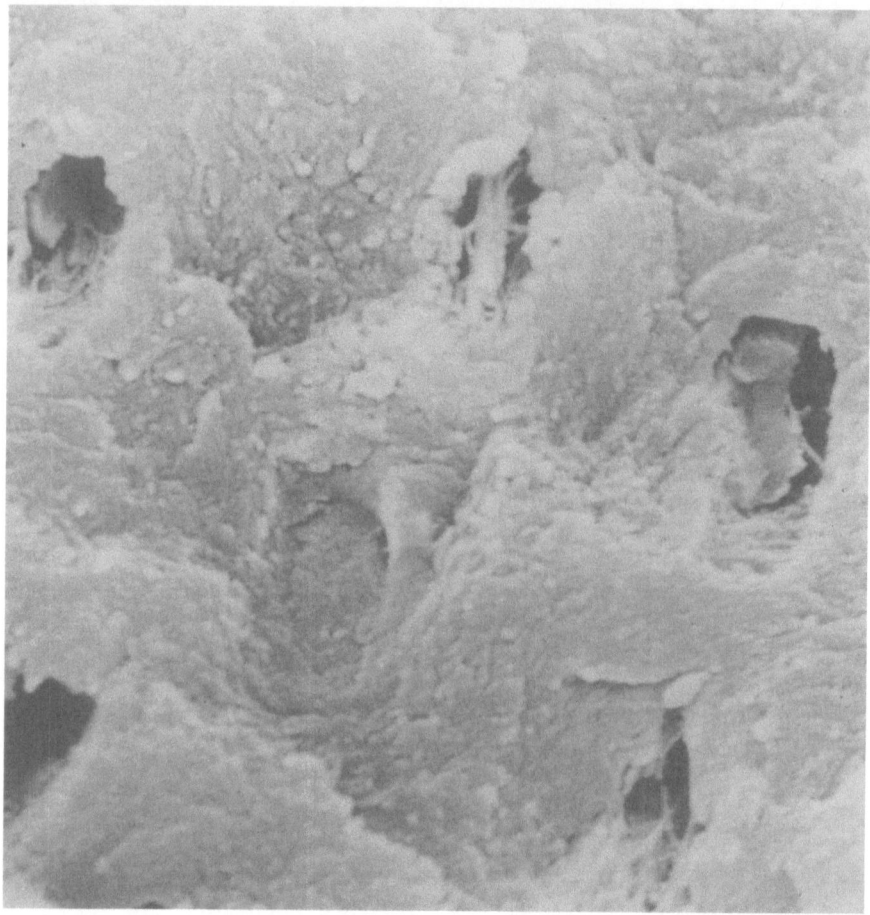

Figure 3. Scanning electron microscopic view of transversely fractured dentineal tubules at the border of the middle and the peripheral third of dentine. Note the thickening of the peritubular dentine constricting the lumen of the dentineal tubules. The odontoblast process can be seen and the intertubular dentine is highly mineralized. (Original magnification × 10 000)

reduction in the widths of predentine and cell-free zones was observed. Initial layers of reparative dentine were detected at the pulpal wall, formed as a response to the lesion [35].

Lesions restricted to the middle third of dentine had a detrimental effect on the metabolism of injured odontoblasts, which appeared as a reduced rate of synthesis and an increased rate of autophagic activity (Figures 1 and 2). Histologically, a reduced width of predentine accompanied by a reduced width of cell-free zone was observed. Thicker layers of reparative dentine were frequently found.

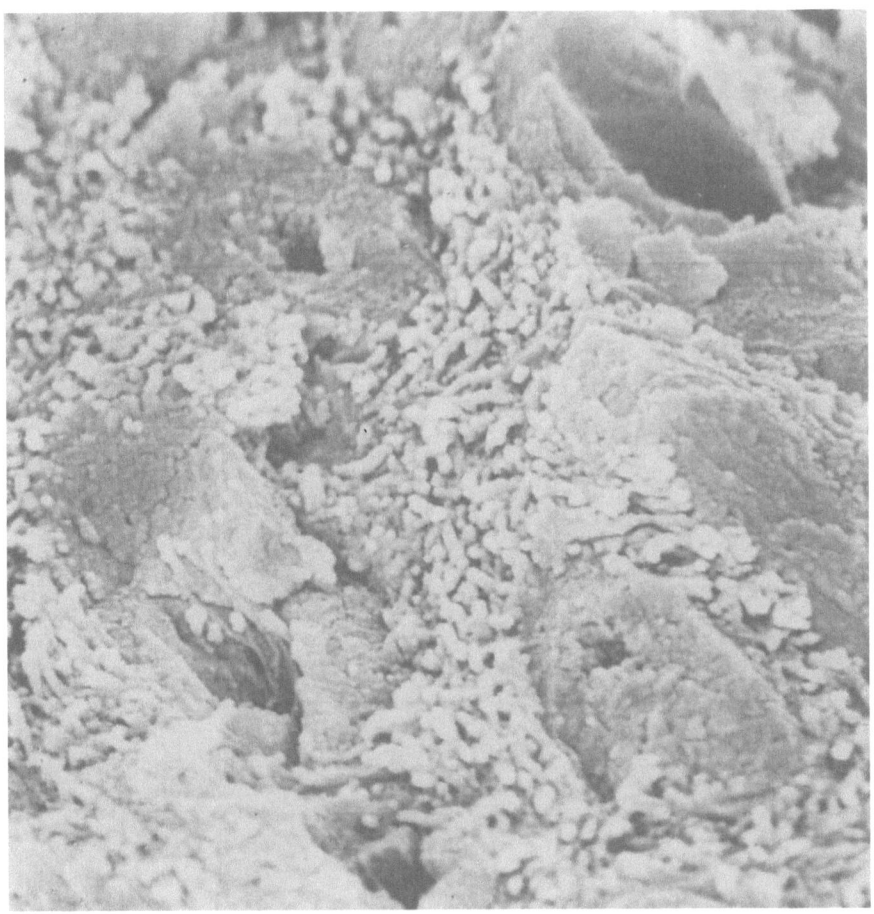

Figure 4. Scanning electron microscopic view of cross-fractured dentineal tubules at the border of the middle and the peripheral third of carious dentine. Note the lumen-obturating depositions and the lack of odontoblast processes. The intertubular dentine is porous. (Original magnification × 10 000)

Two basically different types of reaction may occur in the dentine–predentine complex. Tertiary dentine, often an irregular type as a response to external irritation, may form at the pulp–predentine border. As the second type of reaction, dentinal tubules may become partly or completely obturated by growth of peritubular dentine (Figure 3) or by precipitation of mineral salts within the tubules (Figure 4). The growth of peritubular dentine is a typical vital response, requiring cellular activity. Precipitation of mineral salts within the tubules is considered to be a physical–chemical process.

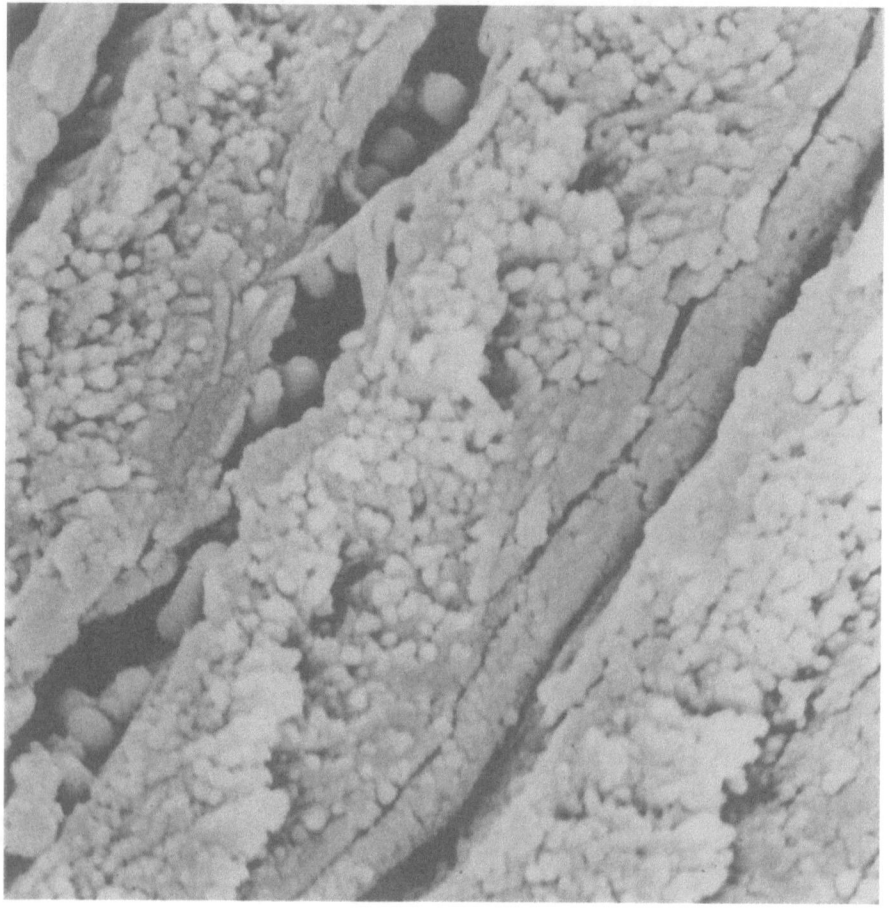

Figure 5. Scanning electron microscopic view of longitudinally fractured dentineal tubules at the middle third of carious dentine. Note the degenerated odontoblast process in one of the tubules, and the bacteria in the lumen of the neighbouring tubules. (Orignal magnification × 10 000)

In addition, dentine exposed to the oral environment may require a hypermineralized surface layer and ground dentine becomes covered by a smear layer. Displacement of the content of the tubules and of the odontoblast nucleus as well as of the cytoplasmic organelles may lead to degeneration of the soft organic components of the dentine. Destruction of odontoblasts will lead to a reduction or lack of predentine formation [42,43].

The generally accepted theory of complete lack of odontoblast processes in the

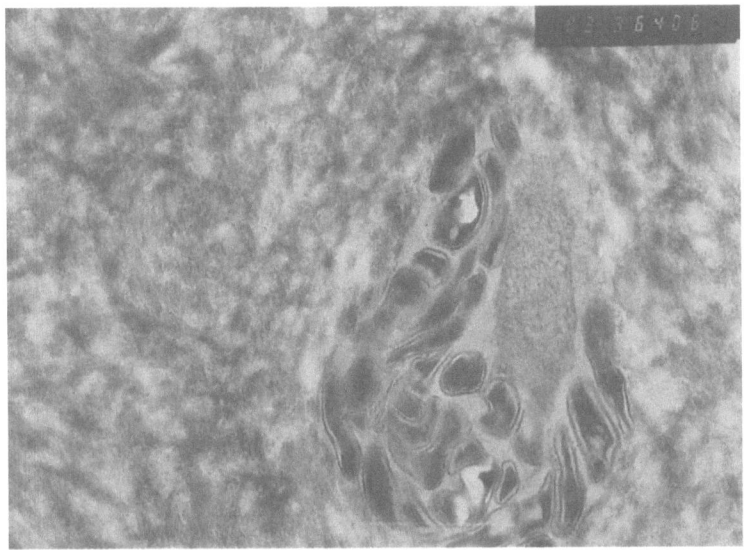

Figure 6. Transmission electron microscopic view of a cross-sectioned dentineal tubule in the middle third of the carious dentine. Note the destroyed structure of collagen fibres and odontoblast process. The lumen of the dentineal tubule is packed with micro-organisms (Original magnification × 36 000)

infected dentine could be debated based on our observations (Figures 5 and 6) and results [42,43].

Because of the lack of detailed understanding of the mechanisms of odontoblast injury caused by microbial invasion of dentinal tubules, further research is necessary, as in the case of investigation of mesenchymal cell responses of soft tissues underlying the injured epithelial layer in other parts of the gastrointestinal system.

REFERENCES

1. Tyldesley WR. Oral Medicine, 2nd edn. Oxford: Oxford University Press; 1981.
2. Valdez IH, Fox PC. Interactions of the salivary and gastrointestinal systems. I. The role of saliva in digestion. Dig Dis. 1991;9:125–32.
3. Eskow RN, Loesche WJ. Oxygen tensions in the human oral cavity. Arch Oral Biol. 1971;16:1127–8.
4. Ower PC, Ciantar M, Newman HN, Wilson M, Bulman JS. The effects on chronic periodontitis of a subgingivally placed redox agent in a slow release device. J Clin Periodontol. 1995;22:494–500.
5. Kenney EB, Ash MM. Oxidation–reduction potential of developing plaque, periodontal pockets and gingival sulci. J Periodontol. 1969;40:630–3.
6. Marsh P, Martin M. Oral Microbiology, 2nd edn. Reinhold; 1984.
7. Smith LDS, Williams BL. Anaerobes and the toxic effect of oxygen. In: The Pathogenic Anaerobic Bacteria, 3rd edn. Springfield; 1984.

8. Finegold SM. Classification and taxonomy of anaerobes. In: Finegold SM, George WL, eds. Anaerobic Infections in Humans. San Diego: Academic Press; 1969:23–36.

9. Müller RF, Künzel W, Szabo J. Scanning and transmission electron microscopy studies of short-term changes in acquired pellicle after two different dietary regimens. Caries Res. 1988;22:98.

10. Müller RF, Künzel W, Szabo J. Pellicle carbohydrates: the initial plaque matrix. Caries Res. 1989;23:108.

11. Müller RF, Künzel W, Szabo J, Luppa H. The effect of natural and artificial surfaces on the nature of salivary deposits. Caries Res. 1989;23:444.

12. Jean A, Kerebel B, Kerebel LM. Scanning electron microscope study of the predentin–pulpal border zone in human dentin. Oral Surg Oral Med Oral Pathol. 1986;61:392–8.

13. Thomas HF. The dentin–predentin complex and its permeability: anatomical overview. J Dent Res. 1985;64:604–12.

14. Szabo J, Trombitas K, Szabo I. The odontoblast process and its branches in human teeth observed by scanning electron microscopy. Arch Oral Biol. 1984;29:331–3.

15. Szabo J, Szabo I, Trombitas K. Inter-odontoblastic fibres in human dentin observed by scanning electron microscopy. Arch Oral Biol. 1985;30:161–5.

16. Frank RM. Electronmicroscopy of undecalcified sections of human adult dentin. Arch Oral Biol. 1959;1:43–56.

17. Isokawa S, Toda Y, Kodama N, Inoue Y. Scanning electron microscope study of human odontoblasts and predentin. J Nihon Univ Sch Dent. 1970;12:54–6.

18. Szabo J, Trombitas K, Szabo I. Scanning electron microscopy of the walls of tubules in human coronal dentin. Arch Oral Biol. 1985;30:705–10.

19. Holland GR. The odontoblast process: form and function. J Dent Res. 1985;64:499–514.

20. Yoshiyama M, Masada J, Uchida A, Ishida H. Scanning electron microscopic characterisation of sensitive versus insensitive human radicular dentin. J Dent Res. 1989;68:1498–502.

21. Szabo J, Merei E, Lazar Gy, Szabo I. A dentin szenzoros beidegzésének vizsgálata fénymikroszkópos autoradiográfiával. Fogorvosi Szemle. 1982;75:302–7.

22. Langeland K, Yagi T. Investigations on the innervation of teeth. Int Dent J. 1972;22:240–69.

23. Darnell J, Lodish H, Baltimore D. Molecular Cell Biology. New York: Scientific American Books, Inc.; 1986:771–813.

24. Garant PR, Szabo J, Nalbandian J. The fine structure of the mouse odontoblast. Arch Oral Biol. 1968;13:857–76.

25. Takuma J, Nagai N. Ultrastructure of rat odontoblasts in various stages of their development and maturation. Arch Oral Biol. 1971;16:993–1001.

26. Driessens FCM, Verbeeck RMH. Metastable states in the system $CaO-P_2O_5-H_2O$ at room temperature. J Crystal Growths. 1981;53:55–62.

27. Johansen E, Parks HF. Electronmicroscopic observations on sound human dentine. Arch Oral Biol. 1962;?:185–93.

28. Symons NBB. The developments of the fibres in the dentine matrix. Br Dent J. 1956;101:255–62.

29. Ten Cate AR. A fine structural study of coronal and root dentinogenesis in the mouse: observations on the so-called 'von Korff fibres' and their contribution to mantle dentine. J Anat. 1978;125:183–97.

30. Pillai MR, Balaram P, Kannan S et al. Interferon activation of latent natural killer cells and alteration in kinetics of target cell lysis: clinical implications for oral precancerous lesions. Oral Surg Oral Med Oral Pathol. 1990;70:458–61.

31. Boisnic S, Frances C, Branchet MC, Szpirglas H, Le Charpentier Y. Immunohistochemical study of oral lesions of lichen planus: diagnostic and pathophysiologic aspects. Oral Surg Oral Med Oral Pathol. 1990;70:462–5.

32. Frank RM, Voegel JC. Ultrastructure of the human odontoblast process and its mineralization during caries. Caries Res. 1980;14:367–80.

33. Fusayama T. Two layers of carious dentin. Diagnosis Treatment Oper Dent. 1979;4:63–70.

34. Fusayama T, Okuse K, Hosada H. Relationship between hardness, discoloration, and microbial invasion in carious dentin. J Dent Res. 1966;45:1033–46.

35. Linde A. Dentin: structure, chemistry and formation. In: Thylstrup A, Leach SA, Qvist V, eds. Dentin and dentin reactions in the oral cavity. Oxford: IRL Press; 1987:17–26.

36. Jolly M, Sullivan HR. The pathology of carious human dentine. Aust Dent J. 1960;5:157–64.

37. Thylstrup A, Qvist V. Principal enamel and dentin reactions during caries progression. In: Thylstrup A, Leach SA, Qvist V, eds. Dentin and dentin reactions in the oral cavity. Oxford: IRL Press; 1987:3–16.

38. Mjör IA. Reaction patterns of dentin. In: Thylstrup A, Leach SA, Qvist V, eds. Dentin and dentin reactions in the oral cavity. Oxford: IRL Press; 1987:27–31.

39. Karjalainen S, Le Bell Y. Odontoblast response in caries. In: Thylstrup A, Leach SA, Qvist V, eds. Dentin and dentin reactions in the oral cavity. Oxford: IRL Press; 1987:85–93.

40. Jones S, Boyde A. In: Dentin and Dentinogenesis. Vol.I. Florida: C.R.C. Press. 1984:81–134.

41. Yamada T, Nakamura T, Iwaku M, Fusayama T. The extent of the odontoblast process in normal and carious human dentine. J Dent Res. 1983;62:798–802.

42. Szabo J, Szabo I. Intratubular structures in carious tooth dentin of human teeth as observed by scanning electron microscopy. Caries Res. 1988;22:91.

43. Szabo J, Szabo I. Transmission and scanning electron microscopic study of morphological changes in dentin under abrasion and root surface caries. Caries Res. 1989;23:460.

G Mózsik et al. Cell Injury and Cytoprotection in the GI Tract. 83–91.

ANALYSIS OF ADRENOCEPTOR- AND RELATED RECEPTOR-MEDIATED GASTRIC CYTOPROTECTION

K. GYIRES

Department of Pharmacology, Semmelweis University of Medicine, Nagyvárad tér 4, H-1089 Budapest, Hungary

ABSTRACT

Clonidine at doses of 0.00625–0.025 mg/kg (given orally) inhibited the gastric mucosal damage induced by either acidified ethanol or indomethacin. At higher doses (0.1–0.2 mg/kg po), the gastroprotective effect of clonidine decreased in the ethanol–ulcer model but remained unchanged against gastric mucosal lesions induced by indomethacin. The gastroprotective effect of clonidine in the ethanol–ulcer model was reversed by the α_2-antagonist, yohimbine (5 mg/kg sc), by the highly selective α_2-antagonist, Ch-38083 (3.5 mg/kg sc), and the α_{2B}-antagonist, prazosin (0.1 mg/kg sc). Clonidine at gastroprotective doses (0.0625–0.025 mg/kg intraduodenally) failed to influence gastric acid secretion in pylorus-ligated rats, while at a higher dose (0.2 mg/kg), it exerted a pronounced antisecretory activity. The antisecretory effect was also reversed by yohimbine and Ch-38083 but not by prazosin. These results suggest that α_{2B}-adrenoceptors are likely to be involved in gastroprotection but not in the antisecretory activity. Since naloxone (1 mg/kg subcutaneously) inhibited the gastroprotective effect of clonidine, interaction between opioid and presynaptic α_2-adrenoceptors might be supposed.

Keywords: clonidine, yohimbine, Ch-38083, prazosin, naloxone, gastroprotection, gastric acid secretion

INTRODUCTION

Gastric acid secretion is mediated by a well-defined receptor population: stimulation of muscarinic histamine and gastrin receptors results in increased gastric acid secretion while the antagonists of these receptors inhibit the gastric acid secretion.

On the other hand, less has been discovered about the possible receptor population involved in gastric mucosal protection. Bertaccini et al. [1] reported that H_3 receptor agonists inhibit the gastric mucosal damage induced by 100% ethanol, an effect which was reversed by the H_3 receptor antagonist, thioperamide, indicating that the H_3 receptor is involved in gastroprotection.

Data on the cytoprotective effect of H_2 receptor antagonists are controversial. Cimetidine and roxatidine were found to exert a protective effect against gastric mucosal damage induced by necrotizing agents [2,3]. However, others failed to confirm the cytoprotective action of H_2-blocking compounds [3,5]. Since only some of the H_2-blocking substances exerted a cytoprotective action, this effect is probably due to a non-specific drug action rather than to a receptor-mediated effect.

Data from the literature and our recent results [6,7] suggest that opioid receptors may be involved in gastroprotection though the opioid receptor subtype(s) involved in the mediation of gastroprotective action has not been clearly defined.

This paper was presented at the Symposium on 'Cell injury and protection in the gastrointestinal tract: from basic science to clinical perspectives', October 8–11, 1995, Pécs, Hungary.

Moreover, presynaptic α_2-adrenoceptor agonists were reported to inhibit different types of the experimental gastric ulcers [8–11]. However, the gastroprotective effect of α_2-antagonists was supposed to be due mainly to their antisecretory effect [12,14]. The aim of the present work was to analyse further possible involvement of receptors – opioid, presynaptic α_2 – in gastroprotection.

MATERIALS AND METHODS

Animals

Male Wistar rats weighing 160–180 g were used. They were fasted for 24 h before experiments but were allowed free access to water. They were kept in individual cages with a metal grid to avoid coprophagy.

Mucosal lesions

Gastric mucosal lesions induced by acidified ethanol

The rats were given 0.5 ml acidified ethanol (98% ethanol in 200 mmol/L HCl) by gavage and killed 1 h later. The gastroprotective compounds were given orally (po) 40 min before the injection of acidified ethanol. The antagonists were injected subcutaneously (sc) 20 min before the administration of gastroprotective compounds.

Gastric mucosal lesions induced by indomethacin

Indomethacin (20 mg/kg) was administered orally in a volume of 5 ml/kg. The animals were killed 4 h after the injection of indomethacin.

The gastroprotective compounds were given orally 30 min before the administration of indomethacin. The antagonists were injected sc 20 min before the administration of the gastroprotective agents.

Measurement of gastric mucosal lesions

The stomachs were removed and opened along the greater curvature. They were rinsed with saline and examined for lesions by an observer who was unaware of the treatment the rats had received. The gross mucosal damage was assessed by calculating a lesion index based on the number and length of sites of haemorrhagic mucosal necrosis, as described previously [7].

Gastric acid secretion in pylorus-ligated rats

Pyloric ligation was performed according to Shay et al. [15]. The surgical procedure and ligation around the pyloric sphincter was carried out under light ether anaesthesia. Four hours after ligation, the animals were sacrificed, the stomach was carefully excised and the gastric content was collected. The volume of gastric juice was measured and the acidity was determined by automatic titration by Universal Recording Titrator (Type OH-407, Radelkis, Hungary). Total acid output was calculated as the product of the acidity and the volume of gastric juice. The test compounds were given either sc or intraduodenally (id) immediately after pylorus ligation.

Materials

Chemicals used were Ch-38083 (7,8-(methylenedioxi)-14-hydroxyalloberbane HCl; Chinoin, Hungary), clonidine (Sigma, USA), indomethacin (Gedeon Richter, Hungary), naloxone (Sigma, USA), prazosin (Sigma, USA) and yohimbine (Sigma, USA).

Drugs were suspended in 1% methylcellulose for oral treatment and dissolved in saline for sc administration. Control animals received the drug solvent.

Statistical analysis

All data are presented as the mean $\pm$ SEM. Statistical analysis of the data was evaluated partly by means of the non-parametric statistical procedure, the Mann–Whitney U test (gastric mucosal damage), and partly by means of the unpaired Student's *t*-test (gastric acid secretion). A probability of $p < 0.05$ was considered statistically significant.

RESULTS

The effect of clonidine on gastric mucosal damage induced by either 100% ethanol or indomethacin (Figure 1)

Clonidine inhibited the gastric mucosal lesions induced by both acidified ethanol and indomethacin at doses of 0.003125–0.025 mg/kg. However, when the dose of clonidine was increased, its gastroprotective effect diminished in the ethanol–ulcer model but remained unchanged against indomethacin-induced gastric mucosal damage.

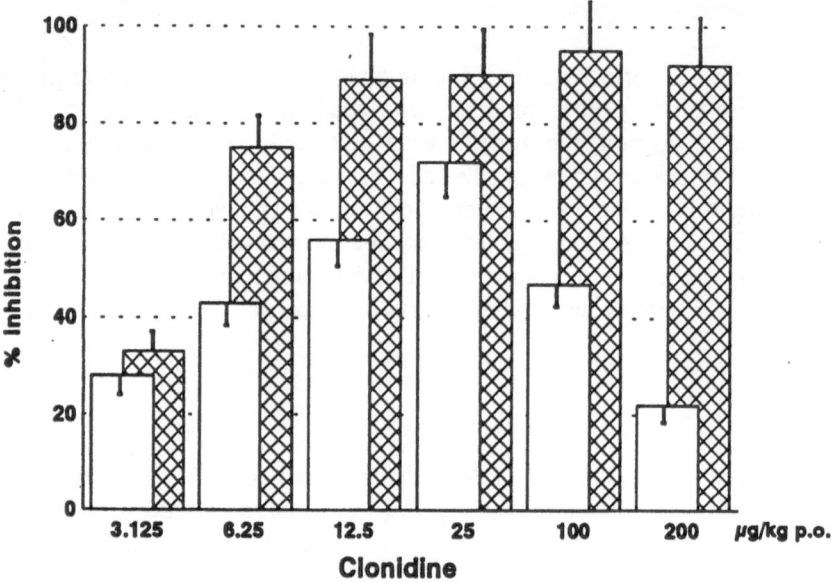

Figure 1. The effect of clonidine against gastric mucosal lesions induced by acidified ethanol (open square) and indomethacin (20 mg/kg po) (hatched squares) in the rat (*n* = 10)

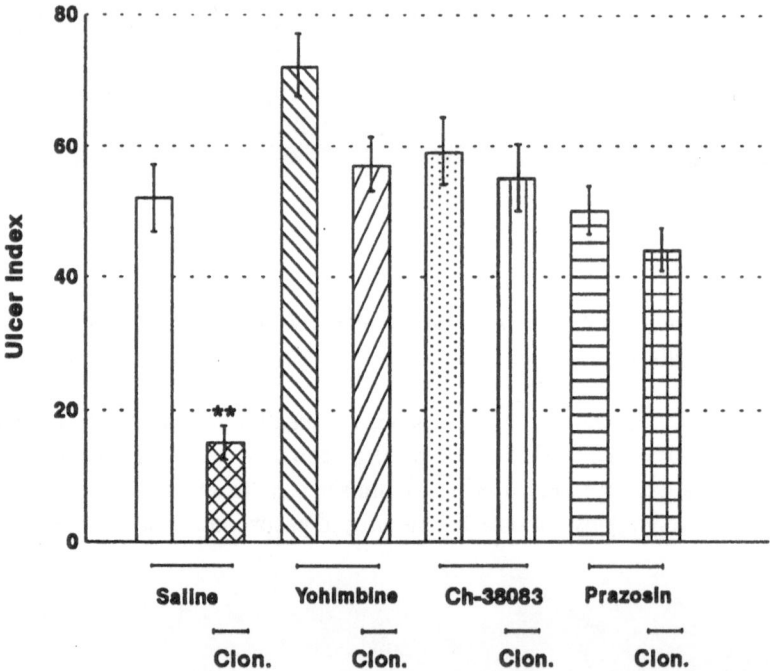

Figure 2. The effect of yohimbine (5 mg/kg sc), Ch-38083 (3.5 mg/kg sc) and prazosin (0.1 mg/kg sc) on the gastroprotective effect of clonidine (0.025 mg/kg po) against acidified ethanol-induced gastric mucosal damage in the rat. **$p < 0.01$ (*n* = 10) (Mann–Whitney U test)

The effect of yohimbine, Ch-38083 and prazosin on the gastroprotective effect of clonidine against acidified ethanol-induced gastric mucosal damage (Figure 2)

Clonidine at 0.025 mg/kg (po) caused a 76% inhibition of acidified ethanol-induced mucosal lesions. Yohimbine (5 mg/kg sc) slightly aggravated, Ch-38083 (3.5 mg/kg sc) failed to influence and prazosin (0.1 mg/kg sc) slightly decreased the ethanol-induced gastric lesions. All the three substances – yohimbine, Ch-38083 and prazosin – antagonized the protective effect of clonidine.

The effect of clonidine on gastric acid secretion in pylorus-ligated rats (Table 1)

Clonidine at doses of 0.0125 and 0.025 mg/kg (id) failed to inhibit gastric acid secretion. A higher dose of clonidine (0.2 mg/kg id) exerted pronounced antisecretory activity: both the volume and acidity of gastric juice was decreased. The antisecretory effect of clonidine was reversed by Ch-38083 (3.5 mg/kg sc), but not by prazosin (0.1 mg/kg sc).

TABLE 1
The effect of Ch-38083 and prazosin on the antisecretory effect of clonidine in rats ($n = 8$)

Compound	Dose (mg/kg)	Volume of secretion (ml)	Concentration (µEq/L)	TAO (µEq/4 h)
Control	–	6.1 ±1.2	70.00±9.0	427.0±68.0
Clonidine	0.0125 id	5.7 ±0.9	70.00±6.0	349.0±40.0
	0.025 id	5.0 ±0.8	62.50±8.0	312.0±45.0
Control	–	6.1 ±0.9	73.50±12.0	448.3±70.0
Clonidine	0.2 id	1.0 ±0.4*	61.50±10.0	61.5±18.0**
Ch-38083	3.5 sc	6.1 ±0.8	77.08±11.0	469.7±65.0
Ch-38083 + clonidine	3.5 sc + 0.2 id	5.98±1.0	76.2 ±15.0	455.6±25.0
Control	–	5.0 ±0.8	76.0 ±7.4	380.0±39.0
Clonidine	0.2 id	0.15±0.03**	58.0 ±9.0	8.7±1.0**
Prazosin	0.1 sc	3.1 ±0.7	70.0 ±8.2	217.0±23.0
Prazosin + clonidine	0.1 sc + 0.2 id	0.2 ±0.04**	60.0 ±9.1	12.0±2.0**

TAO: total acid output; Student's t-test: $*p<0.05$, $**p<0.01$

The effect of naloxone on the gastroprotective effect of clonidine (Figure 3)

Clonidine at 0.025 mg/kg (po) decreased by 80% the gastric mucosal lesions induced by acidified ethanol, while naloxone, at 1 mg/kg (sc) did not influence it. However, the 80% inhibitory effect of clonidine was almost totally reversed when the animals were pretreated with naloxone.

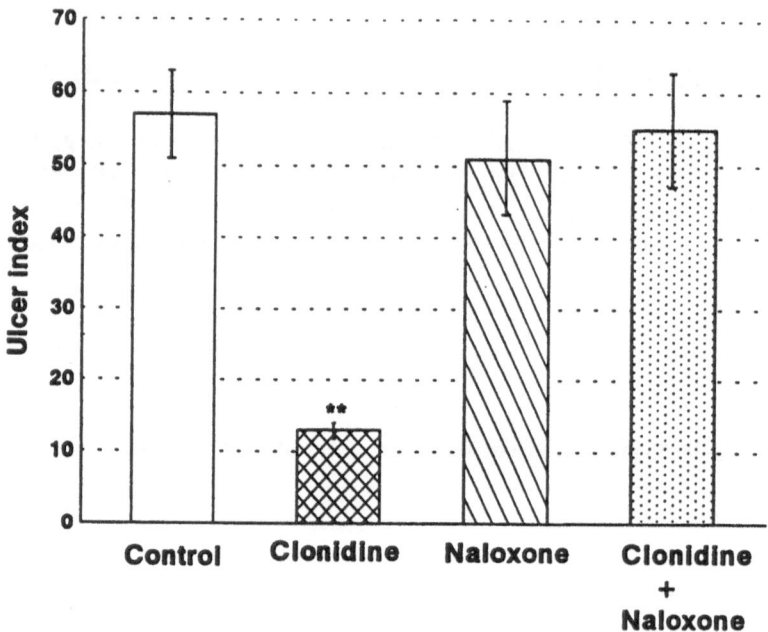

Figure 3. The effect of naloxone (1 mg/kg sc) on the gastroprotective effect of clonidine (0.025 mg/kg po) against gastric mucosal damage induced by acidified ethanol in the rat. **$p < 0.01$ ($n = 10$) (Mann–Whitney U test)

DISCUSSION

Presynaptic α_2-adrenoceptors mediate several responses at different levels in the gastrointestinal tract. They are involved in regulation of gastric acid secretion [12–14] and α_2-agonists also effectively inhibit chemically (aspirin, indomethacin, ethanol, reserpine, cysteamine) and physically (pylorus ligation and stress) induced gastric mucosal lesions [8–11]. Each ulcer model has its own pathophysiological mechanism: some are acid-dependent models (indomethacin-, reserpin-, pylorus ligation- and stress-induced mucosal damage); other models (ethanol- and cysteamine-induced gastric lesions) are independent of gastric acid secretion. The fact that α_2-agonists are active in each of the above models suggests a complex mechanism of gastroprotection and that activation of α_2-receptors can overcome multiple mechanisms of gastric insult.

Our data showed the clonidine, an α_2-receptor agonist, inhibited the gastric damage induced by acidified ethanol at doses of 0.003125–0.025 mg/kg po. In contrast with our data, Kunchandy et al. [8] and Bhandare et al. [11] failed to find clonidine effective against ethanol-induced lesions following oral administration. However, the oral dose used by them was relatively high (0.1 mg/kg) and as demonstrated in the present experimental series, clonidine is ineffective at higher oral doses. Dual action of clonidine following parenteral administration was reported by Del Soldato [10]. Bhandare et al. [11] found that clonidine aggravated mucosal lesions following oral administration at the dose of 0.1 mg/kg, and he suggested that this effect may be due to a local action exerted on the presynaptic imidazoline-preferring receptors in gastric mucosa.

We found that the gastroprotective effect of clonidine was reversed by yohimbine, an antagonist of α_2-adrenoceptor, suggesting that the gastroprotective effect of clonidine is probably mediated through α_2-receptors. However, yohimbine is not selective for α_2-adrenoceptor [16,17]. In order to prove the involvement of α_2-adrenoceptors in gastroprotection, we studied the effect of a highly selective α_2-adrenoceptor antagonist, Ch-38083, a berbane derivative, on the gastroprotective effect of clonidine [16]. The α_1/α_2-adrenoceptor selectivity ratio for yohimbine and Ch-38083 was 4.7 and 1659, respectively. It was found that Ch-38083 reversed the gastroprotective effect of clonidine exerted against both acidified ethanol- and indomethacin-induced gastric damage. At this point, it may be concluded that α_2-adrenoceptors are likely to be involved in gastroprotection.

Data from the literature suggest that there are at least four different subtypes of presynaptic α_2-receptors: α_{2A}, α_{2B}, α_{2C} and α_{2D} [18–20]. This raises the question of whether subtype selectivity for presynaptic α_2-adrenoceptors in gastroprotection can be established. Therefore, we examined the effect of prazosin, an α_{2B}-adrenoceptor antagonist [18] on the anti-ulcer effect of clonidine. It was found that prazosin at a dose of 0.1 mg/kg sc reversed the protective effect of clonidine. This result suggests that α_2-, especially α_{2B}-like, adrenoceptors are involved in gastroprotection.

Though clonidine proved to be active against acidified ethanol-induced lesions – an ulcer model which is independent of gastric acid secretion – to accomplish the criterion of cytoprotection, originally described by Robert et al. [4], we examined the effect of a gastroprotective dose of clonidine on gastric acid secretion in pylorus-ligated rats. It was found that clonidine at doses of 0.0125–0.025 mg/kg injected intraduodenally, failed to influence gastric acid secretion in a significant manner. Higher doses (0.2 mg/kg id) of clonidine caused a very pronounced decrease in gastric acid secretion; it diminished both the volume and the acidity of gastric juice and the total acid output was decreased in a significant manner. These data suggest that the gastroprotective effect of clonidine – even against indomethacin-induced lesions, a model in which gastric acid is involved in the pathomechanism of gastric mucosal lesions – is not likely to be due to its antisecretory effect. This assumption is further supported by the finding that the antisecretory effect of clonidine was antagonized by Ch-38083, but not by the

α_{2B}-adrenoceptor antagonist prazosin, in contrast with the ulcer models. Our data are in agreement with the findings of Blandizzi et al. [21], who suggested that gastric acid secretion is modulated by α_{2A}-like adrenoceptor subtypes.

Data from the literature suggest that there is an interaction between opioid and presynaptic α_2-adrenoceptors in different systems [22,23]. We analysed whether there is a correlation between opioid and α_2-receptors in gastroprotection. It was found that the gastroprotective effect of clonidine is reversed by naloxone (1 mg/kg sc), suggesting a possible interaction between opioid and presynaptic α_2-adrenoceptors.

Summarizing, it can be concluded that stimulation of presynaptic α_2-adrenoceptors may mediate, not only antisecretory action, but also a mucosal protective effect. The gastroprotective effect seems to be subtype specific, namely, α_{2B}-like receptor subtype is thought to mediate the gastroprotective effect, since prazosin reversed the gastroprotective effect of clonidine. Interaction between opioid receptors and presynaptic α_2-adrenoceptors is thought to exist in gastroprotection.

ACKNOWLEDGEMENTS

The author thanks Mrs Szalai and Mrs Barna for technical assistance. This work was supported by Grant OTKA 017794.

REFERENCES

1. Bertaccini G, Coruzzi G, Morini G, Grandi D. Histamine H3 receptors and gastric mucosal protection. Can J Physiol Pharmacol. 1994;72(Suppl 1):237.
2. Moron F, Cuesta E, Bata M, Mozsik Gy. Cytoprotecting-effect of cimetidine: experimental evidence in the rat gastric mucosal lesions induced by intragastric administration of necrotizing agents. Arch Int Pharmacodyn. 1983;265:309–19.
3. Siratuchi K, Fuse H, Hagiwara M, Mikami T, Miyasaka K, Sakuma H. Cytoprotective action of roxatidine acetate HCl. Arch Int Pharmacodyn. 1988;29:295–304.
4. Robert A, Nezamis EJ, Lancaster C, Hanchar JA. Cytoprotection by prostaglandins in rats. Prevention of gastric necrosis produced by alcohol, HCl, NaOH, hypertonic NaCl, and thermal injury. Gastroenterology. 1979;77:433–43.
5. Gyires K, Hermecz I, Knoll J. The effect of some anti-ulcer agents on the early vascular injury of gastric mucosa induced by ethanol in rats. Acta Physiol Hung. 1989;73(2–3):149–54.
6. Ferri S, Speroni E, Candeletti S et al. Protection by opioids against gastric lesions caused by necrotizing agents. Pharmacology. 1988;3:140–4.
7. Gyires K. Morphine inhibits the ethanol-induced gastric damage in rats. Arch Int Pharmacodyn. 1990;36:170–81.
8. Kunchandy J, Khanna S, Kulkarni SK. Effect of alpha$_2$ agonists clonidine, guanfacine and B-HT 920 on gastric acid secretion and ulcers in rats. Arch Int Pharmacdyn. 1985;275:123–38.
9. Dijoseph JF, Eash JR, Mir NG. Gastric anti-secretory and antiulcer effects of WHR 1582A, a compound exerting alpha-2 adrenoceptor agonist activity. J Pharmacol Exp Ther. 1987;241:97–102.
10. Del Soldato P. Gastric lesion-preventing or potentiating action of clonidine in rats. Jpn J Pharmacol. 1986;41:257–79.
11. Bhandare PN, Rataboli PV, D'Souza RSD. Dual action of clonidine on ethanol-induced gastric lesions: is the imidazol-preferring receptor involved? Eur J Pharmacol. 1991;199:243–5.
12. Kaess H, von Mikuliez-Rodecki J. The influence of 2-(2,6-dichloro-phenylamino)-2-imidazoline hydrochloride (Catapressan) on the function of the stomach and pancreas. Eur J Clin Pharmacol. 1971;3:97–101.

13. Cheng HC, Gleason EM, Nathan BA, Lachmann PJ, Woodward JK. Effects of clonidine on gastric acid secretion in the rat. J Pharmacol Exp Ther. 1981;217:121–6.
14. Blandizzi C, Bernardini MC, Natale G, Del Tacca M. α_2-Adrenoceptors-mediated inhibitory and excitatory effects of detomidine on gastric acid secretion. J Pharm Pharmacol. 1988;42:685–8.
15. Shay Y, Sun D, Gruenstein M. A quantitative method for measuring spontaneous gastric secretion in the rat. Gastroenterology. 1954;26:906–13.
16. Vizi ES Jr, Harsing LG, Gaal J, Kapocsi J, Bernath J, Somogyi GT. CH-38083, a selective, potent antagonist of alpha-2 adrenoceptors. J Pharmacol Exp Ther. 1986;238:701–6.
17. Del Tacca M, Tadini P, Blandizzi C, Bernardini MC. Excitatory and inhibitory effect of clonidine on isolated guinea pig small intestine. Pharmacol Res Commun. 1988;20:673–84.
18. Bylund DB. Subtypes of α_2-adrenoceptors. Pharmacological and molecular biological evidence converge. Trends Pharmacol Sci. 1988;9:356–61.
19. Blaxall H, Murphy TJ, Baker JC, Ray C, Bylund DB. Characterisation of the alpha-2C adrenergic receptor subtype in the opossum kidney and in the OK cell line. J Pharmacol Exp Ther. 1991;259:323–9.
20. Remaury A, Paris H. The insulin-secreting cell line, RINm5F, expresses an alpha-2D adrenoceptor and nonadrenergic idazoxan-binding sites. J Pharmacol Exp Ther. 1992;260:417–26.
21. Blandizzi C, Natale G, Colucci R, Carignani D, Lazzeri G, Del Tacca M. Characterization of α_2-adrenoceptor subtypes involved in the modulation of gastric acid secretion. Eur J Pharmacol. 1995;278:179–82.
22. Ali BH, Bashir AA. The effect of some alpha 2-adrenoceptor agonists and antagonists on gastro-intestinal transit in mice: influence of morphine, castor oil and glucose. Clin Exp Pharmacol Physiol. 1993;20(1):11–16.
23. Schnur P, Espinoza M, Flores M, Ortiz S, Vallejos S, Wainwright M. Blocking naloxone-precipitated withdrawal in rats and hamsters. Pharmacol Biochem Behav. 1992;43(4):1093–8.

Section II

CELL INJURY AND PROTECTION IN THE STOMACH

G Mózsik et al. Cell Injury and Cytoprotection in the GI Tract. 95–105.
© 1997 Kluwer Academic Publishers.

THE EFFECT OF INTRAGASTRIC CAPSAICIN AND RESINIFERATOXIN ON INDOMETHACIN-INDUCED GASTRIC MUCOSAL DAMAGE IN RATS

O.M.E. ABDEL SALAM[1], J. SZOLCSÁNYI[2] AND Gy. MÓZSIK[1]*
[1]First Department of Medicine, and [2]Department of Pharmacology, Medical University of Pécs, Ifjúság út, H-7643 Pécs, Hungary
*Correspondence

ABSTRACT

Capsaicin-sensitive sensory nerves have local protective functions in the stomach. In the present study, the effect of capsaicin or its analogue, resiniferatoxin (RTX), on gastric mucosal injury caused by indomethacin was studied in pylorus-ligated rats. Gastric mucosal damage was evoked by the subcutaneous (sc) or intragastric (ig) administration of indomethacin (20 mg/kg) together with the ig administration of 2 ml of physiological saline or 2 ml of 0.15 N HCl. Animals received simultaneously capsaicin or RTX ig at different concentrations and were sacrificed 4 h later. Resiniferatoxin administered ig at a low concentration (40 ng/ml; 0.4 µg/kg) almost totally prevented the development of gastric mucosal injury by sc or ig indomethacin plus ig saline. The protective effect of RTX was not modified by atropine (0.1 mg/kg) or cimetidine (10 mg/kg) treatment, but was not evident after bilateral subdiaphragmatic vagotomy. The sc administration of indomethacin together with ig application of 0.15 N HCl resulted in much more severe gastric mucosal damage than that seen after indomethacin and ig saline. Capsaicin or RTX (both applied at 60 and 120 ng/ml) protected against gastric mucosal injury produced by indomethacin plus ig HCl in a concentration-dependent manner. Data indicate that acid in the stomach has a potentiating effect on the development of the indomethacin-induced gastric injury and that ig capsaicin or RTX at very low concentrations protect against the indomethacin- or indomethacin-plus-acid-induced gastric mucosal injury in rats.

Keywords: capsaicin, resiniferatoxin, indomethacin-induced gastric lesions

INTRODUCTION

Non-steroidal anti-inflammatory drugs (NSAIDs) are widely prescribed medications. Indomethacin, one of the most familiar NSAIDs, is widely used in the treatment of various rheumatic conditions [1]. These drugs are well known to evoke gastrointestinal mucosal damage in man [2,3] and in animal models [4,5]. Several pathogenetic mechanisms are thought to contribute to the gastric mucosal damaging effects of indomethacin, such as prostaglandin inhibition [6,7], reduced mucosal blood flow [8–12] and increased gastric motility [13,14]. The role of acid is, however, not clear. Capsaicin, the pungent constituent in hot red and green peppers of the plant genus *Capsicum* is a selective sensory stimulant of mammalian primary afferent neurones with thin C and A fibres, which, in large doses, produces desensitization to the drug and to other stimuli of sensory neurones [15–17]. Capsaicin-sensitive sensory nerves

---

This paper was presented at the Symposium on 'Cell injury and protection in the gastrointestinal tract: from basic science to clinical perspectives', October 8–11, 1995, Pécs, Hungary.

(CSSN) are involved in local neurogenic defence mechanisms in the stomach [18]. Rats pretreated with large doses of the agent to induce selective and permanent degeneration of thin primary afferent neurones exhibited more pronounced gastric mucosal damage in response to noxious agents than their untreated sensory-intact counterparts [18–20]. On the other hand, administration of capsaicin at low concentrations into the rat stomach exerted a beneficial effect on experimental gastric ulceration [18–22]. Capsaicin-sensitive sensory nerves contain a variety of vasodilator peptides and were demonstrated in the gastric mucosa and submucosa [23,24]. Acute ig administration of capsaicin evokes the release of neuropeptides from the sensory nerve endings [25,26] with consequent enhancement of local microcirculation, a mechanism which plays an important role in the prevention of acute gastric mucusal injury [27].

The present study aimed:

1. To assess the contribution of acid to the injurious effects of indomethacin on the gastric mucosa, and

2. To evaluate the effect of capsaicin or resiniferatoxin, a potent capsaicin analogue [28,29], on the development of gastric mucosal injury by indomethacin in the presence and absence of an exogenous acid load.

MATERIALS AND METHODS

Sprague–Dawley rats of both sexes, 180–200 g body weight, were used in this study and housed under standardized conditions for light and temperature. Rats were kept in cages with wide-meshed floors to prevent coprophagy. Animals were deprived of food for 24 h before the experiments but allowed free access to tap water. Pylorus ligation was performed under light ether anaesthesia, care being taken not to interfere with the blood supply to the stomach and duodenum. Immediately thereafter, gastric mucosal damage was evoked by the subcutaneous (sc) or in some experiments by the oral administration of indomethacin in a single dose of 20 mg/kg. Animals were sacrificed 4 h later by cervical dislocation after being lightly anaesthetized with ether. The oesophagus was ligated and the stomach excised. Gastric juice was collected in graduated tubes after removal of the oesophageal ligature and stomachs were opened along the greater curvature and inspected for the presence of gastric mucosal lesions.

Study design

Indomethacin was dissolved in 5% sodium bicarbonate. In the first experimental series, the drug was given orally as a single dose of 20 mg/kg in 0.2 ml volume together with 1.8 ml of saline with or without RTX (0.4 µg/kg) immediately after pylorus ligation. Control animals received the vehicle.

In the second series of experiments, indomethacin was administered sc as a single dose of 20 mg/kg (0.2 ml volume) immediately after pylorus ligation. At the same time, animals received 2 ml of physiological saline ig alone or with RTX in 40 ng/ml (0.4 µg/ kg). Control animals received the vehicle. In separate experimental groups, the protective effect of RTX 40 ng/ml (0.4 µg/kg) was evaluated in animals treated with atropine or cimetidine or in surgically vagotomized rats. Atropine (0.1 mg/kg) or cimetidine (10 mg/kg) were given sc simultaneously with sc indomethacin and ig RTX (immediately after pylorus ligation). Surgical vagotomy was performed by cutting 3–4 mm from each vagus nerve at the lower end of the oesophagus at the time of pylorus ligation. The effect of atropine and cimetidine in the above doses on gastric acid output in pylorus-ligated rat was also evaluated. The agents were given sc at the time of pylorus ligation and animals received 2 ml of saline orally. Rats were sacrificed 4 h later.

In the last experimental series which aimed to evaluate the effect of acid on indomethacin-induced gastric injury, indomethacin was given sc as a single dose of 20 mg/kg after pylorus ligation. Then, animals were given 2 ml of 0.15 N hydrochloric acid orally with or without capsaicin or RTX (0.6 and 1.2 µg/kg). Control animals received the vehicle. In a separate group, 2 ml of 0.15 N HCl were given orally after pylorus ligation and animals were sacrificed 4 h later.

Assessment of gastric mucosal injury

Stomachs were excised, opened along the greater curvature, briefly rinsed with saline and inspected for the presence of gastric mucosal lesions, including haemorrhagic bands, red streaks and mucosal redness. The number and severity of mucosal lesions were noted. Lesions were scaled as follows: petechial lesions = 1, lesions < 1 mm = 2, lesions between 1 and 2 mm = 3, lesions between 2 and 4 mm = 4, and lesions > 4 mm = 5 [30].

Gastric secretory studies

The volume of gastric contents was measured, the acid output was determined by titration with 0.1 N NaOH to pH 7 (using a Radelkis pH Automatic Titrimeter, Budapest, Hungary) and H^+ output expressed in µEq/rat (mean ± SEM).

Drugs

Indomethacin (Chinoin, Hungary), capsaicin, resiniferatoxin (Sigma, USA), and methylcellulose (Sigma, USA) were used. Stock solutions of resiniferatoxin (250 µg/ ml) and capsaicin (10 mg/ml) contained 10% ethanol, 10% Tween 80 and 80% saline solution. Capsaicin or resiniferatoxin was freshly dissolved in isotonic NaCl immediately before the experiments to obtain the necessary doses.

Statistical analysis

The results were expressed as mean ± SEM. Data were analysed by unpaired Student's *t*-test and values of $p < 0.05$ were regarded as significant. The Mann–Whitney test was applied for mathematical analysis of non-parametric results (ulcer severity).

RESULTS

There was no significant difference in the degree of gastric mucosal damage produced by indomethacin given via the sc or ig routes. The number and severity of gastric mucosal lesions were: 3.2 ± 1.4 and 5.6 ± 0.5 ($n = 7$) vs. 5.0 ± 0.2 and 6.6 ± 0.8 ($n = 6$), respectively. Resiniferatoxin administered ig at a concentration of 40 ng/ml (0.4 µg/kg) almost totally prevented the development of gastric mucosal lesions by sc or ig indomethacin in the 4-h pylorus-ligated rat ($n = 6$–8 per group) (Figures 1 and 2). This dose of RTX had no significant effect on gastric acid output in 4-h pylorus-ligated plus indomethacin-treated rats (data not shown).

Atropine (0.1 mg/kg) or cimetidine (10 mg/kg), given together with sc indomethacin, significantly reduced the indomethacin-induced gastric mucosal damage and did not prevent the protective effect of RTX ($n = 6$ per group) (Figures 3 and 4). Atropine and cimetidine, in the above doses, inhibited gastric acid output in the 4-h pylorus-

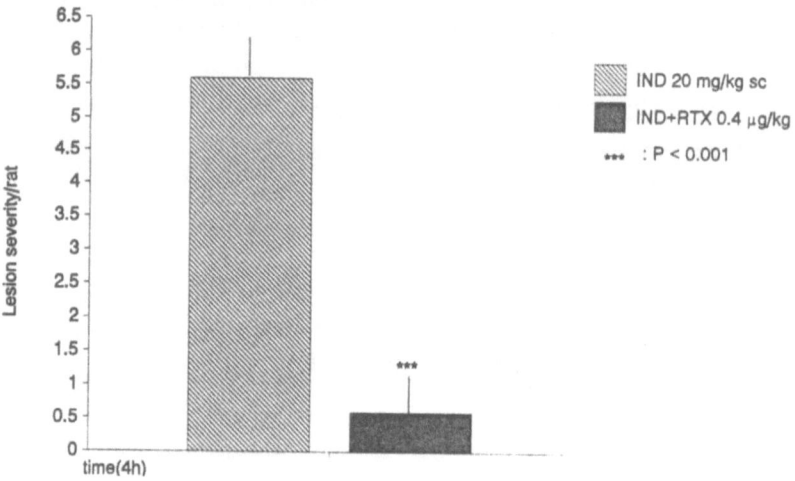

Figure 1. The protective effect of resiniferatoxin (RTX) on the severity of gastric mucosal lesions produced by sc indomethacin (IND; 20 mg/kg) in pylorus-ligated rats with intact vagus nerve. Resiniferatoxin was given orally at a dose of 0.4 µg/kg in 2 ml saline (40 ng/ml) at the time of pylorus ligation and indomethacin administration. Rats were sacrificed 4 h later ($n = 7$–8 per group). Mann–Whitney test

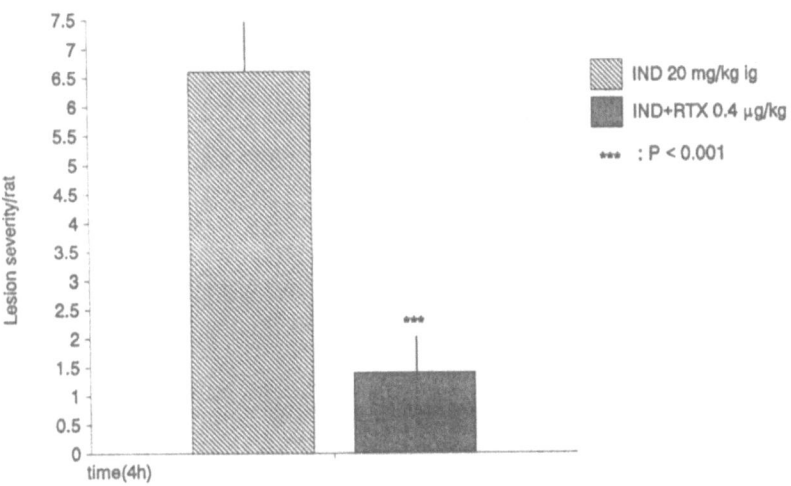

Figure 2. The protective effect of resiniferatoxin (RTX) on the severity of gastric mucosal lesions caused by ig indomethacin (IND) in pylorus-ligated rats. Indomethacin (20 mg/kg) was given orally in a volume of 0.2 ml plus 1.8 ml saline with or without RTX (0.4 μg/kg). Rats were sacrificed 4 h later (*n* = 6 per group). Mann–Whitney test

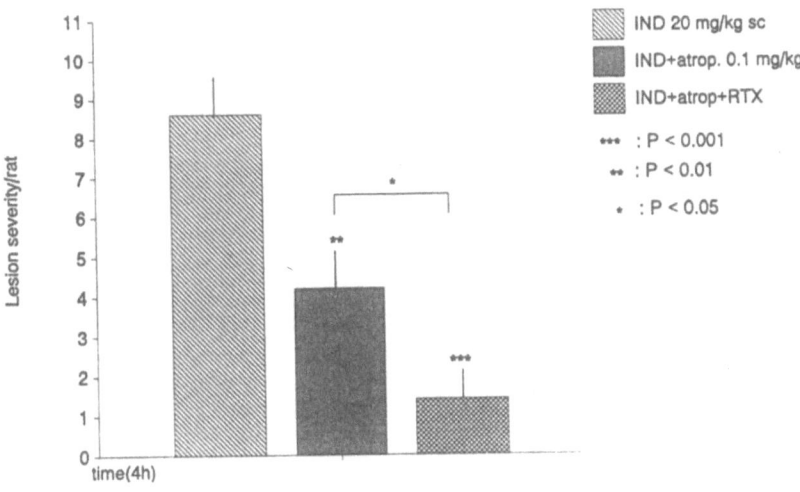

Figure 3. The effect of atropine (atrop; 0.1 mg/kg) on the severity of gastric mucosal lesions produced by sc indomethacin (IND; 20 mg/kg) and on the protective effect of RTX in pylorus-ligated rats. Both atropine and indomethacin were administered simultaneously immediately after pylorus ligation and animals received 2 ml of saline orally with or without RTX (0.4 μg/kg). Rats were sacrificed 4 h later (*n* = 6 per group). Mann–Whitney test

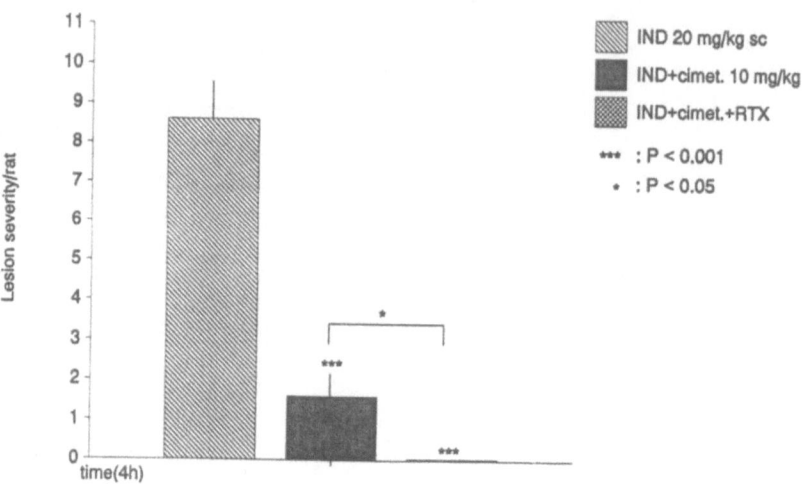

Figure 4. The effect of cimetidine (cimet; 10 mg/kg) on the severity of gastric mucosal lesions produced by sc indomethacin (IND; 20 mg/kg) and on the protective effect of RTX in pylorus-ligated rats. Both cimetidine and indomethacin were administered simultaneously immediately after pylorus ligation and animals received 2 ml saline orally with or without RTX (0.4 µg/kg). Rats were sacrificed 4 h later ($n = 6$ per group). Mann–Whitney test

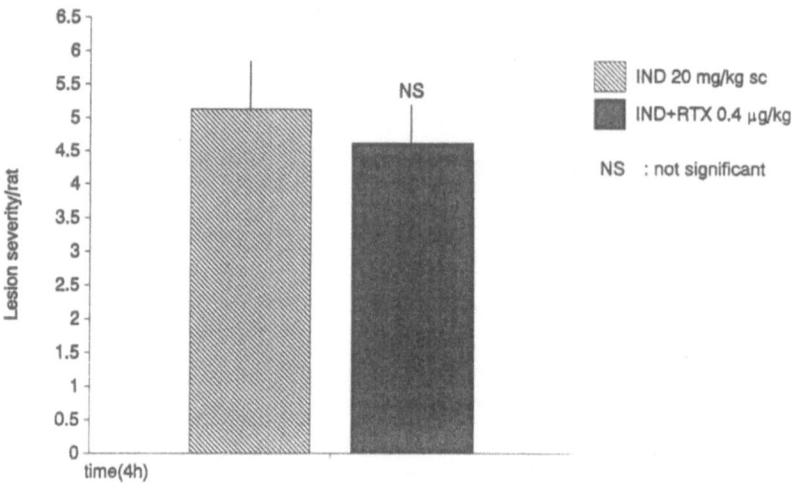

Figure 5. The effect of resiniferatoxin (RTX) on the severity of gastric mucosal lesions produced by sc indomethacin (IND; 20 mg/kg) in surgically vagotomized rats. Bilateral subdiaphragmatic vagotomy was performed at the time of pylorus ligation. Resiniferatoxin was given ig at a dose of 0.4 µg/kg in 2 ml saline (40 ng/ml) after pylorus ligation and at the time of indomethacin administration. Rats were sacrificed 4 h later ($n = 8$ per group). Mann–Whitney test

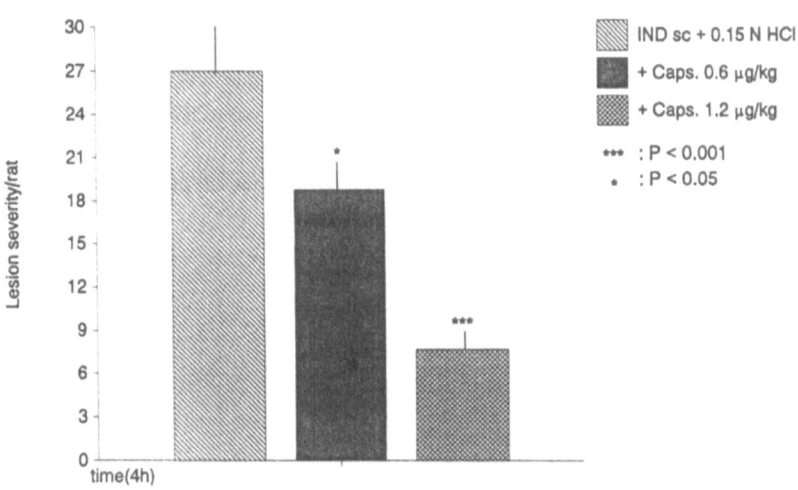

Figure 6. The protective effect of capsaicin (caps.) on the severity of gastric mucosal lesions produced in the pylorus-ligated rat by the sc administration of indomethacin (IND; 20 mg/kg) together with the ig application of 0.15 N HCl. Indomethacin was administered immediately after ligation and rats received 2 ml 0.15 N HCl via an orogastric tube with or without capsaicin (0.6 and 1.2 µg/kg). Rats were sacrificed 4 h later ($n = 6$–9 per group). Mann–Whitney test

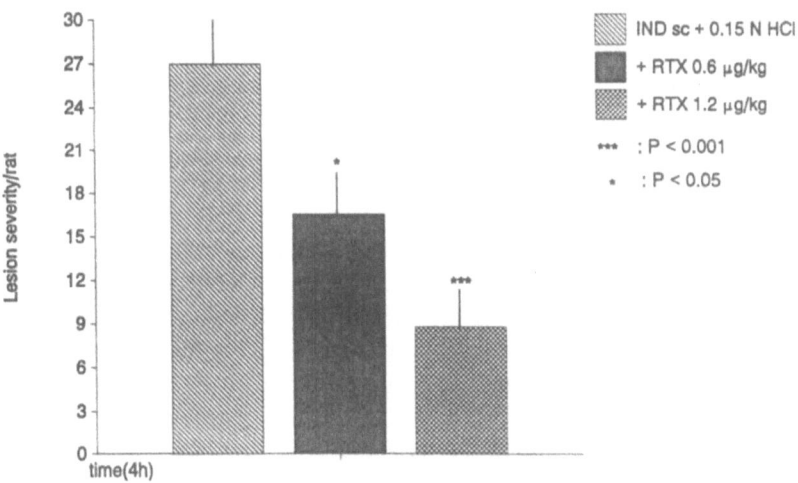

Figure 7. The protective effect of resiniferatoxin (RTX) on the severity of gastric mucosal lesions produced in the pylorus-ligated rat by the sc administration of indomethacin (IND; 20 mg/kg) together with the ig application of 0.15 N HCl. Indomethacin was administered immediately after ligation and rats received 2 ml of 0.15 N HCl via an orogastric tube with or without RTX (0.6 and 1.2 µg/kg). Rats were sacrificed 4 h later ($n = 6$–9 per group). Mann–Whitney test

ligated plus saline-treated (2 ml) rats by 49% and 35.8%, respectively ($n = 5$–6 per group).

In rats in which bilateral subdiaphragmatic vagotomy was performed, RTX (40 ng/ml) did not inhibit the development of indomethacin-induced injury as compared with the control group ($n = 8$ per group) (Figure 5).

In rats that received 2 ml of 0.15 N HCl only, a mild degree of mucosal injury was seen. The number and severity of lesions were 1.8 ± 0.8 and 2.3 ± 1.2, respectively ($n = 5$). On the other hand, the sc administration of indomethacin together with the ig application of 0.15 N HCl (2 ml) resulted in much more severe gastric mucosal damage than that seen after sc indomethacin plus ig saline ($n = 9$). Stomachs exhibited widespread ulceration and frank intragastric bleeding. Deep ulcers were frequent and ulcers about to perforate occurred in 3/9 animals. Capsaicin or RTX applied ig at 0.6 and 1.2 ng/ml protected against gastric mucosal injury by sc indomethacin plus acid in a concentration-dependent manner ($n = 6$) (Figures 6 and 7).

DISCUSSION

The finding that low concentrations of capsaicin, in sensory-stimulant doses, protected against gastric mucosal damage induced by ligating the pylorus in rats (Shay ulcer) [18] represented an important turnpoint in our understanding of the role of sensory nerve endings in local gastric defence mechanisms. Subsequently, the agent has been widely used in experimental ulcer research and has been shown to prevent gastric mucosal damage induced by various noxious agents, provided the concentration in which it is introduced into the stomach is low [18–22]. On the other hand, functional ablation of CSSN by systemic capsaicin pretreatment [18–20] or local desensitization induced by administration of capsaicin at high concentrations into the rat stomach [22] resulted in aggravation of experimental gastric ulcer. Resiniferatoxin is a naturally occurring potent capsaicin-type agent of plant origin [28,29] which possesses a gastroprotective effect similar to that of capsaicin [22,31,32].

The present study provides evidence that ig application of capsaicin or its analogue, RTX, at low concentrations protects against gastric mucosal injury by indomethacin in 4-h pylorus-ligated rats. The protective effect of RTX was not prevented by atropine (0.1 mg/kg) or cimetidine (10 mg/kg) treatment. Further, if an acid load was introduced into the rat stomach, both agents protected against the combined damaging effect of indomethacin plus acid.

Since indomethacin is widely prescribed for the treatment of various rheumatic disorders, the drug-induced gastrointestinal damage is of major importance to clinicians [1,2]. Animal models are therefore used to study the pathogenetic mechanisms of this injury and the possible therapeutic approaches. Several mechanisms have been implicated in the development of gastric mucosal damage by indomethacin. These include: altered mucosal permeability [33], inhibition of prostaglandin synthesis [6,7], increased production of vasoconstrictor leukotrienes [34], increased gastric motility [14,15], reduction in gastric mucosal blood flow [8–13] and vascular endothelial damage [33,34]. Most studies [8–15,35,36] have emphasized the role of microcirculatory derangement in the pathogenesis of indomethacin-induced mucosal injury, while the role of acid received less interest. The present data provide evidence that luminal acid is an important factor in the pathogenesis of indomethacin-induced gastric mucosal injury.

The ig administration of 0.15 N HCl to pylorus-ligated rats, although by itself causing a mild degree of mucosal injury in control rats, markedly potentiated the ulcerogenic effect of sc indomethacin. Work by several investigators has indicated that gastric mucosal blood flow (GMBF) plays a crucial role in maintaining the ability of the stomach mucosa to withstand noxious injury [8,9,37–39]. Ritchie [38] has shown that a reduction in GMBF with vasopressin did not alone produce erosions, but rather potentiated the mucosal damage by taurocholate in acid. Whittle [8] found that a reduction in GMBF produced by indomethacin or an increase in acid back-diffusion induced by sodium taurocholate led to a low incidence of erosions while a combination of both events produced marked mucosal damage. Similarly, Starlinger et al. [37] found that increasing luminal H^+ increased GMBF and that pretreatment with vasopressin prevented the acid-induced increase in GMBF and resulted in gastric mucosal damage. Leung et al. [39] instilled 0.1 N HCl into the stomachs of pylorus-ligated rats and revealed that the gastric mucosal barriers to acid injury break only when arterial blood pressure, and hence GMBF, are reduced to 40% below base line. Indomethacin has been shown in several studies to reduce basal GMBF in intact rats [8,9,11,13,14] and around acetic acid-induced ulcers [10,13]. Therefore, in the present study, it is likely that although a reduction in GMBF and/or inhibition of prostaglandin synthesis by indomethacin only led to a moderate degree of gastric mucosal injury, it made the rat gastric mucosa very susceptible to an acid load. From the present study, it can be concluded that acid plays an important role in the development of indomethacin-induced gastric mucosal injury.

In the stomach, capsaicin evokes the release of vasodilator neuropeptides from sensory nerve endings [25,26], which largely accounts for its gastroprotective action [18,40] and when administered in very low concentrations into the stomach of pylorus-ligated rats, inhibited gastric acid secretion [41,42]. The gastroprotective effects of sensory nerve stimulation therefore involve both enhancement of the local micro-circulation and inhibition of gastric acid secretion [31]. According to the present experiments, the latter might have been involved also in the protective effect of atropine and cimetidine.

ACKNOWLEDGEMENTS

This study was supported by grants from the Hungarian National Research Fund (OTKA T 020098 and T 016945) and the Ministry of Health and Welfare (ETT-03 660/93 and ETT-T 563).

REFERENCES

1. Hart ED, Huskisson EC. Non-steroidal anti-inflammatory drugs. Current status and rational therapeutic use. Drugs. 1984;27:232–55.
2. Pemberton RE, Strand LJ. A review of upper gastrointestinal effects of the newer nonsteroidal antiinflammatory agents. Dig Dis Sci. 1979;24:53–64.
3. Bjarnason I, Smethurst P, Fenn CG, Lee CE, Menzies IS, Levi AJ. Misoprostol reduces indomethacin-induced changes in human small intestinal permeability. Dig Dis Sci. 1989;34:407–11.
4. Djahanguiri B. The production of acute gastric ulceration by indomethacin in the rat. Scand J Gastroenterol. 1969;4:265–7
5. Karádi O, Bódis B, Király À et al. Surgical vagotomy enhances the indomethacin-induced gastrointestinal mucosal damage in rats. Inflammopharmacology. 1994;2:389–99.
6. Whittle BJR, Higgs GA, Eakin KE, Moncada S, Vane JR. Selective inhibition of prostaglandin production in inflammatory exudates and gastric mucosa. Nature. 1980;284:271–3.
7. Rainsford KD, Willis C. Relationship of gastric mucosal damage induced in pigs by antiinflammatory drugs to their effects on prostaglandin production. Dig Dis Sci. 1982;27:624–35.
8. Whittle BJR. Mechanisms underlying gastric mucosal damage induced by indomethacin and bile salts, and the action of prostaglandins. Br J Pharmacol. 1977;60:455–60.
9. Main IHM, Whittle BJR. Investigation of the vasodilator and antisecretory role of prostaglandins in the rat gastric mucosa by use of nonsteroidal antiinflammatory drugs. Br J Pharmacol. 1975;53:217–24.
10. Skarstein A. Effect of indomethacin on blood flow distribution in the stomach of cats with acute gastric ulcer. Scand J Gastroenterol. 1979;14:905–11.
11. Kauffman GL, Aures D, Grossman MI. Intravenous indomethacin and aspirin reduce basal gastric mucosal blood flow in dogs. Am J Physiol. 1980;238:G131–4.
12. Hirose H, Takeuchi K, Okabe S. Effect of indomethacin on gastric mucosal blood flow around acetic acid-induced gastric ulcers in rats. Gastroenterology. 1991;100:1259–65.
13. Ueki S, Takeuchi K, Okabe S. Gastric motility is an important factor in pathogenesis of indomethacin-induced gastric mucosal lesions in rats. Dig Dis Sci. 1988;33:309–16.
14. Takeuchi S, Okada M, Ebara S, Osano H. Increased microvascular permeability and lesion formation during gastric hypermotility caused by indomethacin and 2-deoxy-D-glucose in the rat. J Clin Gastroenterol. 1990;12:S76–84.
15. Szolcsányi J. A pharmacological approach to elucidation of the role of different nerve fibers and receptor endings in mediation of pain. J Physiol (Paris). 1977;73:251–9.
16. Szolcsányi J. Actions of capsaicin on sensory receptors. In: Wood JN, ed. Capsaicin in the Study of Pain. Neuroscience Perspectives. London: Academic Press; 1993:1–23.
17. Holzer P. Capsaicin, cellular targets, mechanisms of action, and selectivity for thin sensory neurons. Pharmacol Rev. 1991;43:143–201.
18. Szolcsányi J. Barthó L. Impaired defense mechanism to peptic ulcer in the capsaicin-desensitized rat. In: Mózsik Gy, Hänninen O, Jávor T, eds. Gastrointestinal Defense Mechanisms. Oxford and Budapest: Pergamon Press and Akademiai Kiadó; 1980:39–51.
19. Holzer P, Lippe IT. Stimulation of afferent neve endings by intragastric capsaicin protects against ethanol-induced damage of gastric mucosa. Neuroscience. 1988;27:981–7.
20. Holzer P, Sametz W. Gastric mucosal protection against ulcerogenic factors in the rat mediated by capsaicin-sensitive afferent neurons. Gastroenterology. 1986;91:975–81.
21. Holzer P, Pabst MA, Lippe IT. Intragastric capsaicin protects against aspirin-induced lesions formation and bleeding in the rat gastric mucosa. Gastroenterology. 1989;96:1425–33.
22. Szolcsányi J. Effect of capsaicin, resiniferatoxin and piperine on ethanol-induced gastric ulcer of the rat. Acta Physiol Hung. 1990;75(suppl):267–8.
23. Sternini C, Reeve JR, Brecha N. Distribution and characterization of calcitonin gene-related peptide immunoreactivity in the digestive system of normal and capsaicin-treated rats. Gastroenterology. 1987;93:852–62.
24. Green T, Dockray GJ. Characterization of the peptidergic afferent innervation of the stomach in the rat, mouse and guinea pig. Neuroscience. 1988;25:181–93.
25. Renzi D, Santicioli P, Maggi CA, Surrenti C, Pradelles P, Meli A. Capsaicin-induced release of substance P-like immunoreactivity from guinea pig stomach in vitro and in vivo. Neurosci Lett. 1988;92:254–8.
26. Holzer P, Peskar BM, Peskar BA, Amann R. Release of calcitonin gene-related peptide induced by capsaicin in the vascularly perfused rat stomach. Neurosci Lett. 1990;108:195–200.

27. Guth PH, Leung FW. Physiology of the gastric circulation. In: Johnson LR, ed. Physiology of the Gastrointestinal Tract. New York: Raven Press; 1987:1031–53.

28. Szallasi A, Blumberg PM. Specific binding of resiniferatoxin, an ultrapotent capsaicin analog, by dorsal root ganglion membranes. Brain Res. 1990;524:109–11.

29. Szolcsányi J, Szallasi A, Szallasi Z, Joo F, Blumberg PM. Resiniferatoxin: an ultrapotent selective modulator of capsaicin-sensitive primary afferent neurons. J Pharmacol Exp Ther. 1990;255:923–8.

30. Mózsik Gy, Móron F, Jávor T. Cellular mechanisms of the development of gastric mucosal damage and of gastric cytoprotection induced by prostacyclin in rats. A pharmacological study. Prostagl Leuk Med. 1982;9:71–84.

31. Abdel-Salam OME, Szolcsányi J, Barthó L, Mózsik Gy. Sensory nerve-mediated mechanisms, gastric mucosal damage and its protection: A critical overview. Gastroprotection. 1994;2:4–12.

32. Abdel-Salam OME, Bódis B, Karádi O, Szolcsányi J, Mózsik Gy. Modification of aspirin and ethanol-induced mucosal damage in rats by intragastric application of resiniferatoxin. Inflammopharmacology. 1995;3:135–47.

33. Chvasta TE, Cooke AR. The effect of several ulcerogenic drugs on the canine gastric mucosal barrier. J Lab Clin Med. 1972;79:302–15.

34. Ohara A, Sugiyama S, Hoshino H et al. Reduction of adverse effects of indomethacin by anti-allergic drugs in rat stomachs. Arzneim-Forsch/Drug Res. 1992;42:1115–8.

35. Nygard G, Hudson HG, Mazure G et al. Procoagulant and prothrombotic responses of human endothelium to indomethacin and endotoxin in vitro. Relevance to non-steroidal anti-inflammatory drug enteropathy. Scand J Gastroenterol. 1995;30:25–32.

36. Rainsford KD. Microvascular injury during gastric mucosal damage by anti-inflammatory drugs in pigs and rats. Agents Actions. 1983;13:457–60.

37. Starlinger M, Schiessel R, Hung CR. H^+ back diffusion stimulating mucosal blood flow in the rabbit fundus. Surgery. 1981;89:232–6.

38. Ritchie WP Jr. Acute gastric mucosal damage induced by bile salts, acid and ischaemia. Gastroenterology. 1975;68:699–707.

39. Leung FW, Itoh M, Hirabayashi K, Guth PH. Role of blood flow in gastric and duodenal injury in the rat. Gastroenterology. 1985;88:281–9.

40. Holzer P, Livingston EH, Saria A, Guth PH. Sensory neurons mediate protective vasodilatation in rat gastric mucosa. Am J Physiol. 1991;260:G363–70.

41. Abdel-Salam OME, Szolcsányi J, Mózsik Gy. Effect of resiniferatoxin on stimulated gastric acid secretory responses in the rat. J Physiol (Paris). 1995;88:353–8.

42. Abdel-Salam OME, Szolcsányi J, Mózsik Gy. Capsaicin and its analogue resiniferatoxin inhibit gastric acid secretion in pylorus-ligated rats. Pharmacol Res. 1995;31:341–5.

G Mózsik et al. Cell Injury and Cytoprotection in the GI Tract. 107–116.
© 1997 Kluwer Academic Publishers.

A COMPARATIVE STUDY ON THE ADENINE NUCLEOTIDE METABOLISM OF ACID-DEPENDENT AND NON-ACID-DEPENDENT ACUTE GASTRIC MUCOSAL INJURY IN THE RAT

B. GASZTONYI, Á. KIRÁLY, G. SÜTŐ, Á. VINCZE, O. KARÁDI AND Gy. MÓZSIK*
First Department of Medicine, Medical University of Pécs, Pécs, Hungary
*Correspondence

This paper was first published in: Inflammopharmacology. 1996;4:351–60.

ABSTRACT

Intragastric (ig) administration of 96% ethanol (EtOH, non-acid-dependent model) and 0.6 mol/L HCl (acid-dependent model) produces acute mucosal lesions in the rat stomach.

Aim: The aim of this study was to compare the EtOH- and HCl-induced biochemical changes and ulcerations of gastric mucosa in the rat examined at different times after administration of the necrotizing agents.

Materials and methods: The observations were carried out on Sprague–Dawley rats weighing 180–210 g. The animals were fasted for 24 h before the experiment but received water freely; 1 ml 96% EtOH or 0.6 mol/L HCl was given ig. The rats were sacrificed at 0, 1, 5, 15, 30 and 60 min after administration of necrotizing agents, when the stomach was removed and the number and severity of mucosal lesions was noted. The mucosa was scraped and its ATP, ADP, AMP and lactate levels were measured enzymatically; the cAMP level was measured by RIA. The ratio of ATP/ADP, adenylate pool (ATP+ADP+AMP) and 'energy charge' [(ATP+0.5ADP)/(ATP+ADP+AMP)] were calculated.

Results:

1. The number and severity of mucosal lesions reached about 50% of total by 5 min after application of the necrotizing agents;

2. The ATP level decreased between 5 and 30 min, but thereafter its level increased (ADP changed in the opposite direction) in both models;

3. The cAMP level increased at 1 and 5 min but decreased later;

4. 'Energy charge' and lactate level did not change.

Conclusions: The biochemical changes in acid- (HCl) and non-acid- (EtOH) dependent gastric ulcer models are similar, but these changes appear earlier in the acid-dependent model.

Keywords: acid-dependent model, non-acid-dependent models, cellular energy systems

---

This paper was presented at the Symposium on 'Cell injury and protection in the gastrointestinal tract: from basic science to clinical perspectives', October 8–11, 1995, Pécs, Hungary.

INTRODUCTION

Different chemicals, applied locally, induce macroscopic gastric mucosal ulcerations in rats [1]. The acid-dependent (HCl) and non-acid-dependent (EtOH) gastric ulcer models are used widely to examine the development of mucosal damage [2–4]. Gastric mucosal ulcers can be produced by per-os administration of 1 ml 96% EtOH or 0.6 mol/L HCl. Different pathways may play a role in the development of induced gastric ulcers by these necrotizing agents, but there may be some common points in the ulcerogenesis of these aggressive agents. The energy state of the mucosal cells plays an important role in the maintenance of the integrity of the mucosa [2].

In the cells, there are two ATP-dependent energy systems: one is the membrane Na^+-K^+-dependent ATPase system [5–7] and the other is the transformation of ATP into cAMP by adenylate cyclase in the presence of Mg^{2+} [5]. Activity of these systems indicates energy turnover. There is a well-determined feedback mechanism between these two energy systems [8].

Different biochemical parameters (ATP, ADP, AMP, cAMP, lactate) were measured to evaluate the 'cross-section' of gastric mucosal biochemistry. The ratio of ATP/ADP, adenylate pool (ATP+ADP+AMP) and 'energy charge' [(ATP+0.5ADP)/(ATP+ADP+AMP)] were calculated [9].

Tissue hypoxia has been suggested by several physiological observations. Biochemically, the existence of tissue hypoxia can be proved by the presence of two factors: a decrease in tissue level of ATP; and a decreased level of ATP due to impaired oxidative phosphorylation (concomitant with increased tissue lactate) [2]. Calculations of the ratio of ATP/ADP and 'energy charge' are widely used biochemical methods for the evaluation of tissue hypoxia [2].

The aims of this study were to compare the HCl- and EtOH-induced (as acid-dependent and non-acid-dependent models) biochemical changes of mucosa and mucosal damage in the rat stomach, and the dependence (of magnitude) on time after administration of necrotizing agents. We compared these changes in mucosal biochemistry in acid-dependent and in non-acid-dependent gastric ulcer models in rats.

MATERIALS AND METHODS

The observations were performed in Sprague–Dawley rats of both sexes weighing 180–210 g. The animals were fasted for 24 h before the experiment but they received water freely. Mucosal damage was produced by po injected administration of 1 ml 96% ethanol or 1 ml 0.6 mol/L HCl. The animals were sacrificed at 0, 1, 5, 15, 30 and 60 min after administration of necrotizing agents, when the number and severity of mucosal lesions were noted. The gastric mucosa was scraped and the ATP, ADP, AMP and lactate levels were determined from total homogenates of gastric mucosa by enzymatic assays using the methods described by the manufacturer (Boehringer, Ingelheim, Germany). The cAMP content of the tissue was determined by RIA (Beckton Dickinson, Orangeburg, USA) [9]. Mucosal protein was assayed by the method of Lowry et al. [10]. The tissue levels of ATP, ADP and AMP were expressed in nanomoles, cAMP in picomoles and lactate in millimoles in 1.0 mg mucosal protein.

The ratio of ATP/ADP, adenylate pool (ATP+ADP+AMP) and 'energy charge' [(ATP+0.5ADP)/(ATP+ADP+AMP)] were subsequently calculated.

Statistical analysis

The results were calculated as means ± SEM. The unpaired Student's *t*-test was used for statistical analysis of results, and the Mann–Whitney U-test for severity of gastric mucosal lesions. Differences were considered significant if $p \leqslant 0.05$.

RESULTS

The extent, i.e. number and severity, of EtOH- and HCl-induced gastric mucosal damage at 5 min was about 50% that at 60 min (= 100%) after administration of necrotizing agents (Figures 1 and 2).

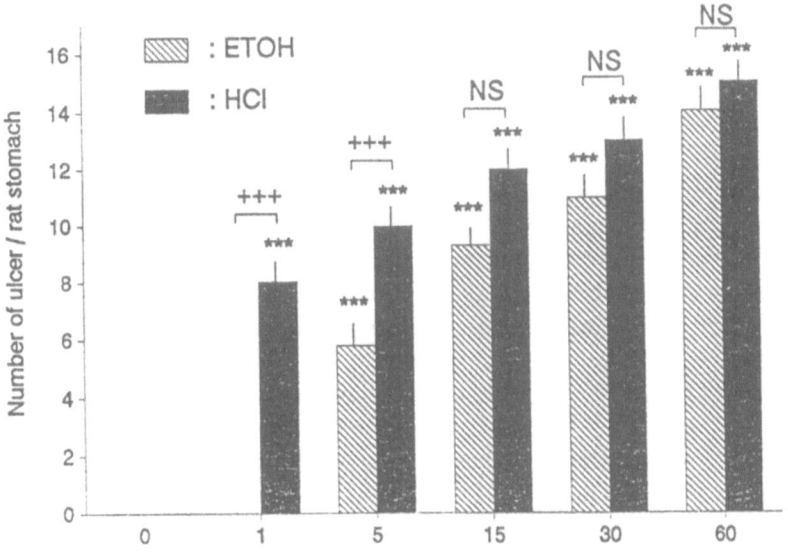

Figure 1. The number of macroscopic gastric mucosal lesions in rats treated with ethanol (1 ml 96% EtOH ig) and HCl (1 ml 0.6 mol/L ig) in relation to time after administration of the necrotizing agent. The results were expressed as means ± SEM of 12 animals. The *p* values were calculated for different times vs. time 0 (denoted *) and results obtained at the same time in the EtOH and HCl models (denoted +). *** and +++: $p < 0.001$. NS = not significantly different compared with respective treatment indicated by bar or control

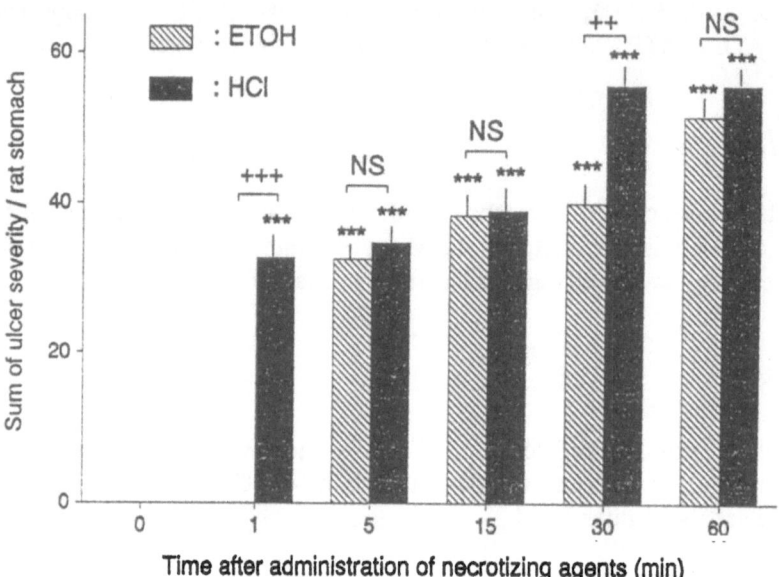

Figure 2. The sum of macroscopic gastric mucosal damage in rats treated with EtOH or HCl. For further explanation, see Figure 1

The tissue level of ATP decreased up to 15 min, then increased significantly up to 60 min, after administration of the necrotizing agents (Figure 3). The opposite change was obtained when gastric mucosal ATP was measured (Figure 4).

Of particular note was that the ratio of ATP/ADP changed significantly 5 min after administration of the necrotizing agent (Figure 5).

The tissue level of AMP decreased from 1 to 60 min after administration of necrotizing agents (Figure 6).

The adenylate pool also decreased after administration of necrotizing agents (Figure 7).

The cAMP concentration increased in an early phase (at 1 and 5 min), then decreased in a late phase (from 15 to 60 min) after administration of the necrotizing agent (Figure 8).

The 'energy charge' was not, however, decreased at 1 or 5 min after administration of the necrotizing agent (Figure 9).

No significant change in lactate level was obtained in the gastric mucosa at any time after administration of necrotizing agents (Figure 10).

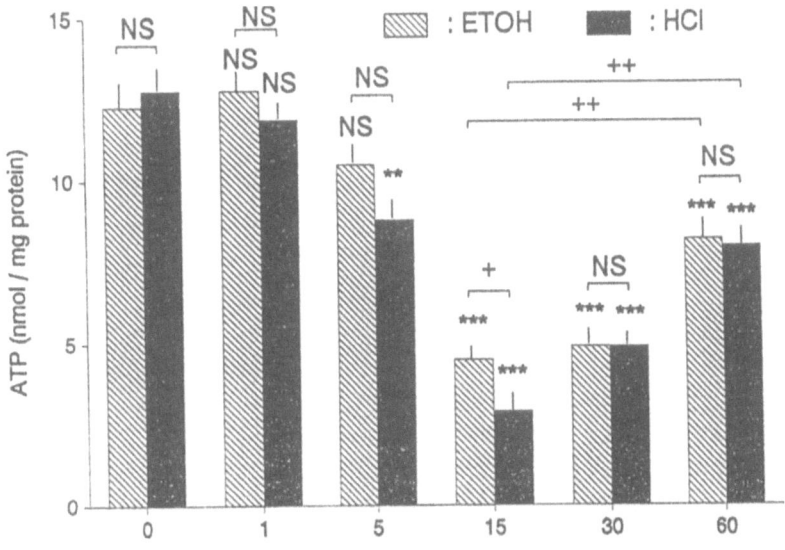

Figure 3. Changes in the gastric mucosal ATP of rats treated with ethanol or HCl in relation to time after administration of the necrotizing agent. For further explanation, see Figure 1. NS, not significant; +, $p < 0.05$; ** and ++, $p < 0.01$; ***, $p < 0.001$

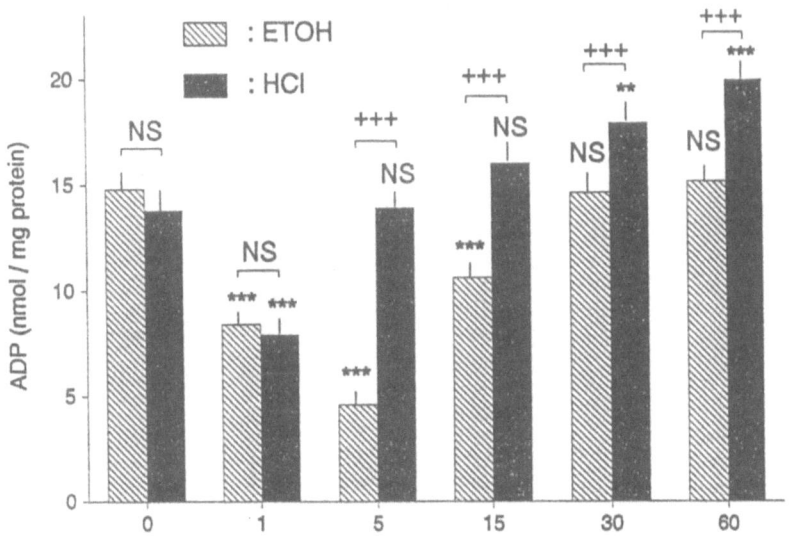

Figure 4. Changes in gastric mucosal ADP of rats treated with EtOH or HCl in relation to time after administration of the necrotizing agent. For further explanation, see Figure 3

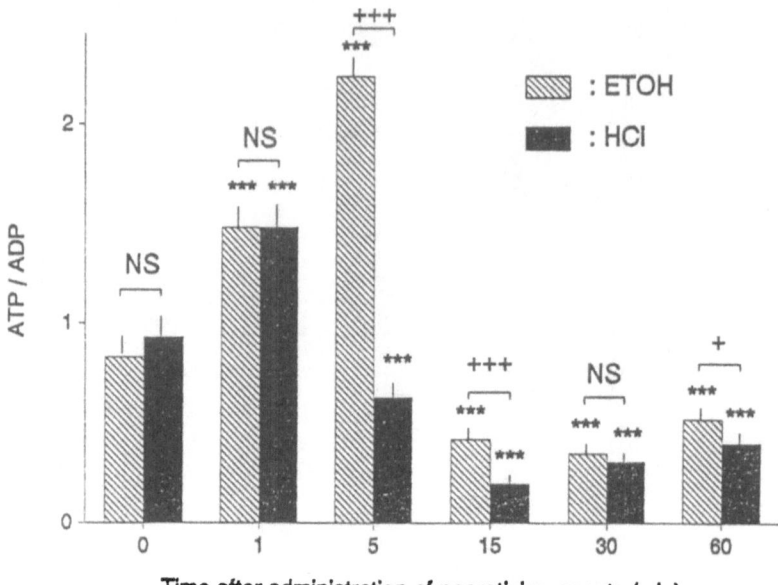

Figure 5. Changes in the ratio of ATP/ADP in the gastric mucosa of rats treated with EtOH or HCl in relation to time after administration of the necrotizing agent. For further explanation, see Figure 1

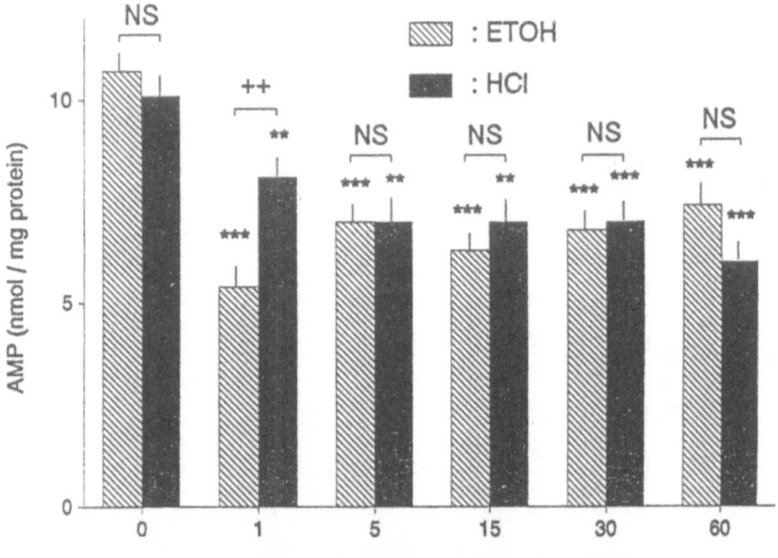

Figure 6. Changes in the gastric mucosal AMP of rats treated with EtOH or HCl in relation to time after administration of the necrotizing agent. For further explanation, see Figure 3

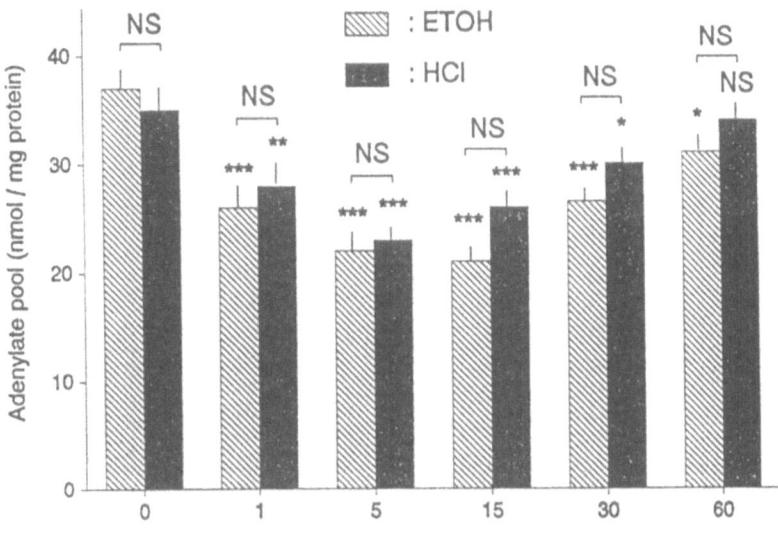

Figure 7. Changes in gastric mucosal adenylate pool (ATP+ADP+AMP) or rats treated with EtOH or HCl in relation to time after administration of the necrotizing agent. For further explanation, see Figures 1 and 3

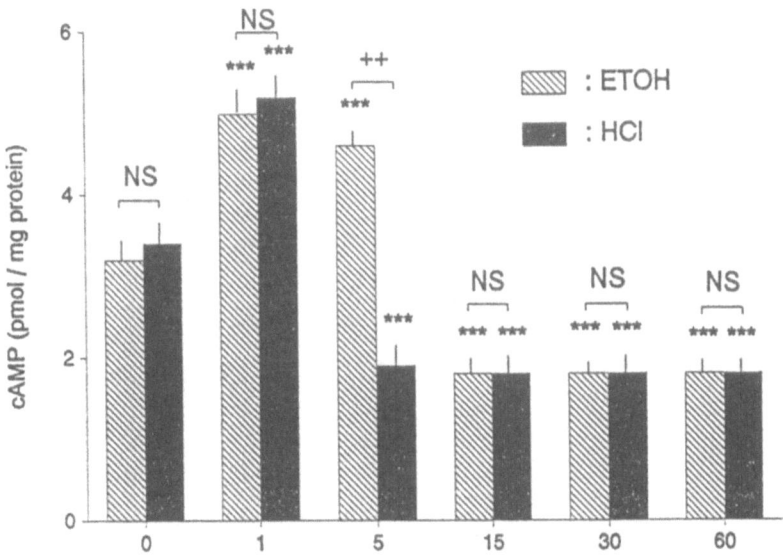

Figure 8. Changes in gastric mucosal cAMP of rats treated with EtOH or HCl in relation to time after administration of the necrotizing agent. For further explanation, see Figures 1 and 3

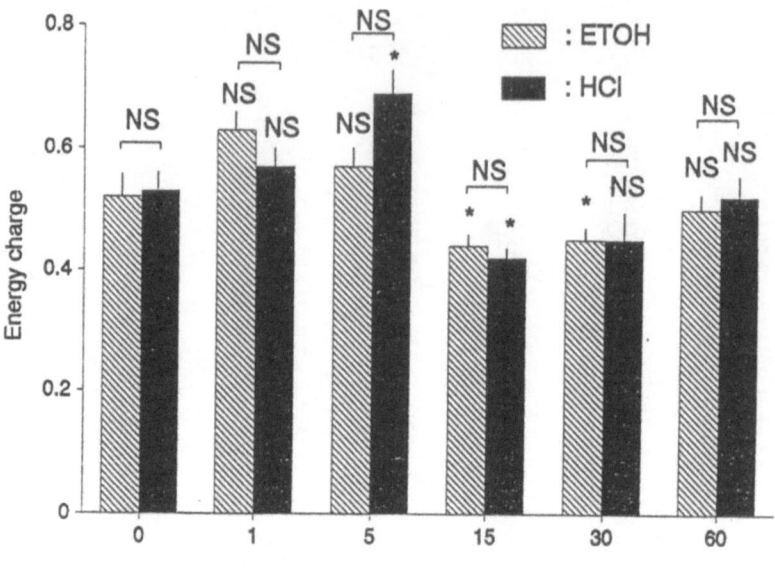

Figure 9. Changes in the gastric mucosal 'energy charge' [(ATP+0.5ADP)/(ATP+ADP+AMP)] of rats treated with EtOH or HCl in relation to time after administration of the necrotizing agent. For further explanation, see Figures 1 and 3

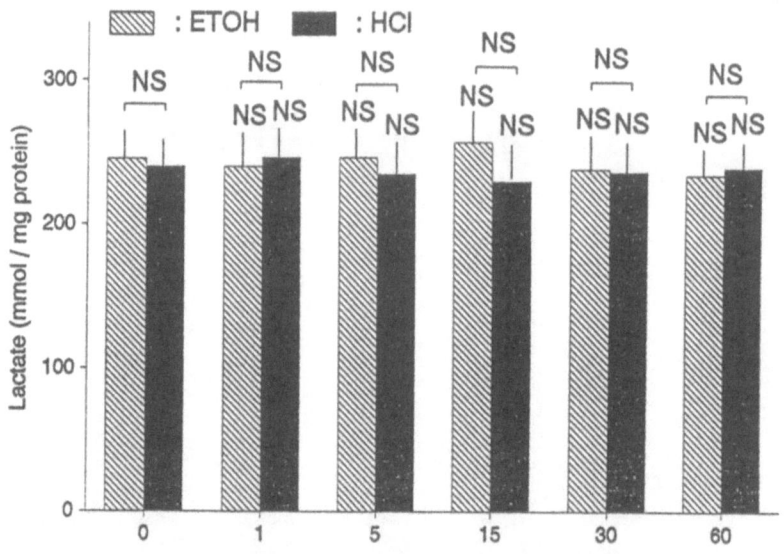

Figure 10. Gastric mucosal level of lactate of rats treated with EtOH or HCl in relation to time after administration of the necrotizing agent. For further explanation, see Figures 1 and 3

DISCUSSION

The aetiology of peptic ulcer disease (PUD) in patients is unknown (excluding drugs, chemicals, various pulmonary or endocrine diseases, etc.); this is why experimental models are frequently used to evaluate the developmental mechanisms of gastric mucosal damage. The measurement of different biochemical parameters is offered to obtain a biochemical profile of the gastric mucosa, which is able to prove or to exclude the presence of hypoxia in the gastric mucosa. Furthermore, the results obtained at different times after administration of necrotizing agents allow time-sequence analysis.

The early appearance of gastric mucosal damage, after administration of different necrotizing agents in acid-dependent and non-acid-dependent models, suggests a direct action of these agents (Figures 1 and 2). It is possible since the changes in vascular permeability precede other events, like alterations in the components of energy metabolism, that changes in mucosal biochemistry are consequences, not causes, of the direct damaging effects of EtOH and HCl.

The transitory decrease and subsequent increase in the level of mucosal ATP in both models excludes the presence (biochemically) of gastric mucosal hypoxia (Figure 3). The increased level of ATP in the later phase of these experiments suggests that oxidative phosphorylation is intact. Oxidative phosphorylation in the cells is impaired in hypoxaemic states, thus resulting in an increased lactate level. The unchanged lactate level found in our experiments (Figure 10) means further evidence for the absence of gastric mucosal hypoxia.

The increase in cAMP directly and indirectly inhibits the extent of ATP–ADP transformation in the early phase (Figures 3, 4 and 8), while, later on, these types of inhibitory effects produced by cAMP disappear from the ATP–ADP transformation [2,5–8].

The results clearly indicate that:

1. The development of EtOH- or HCl-induced mucosal damage is a consequence of active metabolic response of gastric mucosa;

2. The different chemicals produce similar biochemical changes in the gastric mucosa;

3. The time-sequence analysis of the mucosal damage and of changes in mucosal biochemistry suggest a direct injuring effect of necrotizing agents.

ACKNOWLEDGEMENTS

This study was supported by grants from the Hungarian National Research Fund (OTKA-T-020098) and Ministry of Health and Welfare (ETT-03 660/93).

REFERENCES

1. Szabo S, Nagy L. Pathways, mediators and mechanisms of gastroduodenal mucosal injury. Acta Physiol Hung. 1992;80:9–21.
2. Mózsik Gy, Jávor T. A biochemical and pharmacological approach to the genesis of ulcer disease. A model study of ethanol-induced injury to gastric mucosa in rats. Dig Dis Sci. 1988;33:92–105.
3. Frezza M. The mechanisms of ethanol-induced gastric damage. Gastroprotection. 1994;1:4–9.
4. Mózsik Gy, Fiegler M, Garamszegi M et al. Mechanisms of gastric mucosal cytoprotection: Time-sequence analysis of gastric mucosal membrane-bound ATP-dependent energy systems, oxygen free radicals and macroscopic appearance of gastric cytoprotection by PGI_2 and β-carotene in HCl-model of rats. In: Hayaishi O, Niki E, Kondo M, Yoshikawa T, eds. Med Biochem Chem Asp Free Radicals, Proceedings of the 4th Biennial General Meeting of the Society for Free Radicals Research, Kyoto, Japan. Amsterdam: Elsevier Science Publishers; 1989:1421–5.
5. Albers RW. Biochemical aspects of active transport. Annu Rev Biochem. 1967;36:727–56.
6. Robinson GA, Butcher RW, Sutherland EW. Cyclic AMP. New York: Academic Press; 1971.
7. Skou JC. Enzymatical basis for active transport of Na and K across cell membrane. Physiol Rev. 1965;45:596–617.
8. Mózsik Gy, Fiegler M, Nagy L, Patty I, Tárnok F. Gastric and small intestinal energy metabolism in mucosal damage. In: Mózsik Gy, Hanninen O, Jávor T, eds. Advances in Physiological Sciences. Oxford: Pergamon Press–Budapest: Akadémiai Kiadó; 1981;29:213–76.
9. Fiegler M, Jávor T, Nagy L, Patty I, Mózsik Gy. Biochemical background of the development of gastric mucosal damage in pylorus-ligated plus aspirin-treated rats. Int J Tiss React. 1986;8:15–22.
10. Lowry OH, Rosebrough NJ, Farr AL, Randal RJ. Protein measurements with the Folin phenol reagent. J Biol Chem. 1951;193:265–75

G Mózsik et al. Cell Injury and Cytoprotection in the GI Tract. 117–123.
© 1997 Kluwer Academic Publishers.

MORPHOLOGICAL ASPECTS OF BPC-PEPTIDE PROTECTION IN ETHANOL-INDUCED GASTRIC LESIONS IN RATS

S. SEIWERTH*, P. SIKIRIĆ, Ž. GRABAREVIĆ, M. PETEK, R. RUČMAN, M. TUDJA, B. TURKOVIĆ AND D. LJUBANOVIĆ

Center for Digestive Diseases, Institutes of Pathology and Pharmacology, Medical and Veterinary Faculty, University of Zagreb, Pliva Company, Clinical Hospital "Sestre milosrdnice", Zagreb, Croatia
*Correspondence

ABSTRACT

A wide organoprotective action has already been described for the peptide BPC and its synthetic pentadecapeptide BPC 157, including gastroprotection in various ulcer models.

Ethanol-induced gastric lesions are one of the most-often used experimental models in gastroprotection analysis. In the present work, we analysed the morphological aspects of BPC 157 gastroprotection in ethanol-induced gastric damage by using: conventional microscopy, Monastral blue, scanning and transmission electron microscopy. In all experimental periods (1, 5, 60, 180 min and 24 h), we found significant differences between BPC 157-treated animals and controls. The most interesting elements were an apparent microvascular protection exerted by BPC 157 and a prominent mucus-like secretion covering the damaged surface, which appeared early and was more extensive in BPC-treated animals compared with controls.

We conclude that the gastroprotective effect of BPC could be a combination of vascular protection and production of a protective layer preventing further mucosal damage and possibly enhancing re-epithelialization.

Keywords: BPC, pentadecapeptide, organoprotection, ethanol, gastric lesions, morphology, microscopy, electron microscopy

INTRODUCTION

Since the development of the concepts of cytoprotection and organoprotection for prostaglandins and other endogenous substances, such as somatostatin and dopamine [2–4], ethanol-induced gastric injury has been one of the most-often used experimental models, producing much valuable information about the organoprotective mechanisms of different substances.

The gastric juice peptide BPC and its synthetic fragment BPC 157 have been reported to have broad organoprotective activity, including hepatoprotection, pancreas protection, kidney protection, protection of peripheral nerves as well as a prominent anti-inflammatory action [5–8]. One of its most prominent actions is gastroprotection which has been studied in various experimental models [9]. The protective potential of BPC is made even more interesting by its stability in gastric juice [10].

This paper was presented at the Symposium on 'Cell injury and protection in the gastrointestinal tract: from basic science to clinical perspectives', October 8–11, 1995, Pécs, Hungary.

In order to establish the morphological basis and the level of its organoprotective action, in this work, we studied BPC 157 gastroprotection in ethanol-induced gastric lesions by different morphological means – macroscopically, histologically, using Monastral blue and ultrastructurally – using transmission electron microscope and using scanning electron microscope.

MATERIALS AND METHODS

Male albino rats of the Wistar strain, 180–210 g body weight, were used in all experiments. Six to ten animals were assigned to each experimental protocol. In all experiments, animals were fasted 24 h prior to ethanol administration with water ad libitum until 1 h prior to application. Ethanol (1 ml of 96%) was administered by gavage. BPC 157 (10 µg/kg body weight) was given intraperitoneally (ip) 1 h before ethanol. Controls received an equivolume of saline ip (5 ml/kg body weight).

The animals were killed after different time intervals and the lesions analysed by different means:

1 min	–	Monastral blue, light microscopy
5 min	–	Scanning electron microscopy (SEM)
		Transmission electron microscopy (TEM)
60 min	–	TEM, light microscopy
180 min	–	Light microscopy
24 h	–	SEM

Macroscopic changes were analysed at all time intervals.

Macroscopy

Immediately after sacrifice, the abdomen was opened, the duodenum and oesophagus clamped and the stomach distended by saline injection. Thereafter, the stomach was opened along the greater curvature, washed in saline and spread on a board immersed in saline. The lesions were measured using a computer-based image analysis system.

Monastral blue

Four minutes before sacrifice, Monastral blue was applied to the animals (Sigma; 3%, 1 ml/kg body weight iv). The animals were killed 1 min after ethanol application. The stomach was distended and fixed for 24 h in 10% formalin. Thereafter, it was transferred to glycerol for 24 h, mounted in glycerol-gel and analysed under reflected light on a dissection microscope. The area density of blue-labelled blood vessels was assessed using a computer-based image analysis system. The same system was used to assess the area density of haemorrhagic lesions. The results are presented as group means.

Light microscopy

Immediately after the animals were killed, the stomach was removed, distended and fixed for 24 h in 10% formalin. Thereafter, a longitudinal sample, 2 mm thick, including the whole glandular stomach length was taken along the lesser curvature. One oblique sample was taken 2 mm below the forestomach–glandular stomach margin. The specimens were cut semiserially on three levels and the damage assessed concerning superficial epithelial lesions and deep (>0.2 mm) necrosis.

Transmission electron microscopy (TEM)

After the animals were killed, the stomach was distended and fixed in Karnowskys fixative for 24 h. Four samples (1×1 mm) were taken from each side along the lesser curvature. The samples were postfixed in OsO4, dehydrated, embedded in an epoxy resin and cut on an LKB ultramicrotome. Thin sections were mounted on a coated copper grid and viewed under an E9 Opton electron microscope. The morphology and extent of lesions were analysed.

Scanning electron microscopy (SEM)

Samples were taken from the same stomach as for TEM. A sample 8 mm in diameter was taken from the proximal area of glandular stomach (oxyntic mucosa), dehydrated, vacuum dried and coated with colloidal gold. The morphology and extent of damage was assessed under a Cambridge Stereoscan 600 scanning electron microscope.

RESULTS

Macroscopy

After all time intervals, except 1 min, haemorrhagic mucosal defects of different sizes and depths could be observed. The area of these lesions was consistently smaller in BPC-treated animals than in corresponding controls (Figure 1).

Monastral blue

One minute after ethanol application, mucosal vessel damage was clearly observed in controls. BPC-treated animals showed significantly smaller areas of Monastral blue deposition. Correspondingly, the area of macroscopic mucosal lesions was also smaller in treated animals (Figure 2).

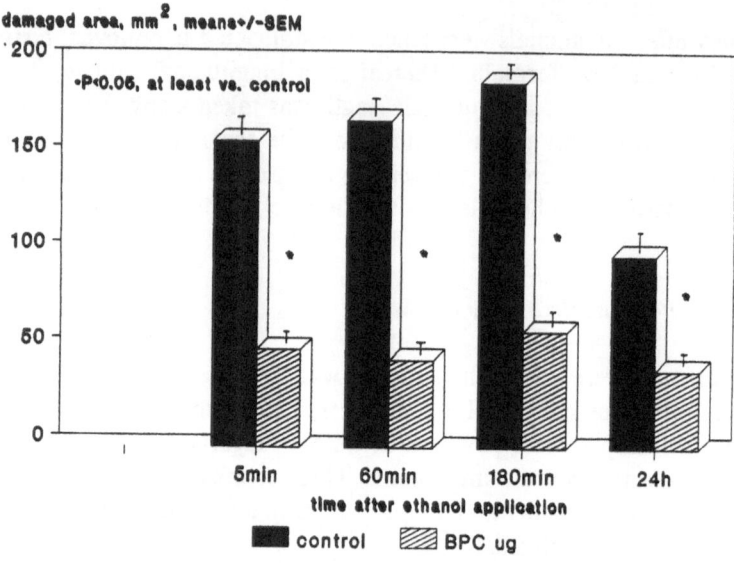

Figure 1. Macroscopic assessment of the effect of BPC application (10 μg/kg ip, 1 h before injury) on ethanol-induced (96% ig) gastric lesions; 6–10 rats per experimental group

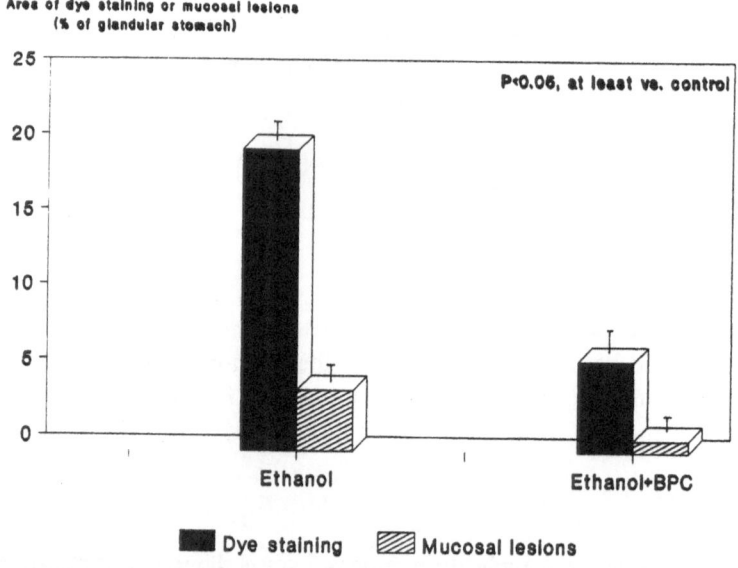

Figure 2. Monastral blue assessment of the effect of BPC application (10 μg/kg ip, 1 h before injury) on ethanol-induced (96% ig) gastric lesions; 6–10 rats per experimental group

Light microscopy

Upon light microscopy, the macroscopic lesions appeared as haemorrhagic erosion with a more or less pronounced inflammatory reaction. At all time intervals, control animals displayed more severe (deep) lesions as well as larger areas of superficial lesions than the corresponding BPC-treated animals.

Transmission electron microscopy

In the early phase (5 min after ethanol), ultrastructurally prominent mucosal blood vessel damage could be observed. In controls, severe erythrocyte deformation and margination as well as thrombosis of small vessels was present. These features were much less pronounced or absent in treated animals. In BPC-treated animals after only 5 min, a thick mucus-like substance was secreted from the depth of the glands, covering the surface epithelium. A similar excretion but not so 'thick' was observed in control animals only at later periods of time.

Scanning electron microscopy

In control animals, mucosal damage was obvious at all time intervals. Five minutes after ethanol administration, abundant lamina propria denudation with massive sloughing of cells was observed. Wide areas were covered by cellular debris. Also the presence of areas displaying only slight superficial injury was noted. In BPC-treated animals, the extent of damage was smaller with only occasional small denuded areas (Figures 3A,B). In large sections the surface was covered with a partly thick mucus-like layer. One hour after ethanol application, controls displayed large denuded areas with occasional signs of epithelial regeneration. Massive cellular debris was present. Occasional deep mucosal 'cracks' (deep defects) were noted. In BPC-treated animals, the signs of regeneration dominated. Large areas of 'sprouting' epithelial cells surrounded the very few denuded areas.

DISCUSSION

In this study, we have demonstrated the morphological features of BPC gastroprotective action. Compared with controls, treated animals showed less damage regardless of the investigative procedure applied. In control animals, the morphology of lesions corresponded to those described in the literature. BPC-treated animals showed on macroscopic and light microscopic examination considerably less damage due to superficial and deep mucosal lesions. One of the most interesting findings was the prevention of endothelial damage as demonstrated in the Monastral blue experiment. Scanning electron microscopy displayed smaller areas of lamina propria denudation and a much earlier and more orderly re-epithelialization of the damaged mucosal

A

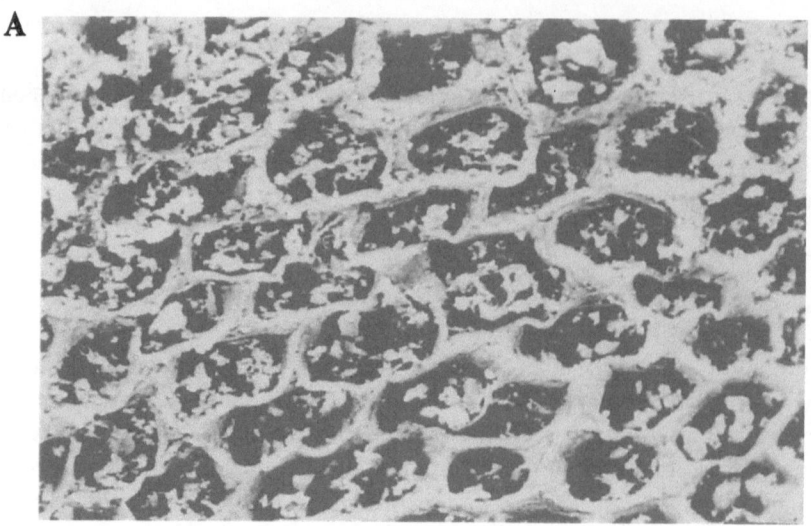

B

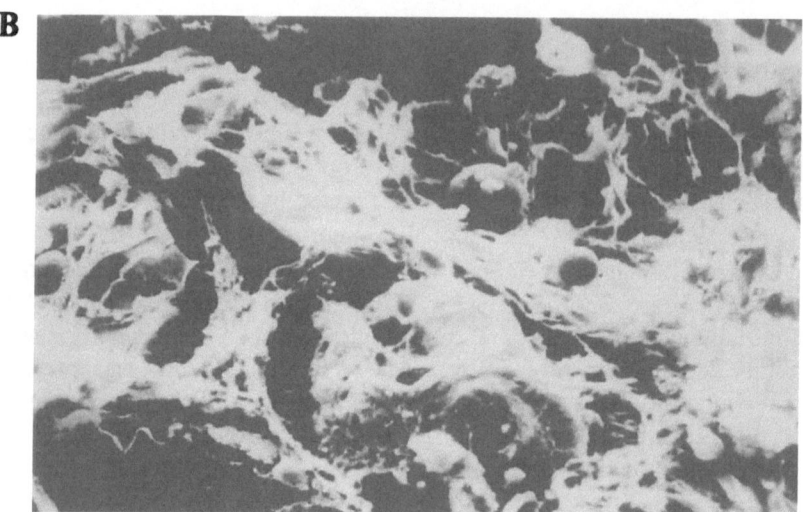

Figure 3. A. Control rat 5 min after ethanol application. Mostly denuded lamina propria with abundant cellular debris (SEM). B. BPC 157-treated animal 5 min after ethanol administration. Abundant mucus-like covering of the mucosal surface is observed (SEM)

surface. Also, at early times, BPC-treated animals had a thick mucus-like substance covering the surface of the glandular stomach.

In our experiments, we used a well-established model and morphological procedures standard in the literature [11,12]. Some of the findings seem to be of interest for elucidating the possible mechanisms of action of BPC gastroprotection. Two experiments showed a lesser extent of mucosal blood vessel damage in treated animals. As microvascular injury seems to be a crucial element in ulcer generation [13], vascular protection may play a very important role in gastroprotection/ulcer healing. BPC-treated animals also consistently showed secretion of a surface-covering mucus-like substance. The importance of endogenously produced coating substances could be to cover the damaged mucosa enabling and speeding up epithelial regeneration, as well as preventing further damage.

From the above-mentioned, it could be hypothesized that the possible mechanisms leading to less initial damage and earlier epithelial regeneration in BPC-treated animals exposed to ethanol are a combination of vascular (endothelium) protection and secretion enhancement of a surface-coating substance.

REFERENCES

1. Robert A, Nezamis JE Lancaster C, Hancher AJ. Cytoprotection prostaglandins in rats. Gastroenterology. 1979;77:433–43.
2. Hernandez DE, Walker CH, Valenzucia JE, Mason GA. Increased dopamine receptor binding in duodenal mucosa of duodenal ulcer patients. Dig Dis Sci. 1989;34:543–7.
3. Hernandez DE. Neuroendocrine mechanisms of stress ulceration: focus on thyrotropin releasing hormone (TRH). Life Sci. 1986;39:279–96.
4. Szabo S, Usadel KH. Cytoprotection by somatostatin: gastric and hepatic lesions. Experientia. 1982;38:254–6.
5. Sikirić P, Rotkvić I, Mise S et al. The influence of dopamine agonists and antagonists on indomethacin lesions in stomach and small intestine in rats. Eur J Pharmacol. 1988;158:61–7.
6. Sikirić P, Petek M, Rucman R et al. A new gastric juice peptide, BPC. An overview of the stomach–stress–organoprotection hypothesis and beneficial effects of BPC. J Physiol. 1993;87:313–27.
7. Sikirić P, Gyres K, Seiwerth S et al. The effect of pentadecapeptide BPC 157 on inflammatory, non-inflammatory, direct and indirect pain and capsaicin neurotoxicity. Inflammopharmacology. 1993;2:121–7.
8. Sikirić P, Seiwerth S, Grabarević Z et al. Hepatoprotective effect of BPC 157, a 15-amino acid peptide, on liver lesions induced by either restraint stress of bile duct and hepatic artery ligation or Cc14 administration. A comparative study with dopamine agonists and somatostatin. Life Sci. 1993;53:PL291–6.
9. Sikirić P, Seiwerth S, Grabarević Z et al. The beneficial effect of BPC 157, a 15-amino acid peptide BPC fragment, on gastric and duodenal lesions induced by restraint stress, cysteamine and 96% ethanol in rats. A comparative study with H2 receptor antagonists, dopamine promoters and gut peptides. Life Sci. 1994;54:PL63–8.
10. Veljaca M, Chan K, Guglietta A. Digestion of h-EGF, h-TGF alpha and BPC 15 in human gastric juice. Pharmacol Res. 1995;31:70.
11. Schmidt KL, Henegan JM, Smith GS, Hilburn PJ, Miller TA. Prostaglandin cytoprotection against ethanol-induced gastric injury in the rat. Gastroenterology. 1985;88:49–59.
12. Tamawski A, Hollander D, Stachura J, Krause WJ, Gergely H. Prostaglandin protection of the gastric mucosa against alcohol injury – a dynamic time-related process. Gastroenterology. 1985;88:334–52.
13. Szabo S, Trier JS, Brown A, Schnoor J. Early vascular injury and increased vascular permeability in gastric mucosal injury caused by ethanol in the rat. Gastroenterology. 1985;88:228–36.

G Mózsik et al. Cell Injury and Cytoprotection in the GI Tract. 125–128.

INHIBITORY EFFECT OF OMENTOPEXY ON EXPERIMENTAL CHRONIC GASTRIC ANTRAL ULCER FORMATION

B.S. DUNJIĆ* AND M. HASHMONAI

Department of Surgery B, Rambam Medical Center, The Bruce Rappaport Faculty of Medicine, Technion–Israel Institute of Technology, Haifa, Israel
*Correspondence

ABSTRACT

Hypoperfusion of the antral mucosa has been suggested as a component contributing to the pathogenesis of indomethacin-induced chronic antral ulcers in the rat. Omentum has been shown to induce angiogenesis, and when fixed to the serosa of the rat intact gastrointestinal tract to stimulate the development of vascular collaterals across the coapted surfaces. We have investigated whether such an enhanced blood supply to the antral mucosa could prevent indomethacin-induced chronic antral ulcers in the rat. Omentum was fastened to the serosa of the anterior wall of the gastric antrum. Six weeks later (period needed for vascular collaterals to develop), chronic gastric ulcers were induced in all animals. Twenty-four hours after the induction of ulcers, rats were sacrificed. The ulcer area was estimated and expressed as the ulcer index. The experimental schedule for control rats was the same as for rats which underwent surgery except initial omentopexy. Compared with control rats, the ulcer index was significantly reduced in rats which underwent omentopexy. In conclusion, omentopexy has the capacity to reduce the extent of indomethacin-induced chronic gastric ulcers in rats. This protection might be partially attributed to vascular ingrowth from omentum into the gastric antrum.

Keywords: omentum, stomach, chronic ulcer, indomethacin, blood flow

INTRODUCTION

Hypoperfusion of the antral mucosa has been suggested as a component contributing to the pathogenesis of indomethacin-induced chronic antral ulcers in the rat [1–6]. Omentum has been shown to induce angiogenesis [7], and when fixed to the serosa of the rat intact gastrointestinal tract, to stimulate the development of vascular collaterals across the coapted surfaces [8].

We have investigated whether such an enhanced blood supply to the antral mucosa could prevent indomethacin-induced chronic antral ulcers in the rat.

This paper was presented at the Symposium on 'Cell injury and protection in the gastrointestinal tract: from basic science to clinical perspectives', October 8–11, 1995, Pécs, Hungary.

MATERIALS AND METHODS

Animals

Twelve male Sprague–Dawley rats, weighing 250 ± 10 g, were obtained from the animal colony of the Department of Experimental Surgery, the Bruce Rappaport Faculty of Medicine, Technion, Israel. They were kept under constant temperature and humidity, and a 12-h light–dark rhythm, with free access to standard rat food pellets (except during starvation) and tap water.

Induction of the gastric mucosal lesions

Chronic ulcers were induced in re-fed rats by subcutaneous injection of indomethacin (Confortid, Dumex, Copenhagen, Denmark). The re-fed rats were allowed access to food pellets for 1 h following a 24-h fast, and indomethacin was given 30 min after re-feeding at a dose of 30 mg/kg body weight [9].

Experimental schedule

Animals were randomly divided into control and experimental groups, each comprising 6 rats. Operative procedures were performed under diethyl ether anaesthesia, through a midline laparotomy. Omentum was fastened to the serosa of the anterior wall of the gastric antrum. Six weeks later (period needed for vascular collaterals to develop), chronic ulcers were induced in all rats. Twenty-four hours after the induction of ulcers, rats were sacrificed with an ether overdose. The ulcer area was estimated and expressed as the ulcer index. The experimental schedule for control rats was the same as for rats which underwent surgery except initial omentopexy.

Evaluation of the gastric mucosal lesions

The stomach was excised, opened along the greater curvature and cleansed with 0.9% saline. To minimize mucosal folding, all specimens were spread and pinned on a cork board. The mucosa was examined for macroscopically evident lesions by using a dissecting microscope (magnification $\times 10$) with a 1-mm square-grid eye piece. The gastric ulcer index was expressed as the sum total of area (mm^2) of individual lesions.

Statistical analysis

Results are expressed as mean $\pm$ SEM. The significance of the difference was determined by the two-sided Student's t-test for unpaired data; $p < 0.05$ was considered significant.

RESULTS

Round, oval or butterfly-shaped gastric antral ulcers were found primarily on the lesser curvature, rarely near the pyloric ring or just distal to the corpus–antrum border on the greater curvature of all indomethacin-treated rats. These ulcers appeared as single lesions or in groups of 2–3 ulcers of different sizes. They were shallow with sharp edges at the same level as the surrounding intact mucosa. Compared with control rats, the ulcer index was significantly reduced in rats which underwent omentopexy (Figure 1).

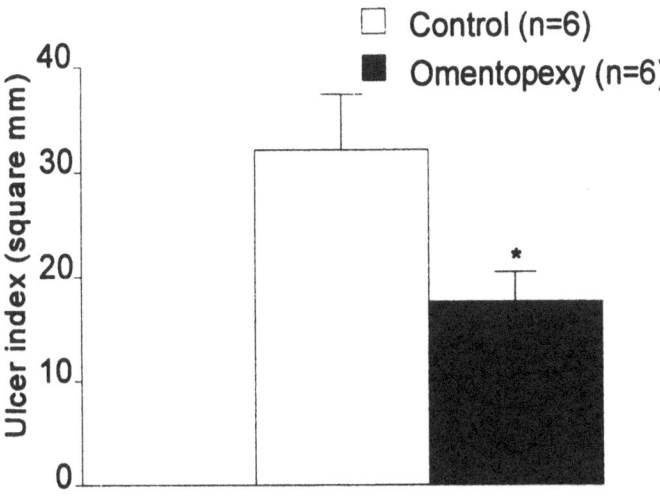

Figure 1. Chronic indomethacin model. Effect of omentopexy on chronic gastric antral ulcers in rats. Values are expressed as mean ± SEM; n = number of rats; *$p < 0.05$ vs control, two-sided Student's t-test for unpaired data

CONCLUSIONS

Omentopexy has the capacity to reduce the extent of indomethacin-induced chronic gastric ulcers in rats. This protection might be partially attributed to vascular ingrowth from omentum into the gastric antrum.

REFERENCES

1. Wallace JL, Arfors KE, McKnight GW. A monoclonal antibody against the CD18 leukocyte adhesion molecule prevents indomethacin-induced gastric damage in the rabbit. Gastroenterology. 1991;100:878–83.
2. Wallace JL. Non-steroidal anti-inflammatory drug gastropathy and cytoprotection: pathogenesis and mechanisms re-examined. Scand J Gastroenterol. 1992;27(suppl 192):3–8.
3. Miura S, Suematsu M, Tanaka S et al. Microcirculatory disturbances in indomethacin-induced intestinal ulcer. Am J Physiol. 1991;261:G213–19.
4. Asako H, Kubes P, Wallace J, Gaginella T, Wolf RE, Granger DN. Indomethacin-induced leukocyte adhesion in mesenteric venules: role of lipoxygenase products. Am J Physiol. 1992;262:G903–8.
5. Piasecki C, Thrasivoulou C, Rahim A. Ulcers produced by ligation of individual gastric mucosal arteries in the guinea pig. Gastroenterology. 1989;97:1121–9.
6. Dunjić BS, Axelson J, Bengmark S. Gastrointestinal blood flow disturbances during development of indomethacin-induced chronic ulcers in rats. Surg Res Commun. 1994;15:311–18.
7. Konturek SJ, Brzozowski T, Pawlik W, Stachura J. Omentum and bFGF in stimulation of healing of chronic gastric ulcerations. Digestion. 1991;49(suppl 1):20.
8. Shoshany G, Cohen E, Mordohovich D, Hayari L, Har-Shai Y, Bar-Maor JA. Creation of the isolated bowel segment in animals by omentoenteropexy. J Pediatr Surg. 1994;29(10):1344–7.
9. Satoh H, Inada I, Hirata T, Maki Y. Indomethacin produces gastric antral ulcers in the refed rats. Gastroenterology. 1981;81:719–25.

G Mózsik et al. Cell Injury and Cytoprotection in the GI Tract. 129–138.

EFFECT OF SURAMIN ON ETHANOL-INDUCED GASTRIC MUCOSAL INJURY: RELATIONSHIP BETWEEN TISSUE DISTRIBUTION AND SEVERITY OF DAMAGE

C. BLANDIZZI[1], R. DANESI[2], G. GHERARDI[3] AND M. DEL TACCA[1*]

[1]Institute of Pharmacology, School of Medicine and Dentistry, University of Pisa, Via Roma 55, I-56126 Pisa, Italy; [2]Superior School of University Studies and Doctoral Research Sant'Anna, Via Carducci 40, I-56127 Pisa, Italy; [3]Department of Pathology, Civil Hospital of Sondrio, Via Stelvio 25, I-23100 Sondrio, Italy
*Correspondence

This paper was first published in: Inflammopharmacology. 1996;4:331–40.

ABSTRACT

Suramin exerts antitumour effects by interfering with the biological activity of several growth factors. It is also known that growth factors, including epidermal growth factor, play a primary role in the protection of gastric mucosa and promotion of ulcer healing. In the present study, the penetration of suramin into the stomach as well as the influence exerted by this drug on ethanol-induced gastric mucosal damage were investigated. Suramin was administered by the intraperitoneal route to male rats every other day for fourteen days. Animals were then used for:

1. Assessment of suramin levels in plasma and tissues;

2. Histomorphometric evaluation of ethanol-induced gastric mucosal damage;

3. Measurement of gastric acid secretion after pylorus ligation.

The concentrations of suramin in plasma, stomach and kidney were $158 \pm 18.8 \, \mu g/ml$, $179.7 \pm 33.0 \, \mu g/g$ and $1480.9 \pm 85.8 \, \mu g/g$ ($n = 6$), respectively. Suramin did not induce gastric mucosal damage under basal conditions. However, the drug markedly enhanced ethanol-induced necrotic damage at all times tested. In addition, suramin significantly enhanced gastric acid output induced by pylorus ligation in conscious rats. Suramin is characterized by an unusually long half-life and a remarkable accumulation in kidney, whereas, in the majority of other organs, the drug reaches levels that are 8–10 times lower than those found in renal tissue. The data obtained in the present study are consistent with this pharmacokinetic profile and suggest that suramin concentration achieved in gastric tissue, which is known to inhibit the proliferation of several cell lines in vitro, is high enough to induce an impairment of mucosal protective mechanisms.

Keywords: suramin, ethanol, mucosal damage, growth factors, delayed repair, distribution, ulcer, acid secretion

This paper was presented at the Symposium on 'Cell injury and protection in the gastrointestinal tract: from basic science to clinical perspectives', October 8–11, 1995, Pécs, Hungary.

INTRODUCTION

Suramin is a polysulphonated naphthylamine derivative of urea endowed with several pharmacological actions [1]. More recently, suramin has been evaluated as an antineoplastic agent [2] and at present it is currently employed in the treatment of hormone-refractory prostate cancer [3]. Although it is likely that different biological activities of suramin participate in its antitumour effect, it is now accepted that this drug is able to affect the proliferation of neoplastic cells by interfering with the activity of various growth factors [1]. Indeed, in-vitro experiments showed that suramin interacts directly with several growth factors, including basic fibroblast growth factor (bFGF) and epidermal growth factor (EGF), thus preventing their binding to specific membrane receptors [4].

Growth factors are involved in a variety of biological processes, including embryogenesis, tissue cell growth and repair, and tumour cell proliferation [5]. Evidence has been provided that some growth factors, as well as their specific receptors, naturally occur throughout the gastrointestinal tract [6], where they play an important role in mucosal protection and repair [7,8]. Several mechanisms appear to account for these protective actions. Indeed, EGF stimulates cell growth and differentiation in the stomach [9], inhibits acid secretion in a variety of mammalian species, including humans [10], and increases gastric mucosal blood flow [11]. In addition, the healing effects exerted by both EGF and bFGF on chronic ulcers were associated with an increase in angiogenesis in the ulcer bed [8,12].

On these bases, it appears conceivable that suramin might interfere with the biological activities of endogenous growth factors at the gastric level. In order to test this hypothesis, the distribution of suramin into the stomach as well as the influence exerted by this drug on ethanol-induced gastric mucosal damage were investigated in the present study. The effects of suramin on gastric acid secretion were also examined.

MATERIALS AND METHODS

Animals and drug treatment

Albino male Wistar rats, 200-220 g body weight, were used throughout the study. They were fed standard laboratory chow and tap water *ad libitum*, and were not used for at least one week after their delivery to the laboratory. The animals were housed, six in a cage, in temperature-controlled rooms on a 12-h light cycle at 22–24°C and 50–60% humidity. Rats were treated with suramin 18 mg/kg or its vehicle (0.5 ml 154 mmol/L NaCl) by the intraperitoneal (ip) route every other day for fourteen days. The dose of suramin was selected on the basis of the treatment schedules currently adopted in clinical practice.

Chromatographic assay of suramin in plasma and tissues

A group of animals was sacrificed 24 h after the last injection of suramin and multiple samples of plasma, stomach, kidney and skeletal muscle were taken. In a portion of the gastric tissue samples, the mucosa and submucosa were separated from the other layers. The reverse-phase ion-pairing liquid chromatographic method used for suramin quantitation has been described in detail by La Rocca et al. [13]. Briefly, protein precipitation and suramin extraction from plasma samples (50 μl) was obtained by the addition of 1 ml of extraction solution (0.05 mol/L tetrabutylammonium phosphate in acetonitrile). Tissue samples (50 mg) were homogenized by few strokes in a Dounce homogenizer containing 1 ml of extraction solution. Samples were centrifuged for 10 min at 15 000 rpm in a microfuge; the supernatants were collected and diluted with an equal volume of ammonium acetate buffer (0.01 mol/L, pH 6.5) and 100 μl were injected into the column. Chromatography was carried out on a 3-μm Lichrosorb C_{18} column (100 × 3 mm internal diameter; Merck, Darmstadt, Germany) using a water–methanol (51:49, v:v) mobile phase containing 0.01 mol/L ammonium acetate buffer (pH 6.5) and 0.001 mol/L tetrabutylammonium phosphate with UV detection at 238 nm. A Gilson HPLC apparatus (Villiers-le-Belle, France) was used throughout the study.

Induction of gastric mucosal damage

Animals underwent the induction of gastric mucosal damage 24 h after the last injection of suramin. Twenty-four hours before the beginning of the experimental procedure, the animals were deprived of food, but free access to water was allowed until 1 h before the experiments started. Mucosal damage was induced with 5 ml/kg of absolute ethanol administered by intragastric (ig) gavage, whereas control rats received an equal volume of tap water. At 1, 2, 4, 8, 12, 24 and 48 h after the treatment, the animals were sacrificed and their stomachs were processed for the quantitative evaluation of necrotic mucosal damage.

Morphometric evaluation of gastric mucosal damage

The stomach was opened along the greater curvature, pinned upon a cork plate with the mucosal surface turned upwards, and fixed in formalin 10% buffered with phosphate (pH 7.4) for 24 h at 4°C. Each stomach was dissected in parallel strips perpendicularly to the lesser curvature and at a distance of 2 mm [14]. The strips from each stomach were sequentially superimposed on a glass slide with the side of each strip distal to the pylorus placed upwards. A 3% solution of melted agar was gently poured on the strips and quickly cooled at 4°C. Thus, the agar block was removed from the glass slide, dehydrated and embedded in paraffin wax (Vogel Histo-Comp, Giessen, Germany). Sections (3-mm thick) were cut with a HM 330 Microm microtome (Heidelberg, Germany) and stained with haematoxylin and eosin (H/E). Sections were observed by light microscopy and the length of both total and damaged mucosa was evaluated by means of a micrometric scale. The lesion index (total damage) was estimated as:

length of damaged mucosa/total length of mucosa × 100.

Moreover, three types of lesions were discriminated, according to the depth of necrotic damage [15]. Type I lesions consisted of lysis of mucosal cells on the luminal free surface; type II lesions consisted of damage to the cells lying on both surface mucosa and gastric pits; type III lesions consisted of damage to gastric glands associated with detachment of whole layers of necrotic superficial mucosa.

Evaluation of gastric acid secretion

The evaluation of gastric acid secretion was carried out 24 h after the last injection of suramin, as previously reported [14]. Twenty-four hours before the beginning of the experimental procedure, the animals were deprived of food but free access to water was allowed until 1 h before the experiments started. During a brief anaesthesia with diethyl ether, the abdomen was opened and the pylorus ligated. The animals were then allowed to recover for 10 min from anaesthesia. Three hours after pylorus ligation, animals were deeply anaesthetized with urethane and laparotomized. The oesophagus was ligated and the whole stomach was removed and opened along the lesser curvature. The accumulated gastric juice was collected in graduated tubes and centrifuged at 3000 rpm for 10 min. Samples with more than 0.5 ml of sediment were discarded. The level of acidity was determined by automatic potentiometric titration to pH 7.0 with 0.01 NaOH, using an Autotitrator pH Meter PHM 82 (Radiometer, Copenhagen) and expressed as both H^+ concentration ($\mu EqH^+/ml$) and output ($\mu EqH^+/3$ h).

Statistics

Results are given as mean ± SEM of n number of experiments. The significance of differences between means was evaluated by Student's t-test for unpaired data; p values less than 0.05 were considered significant.

Drugs

The drugs and chemicals used were: suramin (Bayer AG, Leverkusen, Germany); acetonitrile, tetrabutylammonium phosphate and ammonium acetate (Fluka AG, Buchs, Switzerland); diethyl ether and urethane ethyl carbamate (Sigma Chemicals, St Louis, MO, USA). Other reagents were of analytical grade.

TABLE 1
Concentrations of suramin in rat plasma and tissues. Suramin was administered by the ip route every other day for 14 days; plasma and tissue samples were taken 24 h after the last injection of the drug. Data are represented as mean values obtained from 6 animals ± SEM

Sample	Concentration
Plasma	158.2 ± 18.8 µg/ml
Stomach	179.7 ± 33.0 µg/g
Gastric mucosa plus submucosa	168.4 ± 27.0 µg/g
Kidney	1480.9 ± 85.9 µg/g
Skeletal muscle	57.8 ± 8.9 µg/g

RESULTS

Suramin levels in rat plasma and tissues

The data obtained from the chromatographic assay of suramin in plasma and tissue samples taken from a group of 6 rats are shown in Table 1. The concentrations of suramin in plasma and stomach lumen 24 h after the last injection were 158.2 ± 18.8 µg/ml and 179.7 ± 33.0 µg/g, respectively. The concentration of suramin in gastric mucosa and submucosa (168.4 ± 27.0 µg/g) was not significantly different from that found in whole gastric samples, indicating that selective uptake in gastric tissue did not occur. For comparison, the drug levels in two additional tissues known to accumulate large (kidney) or small (skeletal muscle) amounts of suramin were also measured and found to be 1480.9 ± 85.9 µg/g and 57.8 ± 8.9 µg/g, respectively.

Morphometric evaluation of gastric mucosal damage

In the absence of intraluminal ethanol injection, the histological examination of stomachs dissected from animals receiving the drug vehicle by the ip route revealed the presence of mucosal lesions consisting exclusively of lysis at the level of the surface epithelium (type I lesions) and accounting for 0.52 ± 0.03% ($n = 6$) of the total mucosal extension. Similar findings were obtained in rats treated with suramin over a period of fourteen days (0.48 ± 0.05%, $n = 6$, not significant vs. controls).

The injection of absolute ethanol into the gastric lumen induced gross lesions in the glandular part of the stomach, both in control and suramin-treated animals (data not shown). The histological examination of gastric mucosa showed necrotic lesions of various extension and depth; in the most severe lesions, even the deepest layers of mucosal lamina propria were destroyed (data not shown).

Following the administration of the necrotizing agent to control animals, the morphometric analysis of stomachs revealed that the total mucosal damage reached

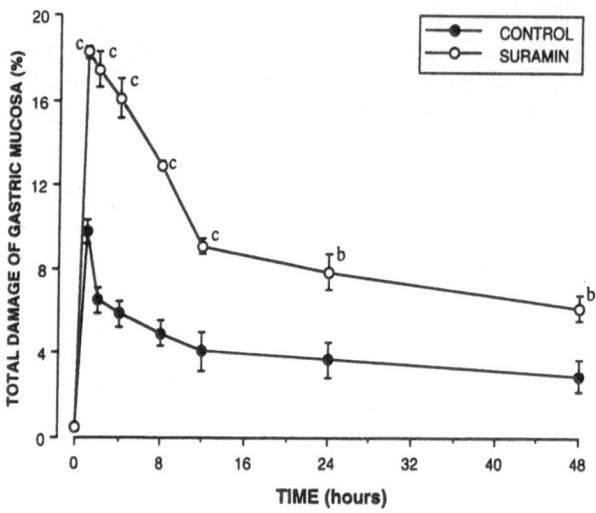

Figure 1. Effect of suramin (18 mg/kg ip every other day for 14 days) on total necrotic damage of gastric mucosa induced by the intragastric injection of absolute ethanol in conscious rats. At time zero, values were obtained in the absence of intragastric ethanol. Each point represents the mean value obtained from 6 experiments $\pm$ SEM (vertical lines). Significant difference from control values: [b]$p < 0.01$; [c]$p < 0.001$

the highest level 1 h after ethanol administration and then declined gradually (Figure 1). Moreover, taking into account the depth of mucosal damage induced by ethanol in control animals, type I and II lesions were usually slightly more frequent than type III lesions after ethanol injection (Figure 2).

Treatment with suramin caused a significant enhancement of ethanol-induced necrotic damage to gastric mucosa. This effect was more pronounced between 1 and 8 h into the experiment and then declined towards the control values (Figure 1). However, 48 h after ethanol administration, the total mucosal damage in suramin-treated animals accounted for $6.15 \pm 0.60\%$ ($n = 6$), this value still being significantly higher than that observed in control stomachs. In addition, when analysing the depth of ethanol-induced gastric damage, it was observed that the potentiating action of suramin consisted mainly of type III lesions (Figure 2).

Evaluation of gastric acid secretion

The short-term treatment of rats with suramin caused a significant enhancement of gastric acid output induced by pylorus ligation in conscious rats. In particular, suramin exerted its enhancing action mainly on the gastric secretory volume, whereas the hydrogen ion concentration in the gastric juice was not significantly affected (Figure 3).

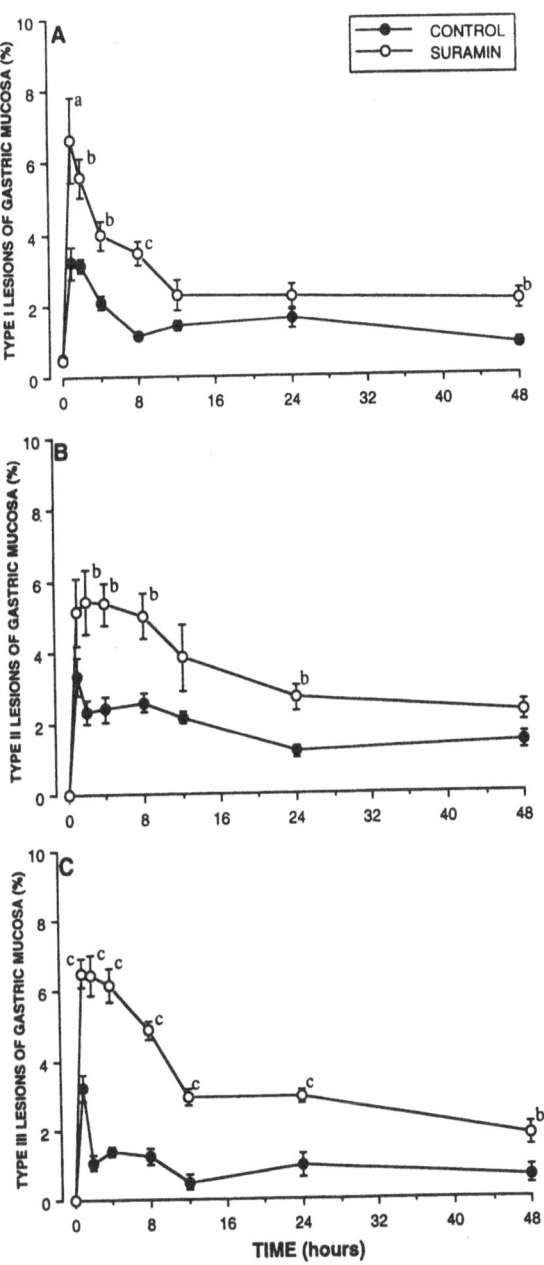

Figure 2. Effects of suramin (18 mg/kg ip every other day for 14 days) on type I (A), type II (B), and type III (C) necrotic damage to gastric mucosa induced by the intragastric injection of absolute ethanol in conscious rats. At time zero, values were obtained in the absence of intragastric ethanol. Each point represents the mean value obtained from 6 experiments ± SEM (vertical lines). Significant difference from control values: [a]$p < 0.05$; [b]$p < 0.01$; [c]$p < 0.001$

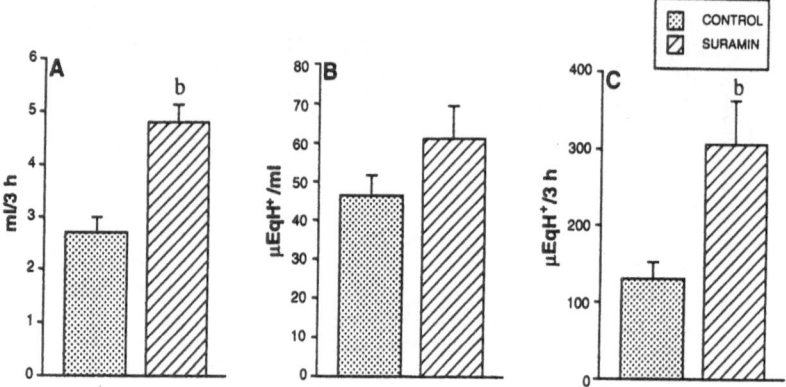

Figure 3. Conscious pylorus-ligated rats. Effect of suramin (18 mg/kg ip every other day for 14 days) on gastric acid secretion in conscious pylorus-ligated rats: (A) total volume (ml/3 h), (B) acid concentration (μEqH$^+$/ml), and (C) acid output (μEqH$^+$/3 h). Columns indicate the mean values obtained from 8 experiments $\pm$ SEM (vertical lines). Significant difference from control values: [b]$p < 0.01$

DISCUSSION

Suramin is currently used in clinical practice as an antitumour agent, mainly due to its ability to interfere with the biological activity of various growth factors [2]. Clinical trials have also indicated that suramin may induce severe toxic effects, including coagulopathy, adrenal insufficiency, peripheral neuropathy, vortex keratopathy and immunosuppression [1]. As far as the gastrointestinal tract is concerned, both vomiting and diarrhoea have been reported following the administration of suramin [1]. However, the possibility that this drug might exert specific toxic effects on gastric mucosa, under either physiological conditions or in the presence of a chemically induced damage, has not yet been investigated. In the present study, evidence was obtained that suramin, after repeated administration, accumulates into the stomach at levels high enough to enhance the mucosal injury elicited by intraluminal injection of absolute ethanol.

Suramin distribution is characterized by its unusually long half-life and remarkable accumulation in kidney. Indeed, in the majority of other organs, the drug reaches levels that are 8–10 times lower than those found in renal tissue. The amount of drug in skeletal muscles is significantly lower than that found in internal organs, and suramin is not detected in central nervous system [1]. The data obtained in the present study are consistent with this pharmacokinetic profile and show that suramin reached a concentration in gastric tissue that was sufficiently elevated to inhibit the proliferation of several normal and transformed cells in vitro through interference with various growth factors including EGF [13]. Moreover, the amount of suramin measured in the stomach is similar to that found in other internal organs, including liver, lung and spleen (data not shown), indicating that the gastric tissue behaves similarly to parenchymal tissues.

The present enhancing effect exerted by suramin on ethanol-induced gastric injury could be detected throughout the whole period of experimental observation, being still significant 48 h after the administration of the necrotizing agent. Since it has been shown that restitution of the gastric mucosa starts within a few minutes after the challenge with ethanol [16], the time-course profile of suramin action suggests that the mechanisms supporting the healing of damaged mucosa were impaired in animals receiving this drug. However, the possibility that suramin might interfere with the physiological factors providing protection to the gastric mucosa against acute chemical injury should be taken into account.

It is known that exogenously administered EGF plays a crucial role in both protection and repair of acute gastric mucosal injury elicited by several necrotizing agents, including ethanol [11], and it seems that both direct and indirect mechanisms participate in these gastroprotective effects. Indeed, EGF was shown to directly stimulate DNA, RNA and protein synthesis as well as angiogenesis at the gastric level [9,12]. On the other hand, EGF was also able to activate some protective factors, including the release of somatostatin [17] and the increase in gastric mucosal blood flow [11]. Interestingly, an involvement of endogenous EGF in both mucosal protection and ulcer healing has also been demonstrated [18]. In particular, the removal of submandibular salivary glands, which results in a remarkable fall in the gastric content of EGF, was shown to increase the susceptibility of gastric mucosa to formation of acute lesions induced by ethanol in the rat [19]. Since suramin was found to inhibit the binding of EGF to its specific receptors [4], it is conceivable that this drug may reproduce in the stomach a condition of reduced availability of EGF, and possibly of other growth factors, similar to that previously observed in sialoadenectomized rats. In support of this view, both the suramin treatment performed in our study as well as sialoadenectomy [18] were not able to induce spontaneous gastric lesions, while they enhanced the damaging action of necrotizing agents.

When tested under basal conditions, suramin did not affect the gastric acid output in anaesthetized rats (Del Tacca, unpublished data), thus suggesting that acid secretion is not involved in the ulcer-promoting effect of this drug. Accordingly, acid secretion was shown not to play a significant role in the damaging action exerted by ethanol on the gastric mucosa [20]. On the other hand, suramin also produced an enhancing effect on the acid output stimulated by pylorus ligation, indicating that, under particular pathophysiological conditions, acid secretion might contribute to the delayed ulcer repair of suramin.

In conclusion, the data obtained in the present study indicate that the suramin concentration achieved in gastric tissue is high enough to induce an impairment of mucosal protective and healing mechanisms. Due to the peculiar pharmacological properties of suramin, it is suggested that an interference with endogenous growth factors might account for the ulcer-enhancing action of this drug.

ACKNOWLEDGEMENTS

The experiments were performed with the technical assistance and collaboration of Mr Bruno Stacchini.

REFERENCES

1. Voogd TE, Vansterkenburg ELM, Wilting J, Janssen LHM. Recent research on the biological activity of suramin. Pharmacol Rev. 1993;45:177–203.
2. La Rocca RV, Stein CA, Meyers CE. Suramin: prototype of a new generation of antitumor compounds. Cancer Cells. 1990;2:106–15.
3. Myers CE, Cooper M, Stein C et al. Suramin: a novel growth factor antagonist with activity in hormone-refractory metastatic prostate cancer. J Clin Oncol. 1992;10:881–9.
4. Gansler T, Vaghmar N, Olson J, Graham S. Suramin inhibits growth factor binding and proliferation by urothelial carcinoma cell cultures. J Urol. 1992;148:910–14.
5. Aaronson SA. Growth factors and cancer. Science. 1991;254:1146–53.
6. Lemoine NR, Leung HY, Gullick WJ. Growth factors in the gastrointestinal tract. Gut. 1992;33:1297–300.
7. Konturek SJ, Dembinski A, Warzecha Z, Brzozowski T, Gregory H. Role of epidermal growth factor in healing of chronic gastroduodenal ulcers in rats. Gastroenterology. 1988;94:1300–7.
8. Folkman J, Szabo S, Stovroff M, McNeil P, Li W, Shing Y. Duodenal ulcer. Discovery of a new mechanism and development of angiogenic therapy that accelerates healing. Ann Surg. 1991;214:414–27.
9. Dembinski A, Gregory H, Konturek SJ, Polanski M. Trophic action of epidermal growth factor in the pancreas and gastroduodenal mucosa in rats. J Physiol (London). 1982;325:35–42.
10. Koffman CG, Elder JB, Ganguli PC, Gregory H, Geary CG. Effect of urogastrone on gastric secretion and serum gastrin concentration in patients with duodenal ulceration. Gut. 1982;23:951–6.
11. Hui WM, Chen BW, Kung AWC, Cho CH, Luk CT, Lam SK. Effect of epidermal growth factor on gastric blood flow in rats: possible role in mucosal protection. Gastroenterology. 1993;104:1605–10.
12. Hase S, Nakazawa S, Tsukamoto Y, Segawa K. Effects of prednisolone and human epidermal growth factor on angiogenesis in granulation tissue of gastric ulcer induced by acetic acid. Digestion. 1989;42:135–41.
13. La Rocca RV, Danesi R, Cooper MR et al. Effect of suramin on human prostate cancer cells in vitro. J Urol. 1991;145:393–8.
14. Blandizzi C, Gherardi G, Marveggio C, Natale G, Carignani D, Del Tacca M. Mechanisms of protection by omeprazole against experimental gastric mucosal damage in rats. Digestion. 1995;56:220–9.
15. Lacy ER, Ito S. Microscopic analysis of ethanol damage to rat gastric mucosa after treatment with a prostaglandin. Gastroenterology. 1982;83:619–25.
16. Ito S, Lacy ER. Morphology of rat gastric mucosal damage, defense, and restitution in the presence of luminal ethanol. Gastroenterology. 1985;88:250–60.
17. Itoh M, Joh T, Imai S et al. Experimental and clinical studies on epidermal growth factor for gastric mucosal protection and healing of gastric ulcers. J Clin Gastroenterol. 1988;10(suppl.1):S7–S12.
18. Olsen SP, Poulsen SS, Kikegaard P, Nexo E. Role of submandibular saliva and epidermal growth factor in gastric cytoprotection. Gastroenterology. 1984;87:103–8.
19. Tepperman BL, Soper BD, Morris GP. Effect of sialoadenectomy on adaptive cytoprotection in the rat. Gastroenterology. 1989;97:123–9.
20. Oates PJ, Hakkinen JP. Studies on the mechanism of ethanol-induced gastric damage in rats. Gastroenterology. 1988;94:10–21.

G Mózsik et al. Cell Injury and Cytoprotection in the GI Tract. 139–145.

EFFECTS OF RANITIDINE, OMEPRAZOLE AND VAGOTOMY ON RAT GASTRIC MUCOSAL PHOSPHOLIPIDS

B.S. DUNJIĆ[1]*, J. AXELSON[2], M.S. DUNJIĆ[3], M. HASHMONAI[1] AND S. BENGMARK[2]

[1]Department of Surgery B, Rambam Medical Center, The Bruce Rappaport Faculty of Medicine, Technion–Israel Institute of Technology, Haifa, Israel; [2]Department of Surgery, Lund University, Lund, Sweden; and [3]Department of Surgery, Institute of Digestive Diseases, Belgrade University School of Medicine, Yugoslavia
*Correspondence

ABSTRACT

Co-ordinate regulation of the gastric acid secretion and production of protective gastric mucosal phospholipids has been suggested. In the present study, the effects of vagotomy, and of equipotent antisecretory doses of ranitidine and omeprazole (with antisecretory effects similar to that of vagotomy) on the gastric mucosal phospholipid composition and content in rats were evaluated. Experimental groups 1, 2 and 3 were given ranitidine (400 μmol/kg), omeprazole (400 μmol/kg) or the vehicle only, by gavage every morning for 14 days, respectively. Groups 4 and 5 were subjected to surgical truncal vagotomy (TV) or surgical TV plus chemoneurolysis (CNL), respectively. Both procedures were performed with a pyloroplasty. Untreated (control) rats, rats in experimental groups 1, 2 and 3, and the rats that underwent surgery were sacrificed at the beginning of the study, 2 h after the last dose of ranitidine, omeprazole or vehicle, and 14 days after surgery, respectively. Biopsy specimens were taken at the lesser curvature of the antrum and corpus, and the lipid analyses were done. The individual phospholipids were identified by thin-layer chromatography. Phosphatidylcholine (PC), phosphatidyl-inositol (PI) and phosphatidylethanolamine (PE) were the main phospholipid classes. The level of PC was higher in the corpus than in the antrum. No differences between corporal and antral total phospholipid content was noticed. Ranitidine decreased the total phospholipid content in the corpus. Omeprazole, surgical TV and surgical TV+CNL decreased the levels of PC, PI and PE, as well as the total phospholipid content, both in the corpus and antrum. In conclusion, ranitidine and omeprazole, in doses that produced inhibition of acid secretion, and vagotomy decreased the content of gastric mucosal protective phospholipids. This may weaken the gastric defence and be of importance in the recurrence of gastric ulcers.

Keywords: gastric barrier, phospholipids, rat, vagotomy, ranitidine, omeprazole

INTRODUCTION

Surfactants are synthesized and secreted by type II pneumocytes, gastric surface mucous and parietal cells, mesothelial cells of periteoneum, epidermal cells etc., i.e. wherever they are needed in vivo, and a common metabolic pathway for producing surfactant has been suggested [1–7]. They have been suggested to have a role according to the specific requirements of the organ or system, such as hydrophobic protective barrier of the skin or protective lining of the stomach, lubricating function in sliding

This paper was presented at the Symposium on 'Cell injury and protection in the gastrointestinal tract: from basic science to clinical perspectives', October 8–11, 1995, Pécs, Hungary.

surfaces of joints and of serosal cells of pericardium, pleural mesothelium or peritoneum, stabilization of the structure of the alveoli and bronchioles allowing optimal gas exchange, modifying membrane permeability etc. [1,3,4,7–12]. The composition of surfactant surface-active phospholipids in different tissues has been reported to vary according to the specific function required, but not to differ appreciably [4,13,14]. It has been suggested that synthesis, secretion and clearance of surfactants are probably regulated in a co-ordinated way [15]. Similarities between gastric and pulmonary phospholipid metabolism have also been proposed [16,17].

In the stomach, surface-active phospholipids have been documented on all surfaces exposed to gastric acid [7,18,19]. They have been suggested to offer a physical basis for the gastric mucosal barrier [7]. Parietal cells have been suggested to produce both gastric acid (natural aggressive agent) and protective surface-active phospholipids, and co-ordinated regulation of the gastric acid secretion and production of protective mucin and phospholipids has been suggested as well [7,20]. Both cholinergic and adrenergic mediators have been documented to regulate the phospholipid secretion in gastric mucus [21].

The suppression of gastric acid secretion by various surgical or pharmacological means has been stressed as an important aspect of peptic ulcer therapy and of other acid-related disorders [22]. Vagotomy, histamine H_2-receptor antagonists and H^+/K^+ ATP-ase inhibitors have been shown to inhibit gastric acid secretion [23–25], but some of them also alter the composition or content of phospholipids in various tissues. In lungs after bilateral cervical vagotomy, structural changes in the type II pneumocytes, loss of lung surface activity and lower relative rate of phospholipids in lung washings have been described [26,27]. Ebrotidine has been shown to increase gastric mucus gel dimension and content of phospholipids [28], while an increase in phospholipids has been documented in both renal basolateral and brush border membranes after ranitidine treatment [29]. It has also been documented that inhibition of acid secretion by various anti-acid secretory agents affects gastric mucus content in different ways [30].

Hence, the reduction of gastric acidity by vagal denervation of the stomach or by agents that inhibit acid secretion may also change the amount of gastric protective phospholipids and consequently make the gastric mucosa more resistant or more vulnerable. The aim of the present work was to study the effects of vagotomy, and of ranitidine or omeprazole treatment on the gastric phospholipid composition and content in rats.

MATERIALS AND METHODS

Animals

Thirty-six intact male Sprague–Dawley rats, weighing 250 ± 10 g, were obtained from the animal colony of the Department of Experimental Surgery, The Bruce Rappaport Faculty of Medicine, Haifa, Israel. They were kept under constant temperature and humidity, a 12-h light–dark rhythm, and had free access to a standard diet of food pellets and tap water.

Experimental schedule

Animals were randomly divided into a control group of untreated rats and 5 experimental groups, each comprising 6 animals. Experimental groups 1, 2 and 3 were given suspensions of ranitidine (Zantac, 400 µmol/kg) or omeprazole (Losec, 400 µmol/kg) in 0.5% methylcellulose (Methocel, 5 ml/kg body weight), or the vehicle only by gavage every morning for 14 days, respectively [31]. A soft polyethylene orogastric tube was used, and suspensions were given to conscious animals. Groups 4 and 5 were subjected to surgical truncal vagotomy (surgical TV) or surgical truncal vagotomy plus chemoneurolysis (surgical TV+CNL), respectively. After vagotomy, the rats were allowed to recover from anaesthesia and given food and water ad libitum throughout the 14-day experimental period. Control rats, rats in experimental groups 1, 2 and 3, and rats that underwent surgery were sacrificed by ether overdose at the beginning of the study, 2 h after the last dose of ranitidine, omeprazole or vehicle, and 14 days after vagotomy, respectively, and the lipids were analysed.

Surgery

All operative procedures were performed under diethyl ether anaesthesia through a midline laparotomy. Instruments were clean but not sterile.

Truncal vagotomy

The gastrohepatic ligament was divided, and the abdominal oesophagus was exposed by passing a mosquito artery forceps behind the oesophagus, keeping well posteriorly. The anterior vagal trunk, running on the ventral surface of the abdominal oesophagus, and the posterior one, identified as a separate nerve on the right side of the oesophagus just below the oesophageal hiatus, were divided as near to the oesophageal hiatus as possible [23].

Truncal vagotomy and chemoneurolysis

The vagal trunks were divided as above. Then the outer surface of the anterior half of the oesophageal circumference was infiltrated with 0.25 ml 30% alcohol as high as possible and the remaining half was similarly infiltrated 0.5 cm distally [23,32].

Pyloroplasty

Both the surgical TV and surgical TV+CNL were performed with a pyloroplasty. The pyloric sphincter was identified as a constriction between the stomach and duodenum, and a 0.5-cm longitudinal incision over the anterior wall of the sphincter was then made, dividing all layers. The wound was closed in the transverse axis using continuous through-and-through sutures of 3/0 Coated VICRYL (polyglactin 910) (Ethicon Ltd, UK) [33].

Lipid analyses

Tissue sampling

The stomach and the duodenum were removed, opened along the greater curvature, and the mucosal surface was examined by using a dissecting microscope (magnification × 10). Biopsy specimens, including the full thickness of the gastric wall, were taken at the lesser curvature of the antrum and corpus, immediately frozen in liquid nitrogen and kept at –20°C until further analyses.

Determination of phospholipids

Tissue samples were homogenized, lipids extracted with chloroform/methanol (2:1, vol/vol), and the lipid extract was analysed for phospholipid classes by thin-layer chromatography (TLC) on silica gel plates. The plates were developed with a solution of chloroform/methanol/ammonium hydroxide (60:35:8, vol/vol/vol). Iodine vapors were used to visualize the lipid spots on the TLC plates using the appropriate standards. The appropriate spots of phospholipid classes were scraped and analysed for their phosphorus content [34]. Phospholipid mass was calculated by multiplying the phosphorus content by 18 for lysophosphatidylcholine (LPC), and by 25 for sphingo-myelin (SPH), phosphatidylcholine (PC), phosphatidylinositol (PI) and phosphatidyl-ethanolamine (PE).

Statistical analysis

Results were expressed as mean $\pm$ SEM. The significance of the differences was determined by the Mann–Whitney U test, and $p < 0.05$ was considered significant.

RESULTS

Phosphatidylcholine, PI and PE were the main phospholipid classes, constituting approximately 45%, 20% and 30%, respectively, of the total phospholipid content (the sum of five individual classes of phospholipids). The level of PC was higher in the corpus than in the antrum. No differences between corporal and antral total phospholipid content was noticed. Ranitidine decreased the total phospholipid content in the corpus. Omeprazole, surgical TV and surgical TV+CNL decreased the levels of PC, PI and PE, as well as the total phospholipid content, both in the corpus and antrum (Table 1).

TABLE 1
Content and composition of gastric phospholipids in control (intact) rats, in rats subjected to surgical TV or surgical TV+CNL, and in rats given omeprazole or ranitidine

Experimental group (n)	Gastric zone	Total phospholipid content†	Individual classes of the gastric phospholipids†				
			LPC	SPH	PC	PI	PE
Control (6)	Antrum	411.5±4.5	9.0±0.4 (2.3±0.2)	26.8±3.4 (6.5±0.8)	165.6±3.4 (40.3±0.9)	83.8±3.9 (20.4±1.0)	126.3±3.0 (30.7±0.6)
	Corpus	418.8±5.9	8.4±0.5 (2.0±0.1)	19.4±0.9 (4.6±0.2)	188.8±3.9 (45.1±0.5)	81.4±3.1 (19.4±0.6)	120.7±2.4 (28.9±0.7)
Surgical TV+CNL (5)	Antrum	↓**			↓**	↓**	↓**
	Corpus	↓**		↓*	↓**	↓**	↓**
Surgical TV (6)	Antrum	↓**			↓**	↓**	↓**
	Corpus	↓**	↓*	↓**	↓**	↓**	↓**
Omeprazole (6)	Antrum	↓**			↓**	↓**	↓**
	Corpus	↓**		↓**	↓**	↓*	↓**
Ranitidine (6)	Antrum	↓*					
	Corpus						

†Gastric phospholipid content is expressed as mean±SEM of the µg P wet wt. Values in parentheses are mean±SEM in %. *p<0.05, **p<0.01 vs. control, Mann–Whitney U test. TV, truncal vagotomy; TV+CNL, truncal vagotomy plus chemoneurolysis

CONCLUSIONS

Ranitidine and omeprazole, in doses that produced inhibition of acid secretion, and vagotomy decreased the content of gastric mucosal protective phospholipids. This may weaken the gastric defence and be of importance in the recurrence of gastric ulcers.

REFERENCES

1. Morgenroth K. The Surfactant System of the Lungs. Berlin: Walter de Gruyter; 1988.
2. Scheiman JM, Kraus ER, Bonnville LA, Weinhold PA, Boland CR. Synthesis and prostaglandin E_2-induced secretion of surfactant phospholipid by isolated gastric mucous cells. Gastroenterology. 1991;100:1232-40.
3. Dobbie JW, Lloyd JK. Mesothelium secretes lamellar bodies in a similar manner to type II pneumocyte secretion of surfactant. Perit Dial Int. 1989;9:215-19.
4. Schmitz G, Müller G. Structure and function of lamellar bodies, lipid–protein complexes involved in storage and secretion of cellular lipids. J Lipid Res. 1991;32:1539-70.
5. Hills BA. The Biology of Surfactant. Cambridge: Cambridge University Press; 1988.
6. Hills BA. The role of lung surfactant. Br J Anaesth. 1990;65:13-29.
7. Hills BA. A physical identity for the gastric mucosal barrier. Med J Aust. 1990;153:76-81.
8. Hills BA, Butler BD, Barrow RE. Boundary lubrication impaired by pleural surfactants and their identification. J Appl Physiol. 1982;53:463-9.
9. Hills BA. Role of surfactant in the Eustachian tube. In: Ekelund L, Jonson B, Malm L, eds. Surfactant and the Respiratory Tract. Amsterdam: Elsevier Science Publishers (Biomedical Division); 1989:343-51.
10. Hills BA. A physical identity for the blood–brain barrier. Proc R Soc NSW. 1989;122:19-26.
11. Hills BA. Oligolamellar lubrication of joints by surface active phospholipid. J Rheumatol. 1989;16:82-91.
12. Ingstrup MH, Svane-Knudsen V, Brofeldt S, Larsen HF, Klintgaard N. Phospholipids in nasal secretion. In: Ekelund L, Jonson B, Malm L, eds. Surfactant and the Respiratory Tract. Amsterdam: Elsevier Science Publishers (Biomedical Division); 1989:311-16.
13. Butler BD, Lichtenberger LM, Hills BA. Distribution of surfactants in the canine gastrointestinal tract and their ability to lubricate. Am J Physiol. 1983;244:G645-51.
14. Arvidson G. Lipid composition of surfactant. In: Ekelund L, Jonson B, Malm L, eds. Surfactant and the Respiratory Tract. Amsterdam: Elsevier Science Publishers (Biomedical Division); 1989:29-31.
15. van Golde LMG, van Iwaarden JF, Batenburg JJ, Verhoef J. Metabolic aspects of pulmonary surfactant: synthesis by alveolar type II cells and possible interactions with alveolar macrophages. In: Ekelund L, Jonson B, Malm L, eds. Surfactant and the Respiratory Tract. Amsterdam: Elsevier Science Publishers (Biomedical Division); 1989:3-13.
16. Wassef MK, Lin YN, Horowitz MI. Phospholipid-deacylating enzymes of rat stomach mucosa. Biochem Biophys Acta. 1978;528:318-30.
17. Wassef MK, Lin YN, Horowitz MI. Molecular species of phosphatidylcholine from rat gastric mucosa. Biochem Biophys Acta. 1979;573:222-6.
18. Goddard PJ, Kao YCJ, Lichtenberger LM. Luminal surface hydrophobicity of canine gastric mucosa is dependent on a surface mucous gel. Gastroenterology. 1990;98:361-70.
19. Kao YCJ, Goddard PJ, Lichtenberger LM. Morphological effects of aspirin and prostaglandin on the canine gastric mucosal surface. Analysis with a phospholipid-selective cytochemical strain. Gastroenterology. 1990;98:592-606.
20. Scheiman JM, Kraus ER, Boland CR. Regulation of canine gastric mucin synthesis and phospholipid secretion by acid secretagogues. Gastroenterology. 1992;103:1842-50.
21. Sengupta S, Piotrowski E, Slomiany A, Slomiany BL. Adrenergic and cholinergic regulation of gastric mucus phospholipid secretion. Scand J Gastroenterol. 1992;27:29-32.
22. Freston JW. Overview of medical therapy of peptic ulcer disease. Gastroenterol Clin N Am. 1990;19:121-40.
23. Salim AS. Surgery or chemoneurolysis for complete vagal denervation of rat stomach. Dig Dis Sci. 1991;36:1074-8.

24. Feldman M, Burton ME. Histamine H_2-receptor antagonists. Standard therapy for acid–peptic diseases. N Engl J Med. 1990;323:1672–80.
25. Maton PN. Omeprazole. N Engl J Med. 1991;324:965–75.
26. Klaus M, Reiss OK, Tooley WH, Piel C, Clements JA. Alveolar epithelial cell mitochondria as source of the surface-active lung lining. Science. 1962;137:750–1.
27. Kunc L, Kuncová M, Holusa R, Soldá F. Physical properties and biochemistry of lung surfactant following vagotomy. Respiration. 1978;35:192–7.
28. Piotrowski J, Yamaki K, Morita M, Slomiany A, Slomiany BL. Ebrotidine – a new H_2-receptor antagonist with mucosal strengthening activity. Biochem Int. 1992;26:659–67.
29. Gill M, Sanyal SN, Sareen ML. Effect of histamine H_2-receptor antagonist, ranitidine on renal brush border and basolateral membranes. Res Exp Med Berl. 1990;190:345–56.
30. Matsumoto A, Asada S, Okumura Y, Takiuchi H, Hirata I, Ohshiba S. Effects of anti-acid secretory agents on various types of gastric mucus. J Clin Gastroenterol. 1992;14(Suppl 1):S94–7.
31. Helander HF, Mattsson H, Elm G, Ottosson S. Structure and function of rat parietal cells during treatment with omeprazole, SCH 28080, SCH 32651, or ranitidine. Scand J Gastroenterol. 1990;25:799–809.
32. Taylor TV, Holt S, Andrews PLR, Heading RC. Vagotomy by chemoneurolysis: an experimental study in the rat. Gut. 1983;24:158–60.
33. Salim AS. The mechanism of vagotomy-induced acute gastric mucosal injury in the rat. Am J Med Sci. 1989;297:343–7.
34. Bartlett GR. Phosphorus assay in column chromatography. J Biol Chem. 1959;234:466–72.

G Mózsik et al. Cell Injury and Cytoprotection in the GI Tract. 147–155.

ARE PHOSPHOLIPIDS INVOLVED IN THE GASTROPROTECTIVE CAPACITY OF AVOCADO?

B.S. DUNJIĆ[*1], J. AXELSON[2], M. HASHMONAI[1] AND S. BENGMARK[2]

[1]Department of Surgery B, Rambam Medical Center, The Bruce Rappaport Faculty of Medicine, Technion–Israel Institute of Technology, Haifa, Israel; and [2]Department of Surgery, Lund University, Lund, Sweden

*Correspondence

ABSTRACT

Replacement and maintenance of gastric protective phospholipids by supplementing exogenous phospholipids as such or in the form of natural food, have been shown to be beneficial in both prevention and treatment of experimentally induced mucosal injuries. Avocado mesocarp has been found to contain high levels of lipids, including phospholipids.

Aims of the present study:
a) To evaluate whether orally given avocado has a gastroprotective effect, and
b) To demonstrate that avocado mesocarp phospholipids are the potentially active ingredients.

Methods: Acute gastric corpus mucosal injury was induced in fasted rats by intragastric administration of absolute ethanol. Avocado mesocarp was mixed with saline and given by gavage, as a pretreatment in a single dose. Lesions were macroscopically evaluated. Avocado phospholipids were demonstrated by transmission electron microscopy, contact angle measurement and thin-layer chromatography.

Results: Avocado pretreatment reduced the extent of acute ethanol-induced gastric mucosal erosions. Various physical forms of phospholipids were seen in the avocado mesocarp. Lysophosphatidylcholine, sphingomyelin, phosphatidylcholine and phosphatidylethanolamine were the main components of the mesocarp phospholipid fraction. Contact angle measurement has shown avocado to be highly surface active at solid interfaces, which avocado renders hydrophobic by adsorption of phospholipids analysed by thin-layer chromatography.

Conclusions: The phospholipid fraction may be the active component responsible for the capacity of the avocado fruit to protect the gastric mucosa against acute ethanol-induced injury. However, the mechanism of the protection afforded by avocado remains to be completely elucidated.

Keywords: avocado fruit, gastric barrier, phospholipids, ethanol, mucosal erosions

INTRODUCTION

Avocado is an edible exotic fruit [1]. Fresh oleaginous mesocarp of the fruit has been found to contain high levels of vitamins, minerals, carbohydrates and unsaturated lipids, including phospholipids [1,2]. Because of such valuable nutritional properties, raw avocado is consumed as a food in many countries.

This paper was presented at the Symposium on 'Cell injury and protection in the gastrointestinal tract: from basic science to clinical perspectives', October 8–11, 1995, Pécs, Hungary.

An oligolamellar lining of phospholipids, produced by gastric surface mucous and parietal cells [3–5], has been demonstrated to cover all gastric surfaces exposed to highly corrosive hydrochloric acid [3,6]. This lining has been suggested to serve as the first extramucosal level in the hierarchically organized gastric mucosal barrier [7–9] and to provide a physical basis for the barrier [3]. Exogenous phospholipids, given as such [10–18] or in the form of natural food [19,20] have been shown to protect the gastric mucosa against injury by replenishing and strengthening the endogenous phospholipid lining of the gastric mucosal barrier.

The present work was undertaken to evaluate the gastric mucosal protective capacity of avocado, and to demonstrate phospholipids, as the potentially active components in avocado.

MATERIALS AND METHODS

The study was divided into two parts:

1. Evaluation of the protective capacity of fresh avocado fruit against acute ethanol-induced gastric mucosal lesions in rats.

2. Demonstration of phospholipids in fresh avocado mesocarp as follows:

   a. Morphological evidence by using transmission of hydrophobic surfaces [3];

   b. Quantification of phospholipids by extracting the lipids from the mesocarp of the fruit, and analysing the lipid extract for its content of the phospholipid classes by thin-layer chromatography (TLC) [21];

   c. Demonstration of surface hydrophobicity by measuring the plateau contact angle of a drop of a hydrophilic liquid (saline) applied to a solid surface. The contact angle has been defined as the angle between the solid–liquid and liquid–air interfaces at the point where all three phases meet. This provides a direct estimation of the degree of hydrophobicity of a non-wettable surface, such as the gastric mucosa which has been shown to have a hydrophobic lining that may be attributed to surface-active phospholipids [22,23].

Evaluation of the gastric mucosal protective capacity of avocado fruit

Animals

Twelve male Sprague–Dawley rats, weighing 250 ± 10 g, were obtained from the animal colony of the Department of Experimental Surgery, the Bruce Rappaport Faculty of Medicine, Technion, Israel. They were kept under constant temperature and humidity and a 12-h light–dark rhythm, with free access to standard rat food pellets (except during starvation) and tap water.

Avocado suspension

Avocado (*Persea americana*) was purchased from local markets. Fresh mesocarp of the fruit was vortexed with saline in a 1:1 (wt/v) ratio, to give a suspension that was sufficiently fluid to administer by orogastric tube.

Induction of the gastric mucosal lesions

Acute mucosal erosions of the gastric corpus were induced in starved rats by intragastric administration of 99.5% absolute ethanol in a dose of 5 ml/kg body weight [24].

Experimental schedule

The animals were randomly divided into control and experimental groups, with six rats each, and starved for 24 h. Two millilitres of avocado suspension were given intragastrically, in a single dose 45 min before absolute ethanol. Control rats received saline in the same volume.

Evaluation of the gastric mucosal lesions

The rats were killed with an ether overdose 45 min after administration of ethanol. The stomach was excised, opened along the greater curvature and cleansed with 0.9% saline. To minimize mucosal folding, all specimens were spread and pinned on a cork board. The mucosa was examined for macroscopically evident lesions by using a dissecting microscope (magnification × 10) with a 1-mm square-grid eye piece. The gastric ulcer index for acute linear erosions was expressed as the sum total of the length, in millimetres, of individual lesions [24,25].

Transmission electron microscopy

The specimens of avocado mesocarp were fixed for 72 h in 2% glutaraldehyde plus 3% tannic acid buffered at a pH of 7.4 with 0.1 mol/L sodium cacodylate at 4°C and rendered isotonic (320 mmol/L) with sodium chloride. Postfixation was effected with 1% osmium tetroxide buffered at pH 7.4 with embedding in Epon. The sections were cut with a diamond knife and examined with an EM 9 A Carl Zeiss electron microscope.

Lipid analysis of fresh avocado mesocarp

The mesocarp was homogenized, lipids extracted with chloroform/methanol (2:1, vol/vol), and the lipid extract was analysed for its content of phospholipid classes by TLC on silica gel plates. The plates were developed with a solution of chloroform/methanol/ammonium hydroxide (60:35:8, vol/vol/vol). Iodine vapors were used to visualize the lipid spots on the TLC plates using the appropriate standards. The appropriate spots of phospholipid classes were scraped and analysed for their phosphorus content. Phospholipid mass was calculated by multiplying the phosphorus content by 18 for lysophosphatidylcholine (LPC), and by 25 for sphingomyelin (SPH), phosphatidylcholine (PC) and phosphatidylethanolamine (PE).

Contact angle measurement

Glass microscope slides were cleaned according to the following procedure: (1) dipping in detergent solution in an ultrasonic bath for 15 min; (2) rinsing with distilled water; (3) boiling in distilled water; (4) dipping in acetone in an ultrasonic bath for 15 min. Very clean, freshly prepared, glass microscope slides were placed on the specimen stage of a goniometer (Model G-1, Kernco Instruments Co. Inc., Horizon City Industrial Park, El Paso, Texas), and the contact angle was measured by applying a droplet of saline to the glass slide surface with a micrometre activated microsyringe. The slides were then left for 2 h immersed in the vortexed avocado suspension, rinsed well with saline, air-dried, and the measurements were repeated. They were then rinsed with chloroform, to remove any adsorbed lipid, and the contact angle readings were made. The washings were evaporated to dryness and stored under nitrogen for subsequent analyses by TLC. The contact angle readings were always made at three different locations on each glass slide surface, averaged for one value per slide, and expressed in degrees as the contact angle for that particular slide.

Statistical analysis

Results were expressed as mean $\pm$ SEM. The significance of the differences in the mean values was determined with a two-sided Student's t-test for unpaired data; $p < 0.05$ was considered significant.

RESULTS

Evaluation of the gastric mucosal protective capacity of avocado

Administration of ethanol in all control rats resulted in diffuse gastric mucosal redness and well-demarcated dark-red stains and streaks situated on the crests of mucosal folds and along the longitudinal axis of the gastric corpus. Avocado suspension reduced ethanol-induced gastric mucosal injury (Figure 1).

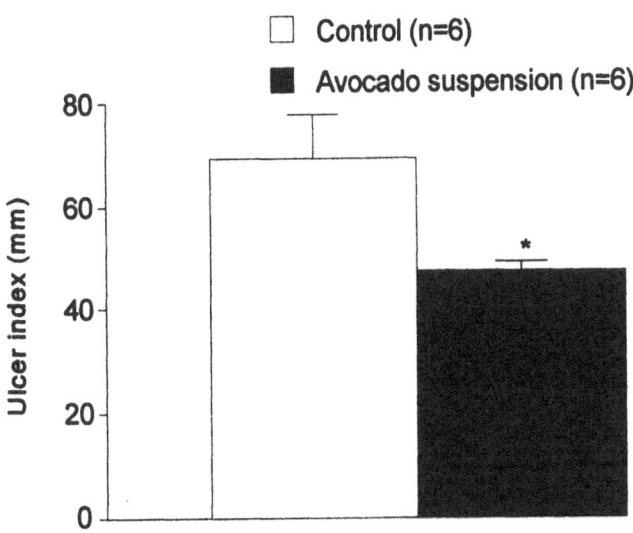

Figure 1. Acute ethanol model. Effect of avocado suspension pretreatment on acute, corporal mucosal lesions in rats. Values are expressed as mean ± SEM; n = number of rats; *$p < 0.05$ vs control, two-sided Student's t-test for unpaired data

Morphological evidence of phospholipids in fresh avocado mesocarp

Electron microscopy showed lamellar layered electron-dense structures, probably representing phospholipids, similar to those found throughout the gastric mucosal barrier and in banana (another natural food with capacity to protect the gastric mucosa) (Figure 2).

Quantification of avocado mesocarp phospholipids

Lysophosphatidylcholine, SPH, PC (the particularly surface-active phospholipid) and PE were the main components of the mesocarp phospholipid fraction (Table 1).

Demonstration of surface hydrophobicity

Contact angle measurement

The glass slides were highly hydrophobic upon removal from the avocado suspension. Upon washing with chloroform, the mean contact angle was reduced (Figure 3).

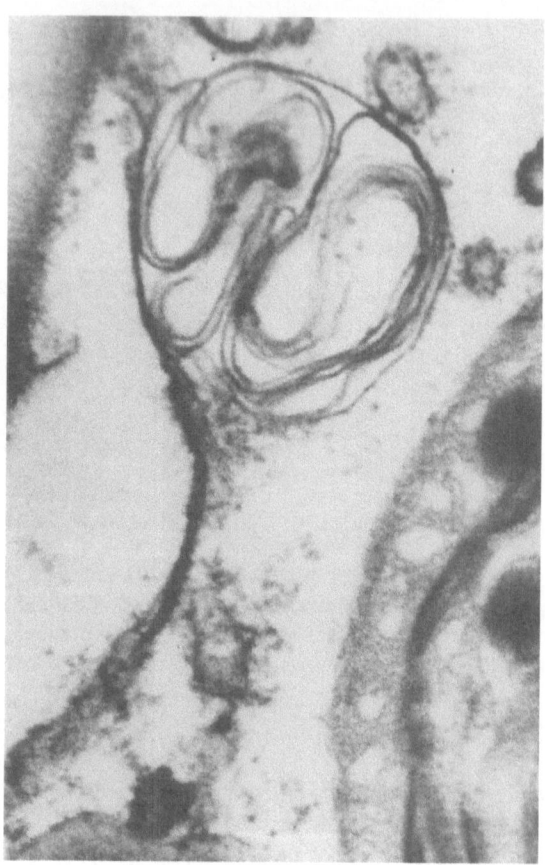

Figure 2. An electron micrograph of the avocado mesocarp showing lamellar layered electron-dense structures (phospholipids)

TABLE 1
Phospholipid classes isolated from fresh avocado mesocarp

Phospholipid classes	Phospholipid content (%)
Lysophosphatidylcholine	3
Sphingomyelin	5
Phosphatidylcholine	41
Phosphatidylethanolamine	51

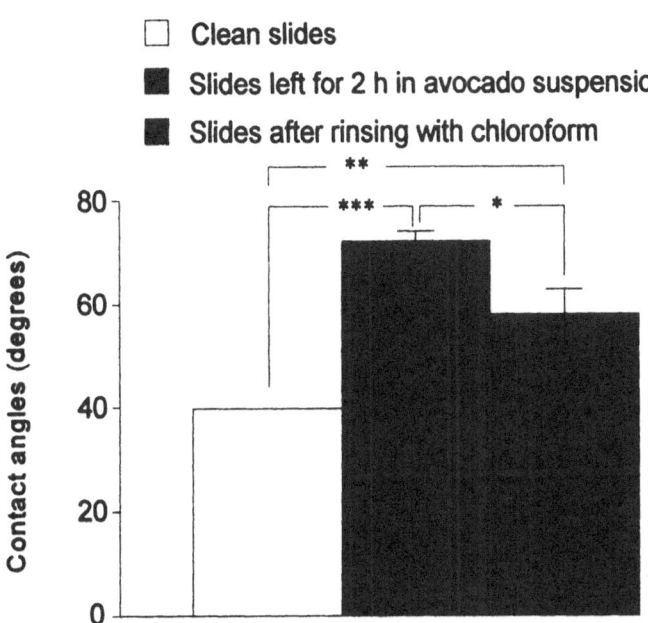

Figure 3. Contact angle before and after immersing glass microscope slides into avocado suspension, and after rinsing slides with chloroform. Values are expressed as mean ± SEM. *$p < 0.05$, **$p < 0.01$, ***$p < 0.001$ vs control (clean slides), two-sided Student's t-test for unpaired data

TABLE 2
Phospholipid classes isolated from glass slide washings

Phospholipid classes	Phospholipid content (%)
Lysophosphatidylcholine	3
Sphingomyelin	8
Phosphatidylcholine	41
Phosphatidylethanolamine	48

Thin-layer chromatography analyses of the washings

This demonstrated that the adsorbed lipids removed by chloroform were phospholipids, mainly LPC, SPH, PC and PE (Table 2). The same classes were found in the avocado mesocarp (Table 1).

CONCLUSIONS

The phospholipid fraction may be the active constituent responsible for the capacity of the avocado fruit to protect the gastric mucosa against acute ethanol-induced injury. However, the mechanism of protection afforded by the avocado has yet to be completely elucidated.

REFERENCES

1. Herrmann K. Review on chemical composition and constituents of some important exotic fruit. Z Lebensm Unters Forsch. 1981;173:47–60.
2. Lewis CE, Morris R, O'Brien K. The oil content of avocado mesocarp. J Sci Food Agric. 1978;29:943–9.
3. Hills BA. A physical identity for the gastric mucosal barrier. Med J Aust. 1990;153:76–81.
4. Scheiman JM, Kraus ER, Bonnville LA, Weinhold PA, Boland CR. Synthesis and prostaglandin E$_2$-induced secretion of surfactant phospholipid by isolated gastric mucous cells. Gastroenterology. 1991;100:1232–40.
5. Schmitz G, Müller G. Structure and function of lamellar bodies, lipid–protein complexes involved in storage and secretion of cellular lipids. J Lipid Res. 1991;32:1539–70.
6. Hills BA. A mucosal barrier of gastric surfactant identified in the human stomach. Aust NZ J Med. 1992;22:441–4.
7. Hills BA, Butler BD, Lichtenberger LM. Gastric mucosal barrier: hydrophobic lining to the lumen of the stomach. Am J Physiol. 1983;244:G561–8.
8. Butler BD, Lichtenberg LM, Hills BA. Distribution of surfactants in the canine gastrointestinal tract and their ability to lubricate. Am J Physiol. 1983;244:G645–51.
9. Wallace JL. Gastroduodenal mucosal defense. Curr Opin Gastroenterol. 1991;7:870–5.
10. Lichtenberger LM, Graziani LA, Dial EJ, Butler BD, Hills BA. Role of surface-active phospholipids in gastric cytoprotection. Science. 1983;219:1327–8.
11. Leyck S, Dereu N, Etschenberg E et al. Improvement of the gastric tolerance of non-steroidal anti-inflammatory drugs by polyene phosphatidylcholine (Phospholipon 100). Eur J Pharmacol. 1985;117:35–42.
12. Szelenyi I, Engler H. Cytoprotective role of gastric surfactant in the ethanol-produced gastric mucosal injury of the rat. Pharmacology. 1986;33:199–205.
13. Dial EJ, Lichtenberger LM. Milk protection against experimental ulcerogenesis in rats. Dig Dis Sci. 1987;32:1145–50.
14. Swarm RA, Ashley SW, Soybel DI, Ordways FS, Cheung LY. Protective effect of exogenous phospholipid on aspirin-induced gastric mucosal injury. Am J Surg. 1987;153:48–53.
15. Kiviluoto T, Paimela H, Mustonen H, Kivilaakso E. Exogenous surface-active phospholipid protects Necturus gastric mucosa against luminal acid and barrier-breaking agents. Gastroenterology. 1991;100:38–46.
16. Kivinen A, Tarpila S, Salminen S, Vapaatalo H. Protective effect of milk phospholipids on aspirin-induced gastric mucosal injury [abstract]. Digestion. 1991;49(1 Suppl):40.
17. Kivinen A, Tarpila S, Kiviluoto T, Mustonen H, Kivilaakso E. Exogenous milk phospholipids protect the gastric mucosa against intracellular acidosis induced by luminal acid. Eur Surg Res. 1993;25(1 Suppl):50.
18. Dunjić BS, Axelson J, Ar'Rajab A, Larsson K, Bengmark S. Gastroprotective capability of exogenous phosphatidylcholine in experimentally induced chronic gastric ulcers in rats. Scand J Gastroenterol. 1993;28:89–94.
19. Hills BA, Kirwood CA. Surfactant approach to the gastric mucosal barrier: protection of rats by banana even when acidified. Gastroenterology. 1989;97:294–303.
20. Dunjić BS, Svensson I, Axelson J et al. Green banana protection of gastric mucosa against experimentally induced injuries in rats. A multicomponent mechanism? Scand J Gastroenterol. 1993;28:894–8.
21. Bartlett GR. Phosphorous assay in column chromatography. J Biol Chem. 1959;234:466–72.

22. Pesach D, Marmur A. Marangoni effects in the spreading of liquid mixtures on a solid. Langmuir. 1987;3:519–24.
23. Spychal RT, Marrero JM, Saverymuttu SH, Northfield TC. Measurement of the surface hydrophobicity of human gastrointestinal mucosa. Gastroenterology. 1989;97:104–11.
24. Guth PH, Paulsen G, Nagata H. Histologic and microcirculatory changes in alcohol-induced gastric lesions in the rat: effect of prostaglandin cytoprotection. Gastroenterology. 1984;87:1083–90.
25. Whittle BJR. Relationship between the prevention of rat gastric erosions and the inhibition of acid secretion by prostaglandins. Eur J Pharmacol. 1976;40:233–9.

G Mózsik et al. Cell Injury and Cytoprotection in the GI Tract. 157–161.

TRANSMUCOSAL POTENTIAL DIFFERENCE AS A MARKER OF *HELICOBACTER PYLORI*-INDUCED GASTRIC MUCOSAL BARRIER DAMAGE

I. RÁCZ*, Gy. PÉCSI, A. SZABÓ AND D. VARGA

First Department of Medicine, Petz Aladár Teaching Hospital, Győr, Hungary
*Correspondence

ABSTRACT

High local concentrations of ammonia within the gastric mucus layer, generated by *Helicobacter pylori* (*H. pylori*) urease, changes the pH profile of the mucosa and may even augment acid back diffusion into the gastric mucosa. This is known to damage the mucosa and decrease gastric mucosal barrier function. Gastric transmucosal potential difference (PD) is a sensitive and numerical marker of gastric mucosal barrier.

The aim of the study was to evaluate gastric PD in 15 *H. pylori*-positive antral gastritis patients before and after eradication therapy. Gastric PD was measured by an endoscopic method. *H. pylori* status was tested by a rapid urease test as well as by histology. Eradication therapy consisted of 20 mg omeprazole od, 2×250 mg clarithromycin bid, 2×500 mg tinidazole bid for a week. *H. pylori* status, histology and gastric PD level were reconsidered 4 weeks after completion of eradication therapy.

Mean antral gastric PD was 15.3 ± 2.4 mV in the antrum and 37.4 ± 4.3 mV in the gastric body before therapy. In the successfully eradicated group ($n = 12$), mean antral PD was significantly ($p < 0.05$) elevated (22.3 ± 3.1 mV), while, in those who remained *H. pylori* positive ($n = 3$), the mean antral PD was unchanged (16.8 ± 3.2 mV). No significant PD change was observed in the gastric body irrespective of antral *H. pylori* status.

It is concluded that *H. pylori* eradication had a rapid and markedly beneficial effect on gastric mucosal barrier function, which is easily detectable by gastric PD measurement.

Keywords: H. pylori, mucosal, gastritis, transmucosal potential difference

INTRODUCTION

The rediscovery of *Helicobacter pylori* (*H. pylori*) by Barry Marshall and Robin Warren [1] in 1983 opened the way for major medical progress in the understanding of upper gastrointestinal disease conditions. Several studies confirmed a close relationship between gastric *H. pylori* infection and chronic active gastritis [2,3].

One of the most characteristic properties of *H. pylori* is urease enzyme production [4]. A high local concentration of ammonia within the gastric mucus layer, generated by *H. pylori* urease, changes the pH profile of the mucosa and may even augment acid back diffusion into the gastric mucosa. This is known to damage the mucosa and decrease gastric mucosal barrier function. Chronic gastritis also parallels the mucosal barrier alteration [5].

This paper was presented at the Symposium on 'Cell injury and protection in the gastrointestinal tract: from basic science to clinical perspectives', October 8–11, 1995, Pécs, Hungary.

Gastric transmucosal potential difference (PD) is a very sensitive and numerical marker of gastric mucosal barrier [6,7].

The aim of the present study was to measure gastric PD in *H. pylori*-positive antral gastritis patients before and after eradication therapy and, with this method, we tested the interaction of *H. pylori* with the gastric mucosal barrier.

PATIENTS AND METHODS

A total number of 15 histologically confirmed antral gastritis patients were included (age: 48.7 ± 16.6 years, range 24–72); ulcer patients and NSAID users were excluded from the study. *H. pylori* status was tested by rapid urease test as well as by histology using haematoxilin–eosin, Giemsa and Warthin–Starry stainings simultaneously. *H. pylori* positivity or negativity was accepted only when there was concordance of urease test and histology. Two biopsies were taken from the prepyloric antral region and also from the gastric body in each patient. The histological result was evaluated in accordance with the Sydney system [8]. The two parameters, density of *H. pylori* colonization, and activity of gastritis, were graded semiquantitatively, applying criteria described elsewhere [9].

Gastric PD was measured by an endoscopic method [7]. The reference electrode was placed on the forearm prepared by intradermal injection of 0.1 ml physiological sodium chloride to reduce the PD between skin and blood. One advantage of the endoscopic method is that PD can be recorded in any desired area of the stomach under direct vision (Figure 1).

Eradication therapy consisted of 20 mg omeprazole od, 2×250 mg clarithromycin bid and 2×500 mg tinidazole bid for a week. *H. pylori* status, histology and gastric PD levels were monitored for 4 weeks after completion of eradication therapy. All patients remained therapy free during this 4-week period. Statistical significance was analysed by the *t*-test. All patients gave informed consent before enrollment in the study.

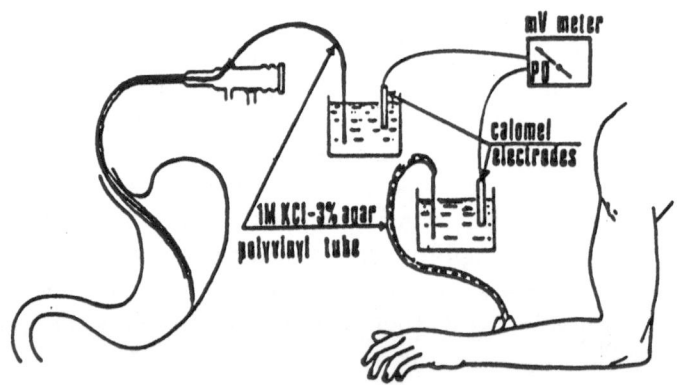

Figure 1. Diagramatic representation of method used to measure gastric transmucosal potential difference (PD) during endoscopy

TABLE 1

H. pylori colonization and gastritis activity grades before and after eradication therapy

	H. pylori colonization grade				Activity of gastritis		
	I	II	III	IV	Mild	Moderate	Severe
Inclusion							
Antrum	–	2	8	5	2	9	4
Corpus	2	1	–	–	1	1	–
Control							
Antrum	2	1	–	–	4	2	1
Corpus	1	–	–	–	1	–	–

RESULTS

The grading of *H. pylori* colonization and the activity of gastritis at the time of inclusion and at control investigations are shown in Table 1.

It can be recognized that there is a parallel between bacterial colonization and gastritis activity grades in the antral mucosa at the time of inclusion as well as after eradication therapy. Out of 15 *H. pylori*-positive antral gastritis patients, only 3 corpus biopsy specimens showed *H. pylori* positivity, indicating the low co-infection frequency. Regarding antral biopsies, we found that 80% (12/15) had eradication of *H. pylori* 4 weeks after cessation of therapy, and, in only 3 patients out of the initial 13 did the gastritis activity grade remain moderate or severe. Among those with successful eradication of *H. pylori*, the gastritis was considered to be healed or mildly active. Mean antral gastric PD was 15.3 ± 2.4 mV in the antrum and 37.4 ± 4.3 mV in the gastric body before therapy. In the successfully eradicated group, mean antral PD was significantly elevated (22.3 ± 3.1 mV), while, in those who remained *H. pylori* positive, the mean antral PD was unchanged (16.8 ± 3.2 mV). No significant PD change was observed in the gastric body irrespective of antral *H. pylori* status (Figure 2).

DISCUSSION

Gastric mucosal integrity is preserved due to an equilibrium between exogenous and endogenous aggressive factors and protective mechanisms operating within pre-epithelial, epithelial and post-epithelial compartments. The mucus layer is considered a core component of pre-epithelial mucosal defence [10]. The mucus layer maintains a concentration gradient for hydrogen ions [11]. It is generally believed that the mucus layer provides a unique biological niche for colonization of *H. pylori* [10].

The ability of *H. pylori* to produce urease and phospholipase may be factors

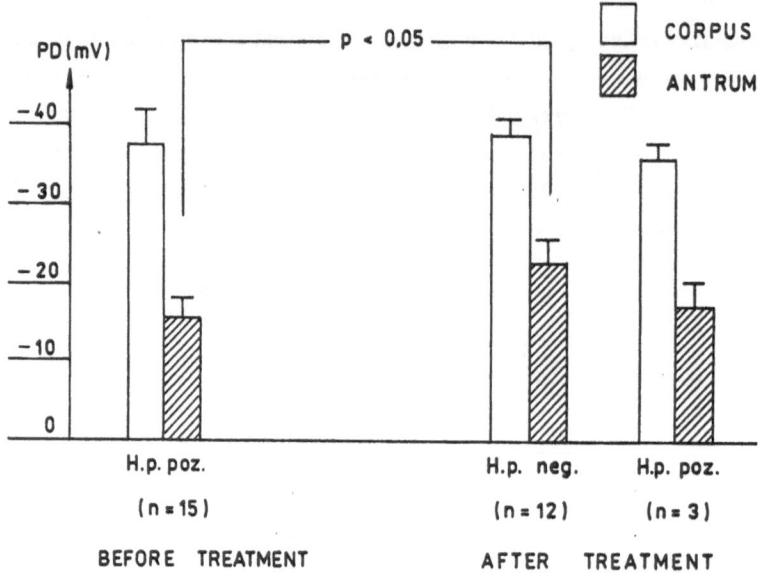

Figure 2. Gastric transmucosal potential difference (PD) results before and after *Helicobacter pylori* (H.p.) eradication therapy

determining the virulence of the organism [4]. A high local concentration of ammonia within the gastric mucus layer, generated by *H. pylori* urease, changes the pH profile of the unstirred adherent gel layer and may even augment acid back diffusion into the gastric mucosa, while phospholipase weakens the epithelial cell membrane and leads to cell damage [12]. All these processes damage the gastric mucosal barrier, the unique ability of mucosa to protect itself against hydrogen rediffusion and consequently gastritis [13].

Gastric PD is a very sensitive, numerical and cumulative index of gastric mucosal barrier [6]. The luminal surface of the mucosa is electrically negative when compared with the serosal surface. There is a prominent lumen negative PD in the stomach [14]. The net effect of gastric mucosal barrier disruption is a drop in electrical PD. Earlier studies indicated a significant PD decrease in the presence of acute and chronic gastritis as well [15], but, up to now, no special interest has been focused on the mucosal electrophysiological effect of *H. pylori* infection.

The aim of our study was to evaluate gastric mucosal barrier integrity by PD measurement in *H. pylori*-positive antral gastritis patients before and after eradication therapy. In other words, we studied not only the morphological aspects of *H. pylori*-induced pathological processes but we proposed to estimate the pathophysiological background as well.

At the antral mucosal barrier, a significant decrease in the PD measurement was clearly detected in *H. pylori*-induced antral gastritis patients. However, after eradication of *H. pylori*, antral PD rose significantly reflecting the restoration of the mucosal barrier. All these pathophysiological processes were in close correlation with the histomorphological picture.

It is concluded that *H. pylori* eradication has a rapid and markedly beneficial effect on gastric mucosal barrier function, which is easily detected by gastric PD measurement. Furthermore, gastric transmucosal PD measurement provides valuable information regarding *H. pylori*-induced gastric processes.

ACKNOWLEDGEMENTS

This study was supported by grant T-02 499/93 from the Hungarian Ministry of Welfare.

REFERENCES

1. Warren JR, Marshall BJ. Unidentified curved bacilli on gastric epithelium in active chronic gastritis (letter). Lancet. 1983;1:1273.
2. Sipponen P, Seppälä K. Long-term consequences of H. pylori infection: time trends in H. pylori gastritis, gastric cancer and peptic ulcer disease. In: Hunt RH, Tytgat GNJ, eds. Helicobacter pylori. Dordrecht, Boston, London: Kluwer Academic Publishers; 1994:372–80.
3. Valle J, Seppälä K, Sipponen P, Kosunen T. Disappearance of gastritis after eradication of Helicobacter pylori: a morphometric study. Scand J Gastroenterol. 1991;26:1057–65.
4. Marshall BJ. Helicbacter pylori. Am J Gastroenterol. 1994;89:S116–28.
5. Schade C, Flemström G, Holm L. Hydrogen ion concentration in the mucus layer on top of acid-stimulated and -inhibited rat gastric mucosa. Gastroenterology. 1994;107:180–8.
6. Andersson S, Grossman MI. Profile of pH, pressure and potential difference at gastroduodenal junction in man. Gastroenterology. 1965;49:364–72.
7. Rácz I. Transmucosal potential difference. In: Cheli R, ed. Gastric Protection. New York: Raven Press; 1988:65–86.
8. Price AB. The Sydney System: histological division. J Gastroenterol Hepatol. 1991;6:209–12.
9. Rácz I, Horváth O, Pécsi Gy, Goda M. Helicobacter pylori infection in the chronic erosions of antral mucosa; a therapeutical approach. Gastroprotection. 1994;4:4–8.
10. Sarosiek J, Namiot Z, Marshall D et al. Breakdown of the mucus layer by H. pylori. In: Hunt RH, Tytgat GNJ, eds. Helicobacter pylori. Dordrecht, Boston, London: Kluwer Academic Publishers; 1994:123–38.
11. Ó'Morain CA. Helicobacter pylori – introduction. In: Ó'Morain CA, O'Connor H, eds. Helicobacter pylori: Implications and Practice. Bad Homburg, Madrid, Englewood, NJ: Normed Verlag; 1994:1–12.
12. Kreiss C, Blum AL, Malfertheiner P. Peptic ulcer pathogenesis. Curr Opin Gastroenterol. 1995;11:S25–S31.
13. Desai MA, Vadgama PM. Enhanced H^+ diffusion by NH_4^+/HCO_3^-: implications for Helicobacter pylori-associated peptic ulceration. Digestion. 1993;54:32–9.
14. Iyey KJ, Baskin W, Jeffery G. Effect of cimetidine on gastric potential difference in man. Lancet. 1978;2:1072–6.
15. Hossenbocus A, Fitzpatrick P, Colin-Jones DG. Measurement of gastric potential difference at endoscopy. Gut. 1975;14:410–14.

G Mózsik et al. Cell Injury and Cytoprotection in the GI Tract. 163–173.

IMPAIRED GASTRIC MUCOSAL DEFENCE IN *HELICOBACTER PYLORI*-RELATED CONDITIONS

M. JABLONSKÁ* AND A. CHLUMSKÁ

Fourth Medical Clinic and Second Pathology and Anatomy Institute, Charles University, Prague, Czech Republic

*Correspondence

ABSTRACT

Helicobacter pylori (*H. pylori*) infection of the stomach may be harmful both to the mucus layer and the underlying cells which might impair defence against noxious agents such as NSAIDs. The aim of this study was to evaluate the prevalence of *H. pylori* and gastric lesions in NSAID-treated patients.

Methods: In 132 patients treated with NSAID and upper gastrointestinal symptoms (63 males, 69 females, mean age 49 years, range 28–59), endoscopic investigation of the antral and corporal mucosa, including *H. pylori* testing (urease and histology) was performed.

Results:

1. *H. pylori* was found in 95 patients (72%);

2. In this group, ulcers were found in 73 cases (77%), 33 in the duodenal bulb (35%), 27 in the prepyloric region (29%) and 13 (13%) in the gastric body.

3. In the *H. pylori*-negative group (37), ulcers were found in 19 patients (51%), 7 (19%) in the duodenal bulb, 8 (21.6%) in the prepyloric region and 4 (10.8%) in the gastric body.

4. In the *H. pylori*-positive group, a predominant finding was chronic superficial active gastritis, with focal intestinal metaplasia (mostly complete) and atrophy in 25 (24%) of ulcer and in 26 (23%) of non-ulcer cases; in 33 (29%) in prepyloric and in 38 (53%) in gastric body ulcer.

5. Chronic superficial gastritis was not found in the *H. pylori*-negative group.

6. Endoscopic findings in non-ulcer cases showed a higher proportion of more-severe lesions – bleeding areas – in the *H. pylori*-positive group, whereas less-severe lesions (erosions, bleeding, spots) were more often present in the *H. pylori*-negative group. Frank bleeding occurred in 20% of the *H. pylori*-positive and in 19% of the *H. pylori*-negative group, in the first group predominantly due to ulcer.

Conclusions: NSAID-related ulcers occur more frequently in *H. pylori*-positive cases, probably due to impaired defence. This seems to justify *H. pylori* testing and adequate treatment of positive cases in NSAID gastropathy.

Keywords: Helicobacter pylori, NSAID gastropathy, impaired defence, ulcer, bleeding

This paper was presented at the Symposium on 'Cell injury and protection in the gastrointestinal tract: from basic science to clinical perspectives', October 8–11, 1995, Pécs, Hungary.

INTRODUCTION

In 1982, Marshall and Warren isolated a spiral urease-producing organism, later identified as *Helicobacter pylori*, nestled in the narrow interface between the gastric epithelial cell surface and the mucus layer. A very strong association between this organism and upper gastrointestinal disease has been reported. A causal relationship between *H. pylori* and chronic superficial gastritis has been well established. This gastritis has been produced by intragastric administration in some animal models and by oral administration in two humans [1].

A causal relationship between *H. pylori* and peptic ulcer disease is more difficult to establish. However, since nearly all patients with duodenal ulcer have *H. pylori* gastric infection, the organism may be a prerequisite for the occurrence of almost all duodenal ulcers in the absence of other precipitating factors (NSAIDs, Zollinger–Ellison syndrome). The association between *H. pylori* infection and gastric ulcer is slightly less strong; nevertheless, since the majority of *H. pylori*-infected individuals do not develop peptic ulcers, strain variability or other factors must play a role in the pathogenesis of peptic ulcer disease [2].

In peptic ulcer disease, the strongest evidence for a pathogenetic role of *H. pylori* is the decrease in recurrence rate following the eradication of *H. pylori*. An interesting result of recent studies has questioned the mechanism by which an antral organism causes a duodenal lesion. This includes bacterial colonization of gastric metaplasia in the duodenum (secondary to acid). Further studies are needed to clarify the question of whether perhaps other trends of *H. pylori*, associated with prepyloric and gastric body ulcer, are more likely to be associated with gastric atrophy and intestinal metaplasia (a possible link to carcinogenesis).

Non-ulcerative dyspepsia has not yet been shown convincingly to be associated with *H. pylori* infection. On the other hand, a disturbing epidemiological relationship between *H. pylori* infection and gastric cancer has been reported [1,2]. This aspect addressed both the problem of development of gastric atrophy and intestinal metaplasia and some biochemical results showing a higher potential of malignancy in *H. pylori* stomachs. A rare disorder, non Hodgkin's lymphoma of the stomach, may be linked to this malignancy as well as to a subset – mucosa-associated lymphoid tissue lymphomas of stomach. On the whole, it appears that, if there is any causal relationship between *H. pylori* infection and gastric cancer, clearly other factors are also important in gastric carcinogeneis and *H. pylori* eradication to prevent gastric cancer is not generally recommended at present [1].

VIRULENCE AND PATHOGENECITY OF *H. PYLORI*

The flagella of *H. pylori* give its motility in the gastric juice and gastric mucus. Its safe passage through the gastric acid barrier and arrival at the protective mucus layer is achieved by means of its sufficient generation of bicarbonate and ammonium ions.

Ammonia raises the pH of the gastric mucus layer from about 6 to 7 and depletes aerobic cells of α-ketoglutarate. Hypergastrinaemia in patients with *H. pylori* may be due to ammonia since gastrin RNA message in rat gastric mucosa exposed to ammonia and inflammatory agents is increased. This may account for increased *H. pylori* urease in duodenal ulcer patients due to a greater *H. pylori* density. Moreover, ammonia induces, at high concentrations, vacuoles just the same as those induced by VAC A toxin of *H. pylori*. Thus, one effect of VAC A may be a potentiation of the effect of ammonia [3,4].

In the gastric mucus, *H. pylori* is able to attach to phospholipids (phosphatidyletha-nolamine) sialated glycoproteins and Lewis B antigens (in blood group O). Its delivery of soluble proteases and phospholipase may be harmful to both the mucus layer and the underlying cells. Thus, impaired mucus strength may allow more hydrogen ion to penetrate the mucosa [5].

CYTOTOXIN OF *H. PYLORI*

The 'vacuolating cytotoxin' (an 87-kDa protein), expressed in about 65% of *H. pylori* strains, causes vacuoles in epithelial cells, present in most cases of duodenal ulcer. The gene for this cytotoxin, VAC A (cloned by Cover), is always present in *H. pylori* with production of an active protein in 65%; cytotoxin CAGA, a second protein at 127 kDa, is a marker for vacuolating toxic effect; its gene is present only in the presence of VAC A cytotoxic effect. Clinically, it seems important that antibodies to the toxin are present in nearly all duodenal ulcer patients; however, the exact function of CAG A is still unknown [2,6].

Immunological responses

Large numbers of neutrophils and lymphocytes are attracted to *H. pylori* due to its chemotactic proteins. Interleukins (C II 2) tumour necrosis factor and oxygen free radicals are released in response to *H. pylori*. VAC A toxin may be linked to a more intensive neutrophil reaction (active gastritis) with increased tissue damage [7,8].

Due to production of superoxide dismutase (SOD) and catalase, *H. pylori* is protected from neutrophil phagocytosis (SOD and catalase interrupting the usual chain of events).

IgG and IgA, secreted by lymphocytes and plasma cells in *H. pylori* infection, may be useful for diagnosis; IgG is more sensitive but IgA levels fall faster after eradication [9].

The technique of generating *H. pylori*-specific antibody is able to detect an immunological history long after disappearance of *H. pylori*. This seems to be useful in cases without current *H. pylori* infection (in advanced chronic gastritis with atrophy and intestinal metaplasia and gastric cancer) [10].

Inflammation and carcinogenesis

Tissue damage due to *H. pylori* actions may be linked to non-gastric (intestinal) type epithelium growth in the stomach. This leads to colonization by other bacteria, reducing nitrate with predisposition to the formation of carcinogenic nitrosamines [11]; on the other hand, chronic inflammation may generate superoxide and nitric oxide, forming reactive oxygen species and nitrosamine [12]; the carcinogenetic pathway is modulated by other factors (diet, environment, epidemiology) [13].

AIM OF THE STUDY

Besides the actions mentioned above, *H. pylori* infection interferes also with regulatory mechanisms of gastric secretion, leading to a decrease in somatostatin cells in the antral mucosa and elevation of serum gastrin. This factor may also contribute to impaired defence mechanisms of the gastric mucosa produced by the broad spectrum of *H. pylori* actions.

Clinically, it appears to be important to consider implications of a combination of *H. pylori* infection with mucosal damage caused by non-steroidal anti-inflammatory drugs (NSAIDs). According to incontrovertible evidence, the use of these drugs is associated with various types of gastroduodenal lesions (ulcer, ulcer complications, life threatening situations). NSAID, as cyclo-oxygenase inhibitors, interfere with most identified gastroduodenal defence mechanisms and produce or enhance mucosal injury, including reduction of the thickness of the mucosa, inhibition of duodenal bicarbonate secretion, vasoconstriction and a variety of factors linked to inhibition of prostaglandin synthesis [14–16].

The possible interaction of *Helicobacter*-associated lesions of the upper GI tract with actions of NSAIDs has not yet received major attention, probably for the rapid increase of knowledge concerning *H. pylori* during a relatively short period; however, it seems that the interaction between *H. pylori* actions and NSAID damage and its mechanisms might be of considerable clinical importance although both experimental and clinical evidence are incomplete as well as proposals to prevent combined damage; thus, the aim of this study was the evaluation of prevalence and type of *H. pylori*-related upper gastrointestinal lesions in NSAID-treated patients.

GROUPS OF PATIENTS AND METHODS

One hundred and thirty-two patients (mean age 48 years) treated with NSAIDs and with upper gastrointestinal symptoms were studied (63 males, mean age 51, range 32–59; 69 females, mean age 45, range 28–56); in all patients, upper gastrointestinal endoscopy was performed, including testing for *H. pylori* in samples from the antral mucosa both with the rapid urease test and histological examination (Warthin–Starry strains). Endoscopic findings were recorded (ulcer and non-ulcer lesions according to OMGE terminology) and histological findings were assessed conforming with the

TABLE 1

Endoscopic findings (ulcers and other lesions) in the *H. pylori*-positive (group I) and *H. pylori*-negative (group II) groups

	Group I Number	%	Group II Number	%
Ulcer(s)	73	77	19	51
Other lesions	19	20	12	32
No lesion	3	2	6	15
All	95		37	

Sydney classification of chronic gastritis. Relationships between mucosal damage due to NSAIDs and grades of *H. pylori* inflammation, colonization and activity were analysed (semiquantitatively); treatment prior to clinical manifestation of lesions was also analysed. Results were evaluated for comparison between *H. pylori*-positive and -negative cases.

RESULTS

H. pylori characteristics and endoscopic findings

H. pylori positivity was found in 95 (72%) of the patients, 41 males and 54 females, mean age 49 ± 14 (group I). In 37 cases, *H. pylori* was negative (28%), 22 males, 15 females, mean age 45 ± 12 (group II).

Endoscopy showed ulcers in 73 cases (77%) in group I and in 19 (51%) in group II; other lesions were present in 19 (20%) of group I and in 12 cases (32%) of group II. No lesions were found in 3 cases (2%) from group I and in 6 (15%) from group II (see Table 1).

Ulcers

In the patients with ulcers, these lesions were in the duodenal bulb in 33 (35%) of group I and in 7 cases (19%) of group II. Prepyloric ulcers were found in 27 cases (29%) in group I and in 8 cases (21.6%) in group II. Gastric body ulcers were found in 13 cases (13%) in group I and in 4 cases (10.8%) in group II.

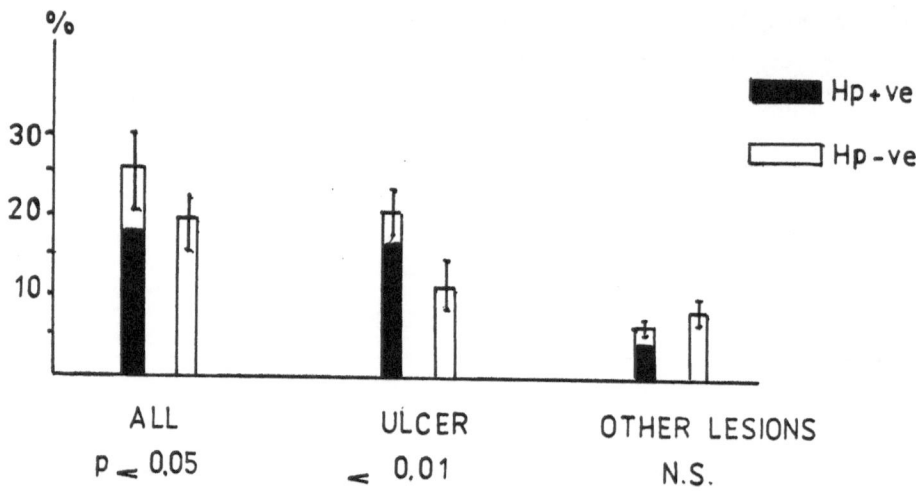

Figure 1. Occurrrence of frank bleeding in the *H. pylori*-positive and -negative groups – in patients with ulcer, patients with other lesions, and all patients

Other lesions

Erosions were found in 10 cases (10.5%) in group I and in 8 cases (21.6%) in group II. Bleeding spots occurred in 5 cases (5.2%) in group I and in 4 cases (10.8%) in group II. Bleeding areas (more severe lesions) were found in 4 cases (4.2%) in group I and in no case in group II.

Frank bleeding (Figure 1)

Frank bleeding occurred in 25 cases (26%) of the patients in group I (*H. pylori* positive) and in 7 (19%) in group II (*H. pylori* negative). In 19 cases (20%) in group I and in 4 cases (10.8%) in group II, bleeding was caused by ulcers; in 6 (6%) in group I and 3 (8%) in group II, it was caused by other lesions.

Thus, peptic ulcers (duodenal and prepyloric) occurred significantly more frequently in *H. pylori*-positive NSAID takers and also more severe bleeding lesions (seen endoscopically) and frank bleeding were more frequent in *H. pylori*-postive NSAID takers.

TABLE 2
The prevalence of intestinal metaplasia (IM) and atrophy in various types of ulcer in *H. pylori*-positive patients

Ulcer (*n*)	Intestinal metaplasia		Atrophy	
	Number	%	Number	%
Duodenal (33)	4	12	2	6
Prepyloric (27)	9	33	8	29
Gastric body (13)	5	38	7	53
Total	18		17	

Histological findings

In group I, chronic superficial gastritis was present in all the cases with ulcer (73) and without ulcer (22); atrophic changes occurred in 17 (24%) cases with ulcer and in 5 (23%) without ulcer. Intestinal metaplasia (IM) showed a similar pattern with 19 (25%) in ulcer cases and 7 (26%) without ulcer.

Prevalence of IM and atrophy (Table 2)

An analysis of the prevalence of IM and atrophy in various types of ulcer (group I) showed a low proportion of IM and atrophy in duodenal ulcer (4 cases of IM (11%) and 2 cases of atrophy (6%)); a considerably higher proportion in prepyloric ulcer (9 cases of IM (33%) and 8 cases of atrophy (29%)) and an even higher proportion in gastric body ulcer (5 cases of IM (38%) and 7 of atrophy (53%)).

Intestinal metaplasia (Table 3)

Evaluation of complete and incomplete intestinal metaplasia (staining technique) in group I showed no cases of incomplete intestinal metaplasia in duodenal ulcer, a small proportion in prepyloric ulcer and nearly the same numbers as for complete IM in gastric body ulcers and other lesions. Incomplete IM is thought to be the result of rather advanced chronic gastritis, possibly linked to carcinogenesis.

Histological findings in group II

These showed chronic superficial gastritis in only 3 cases (8.1%), focal gastritis in 9

TABLE 3

Evaluation of complete and incomplete intestinal metaplasia in the *H. pylori*-positive group with various types of ulcer

Ulcer (*n*)	Complete	Incomplete
Duodenal (12)	3	0
Prepyloric (8)	5	2
Gastric body (7)	4	3
Other lesions (15)	5	4
Total	17	9

(24.3%), uncharacteristic changes in 11 (29.6%) and no gastritis in 14 (37.8%). IM and atrophy were found in only one case.

On the whole, histological changes in *H. pylori*-infected cases showed the whole spectrum of *H. pylori*-associated chronic gastritis, including IM and atrophy. However, these changes were rare in duodenal ulcer patients and more frequent in other types of ulcer, possibly pointing to different strains of the organism.

Relationship between mucosal damage, inflammation and H. pylori (Figure 2)

The relationship between the grade of mucosal damage due to NSAIDs and grade of inflammation, *H. pylori* colonization and activity (semiquantitatively) in *H. pylori*-positive NSAID takers showed a positive correlation between the grade of inflammation and the grade of mucosal damage; an inverse correlation between the grade of *H. pylori* colonization and mucosal damage. This seems to support the observation that, in advanced chronic gastritis with IM and atrophy, *H. pylori* colonization decreases and may account (in part) for the development of NSAID *H. pylori*-positive takers showing only moderate grades of colonization; thus, the grade of mucosal damage seems to be more closely related to the progression of gastritis than to the actual grade of *H. pylori* colonization.

Medical treatment

Medical treatment received by the patients taking NSAID with *H. pylori* positivity or negativity prior to clinical manifestation of lesions was divided into maintenance anti-ulcer treatment (I), intermittent treatment (II) and no anti-ulcer treatment. Only a minority of patients had maintenance treatment (11 out of 92 in the *H. pylori*-positive group, and 4 out of 31 in the negative group). Intermittent treatment was given more

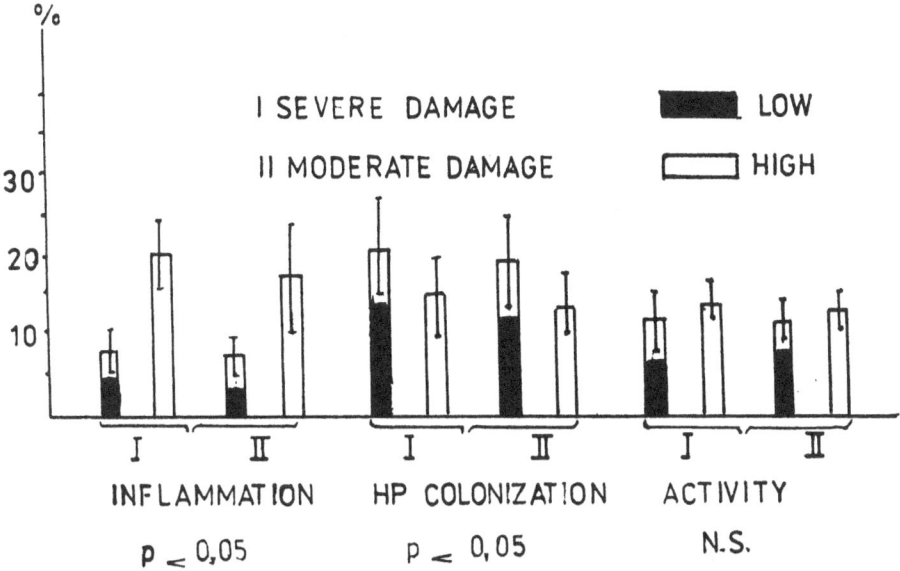

Figure 2. Relationship between mucosal damage due to NSAIDs and grade of *H. pylori* inflammation, colonization and activity (semiquantitatively assessed)

frequently (34 and 9 patients, respectively). However, in most cases, no anti-ulcer treatment was used at all (47 and 18 patients, respectively). Important clinical manifestations – frank bleeding (particularly) and ulcer – were considerably more frequent in this untreated group, whereas these complications were rather infrequent (5 of 69) or even absent in patients on maintenance treatment, even with *H. pylori* positivity.

DISCUSSION

The mechanisms of development of upper gastrointestinal damage due to *H. pylori* and NSAIDs appear to be rather different, and it does not seem easy to detect common pathways. Substantial differences appear from the typical ability of *H. pylori* to produce chronic inflammation with a variety of host reactions causing mucosal incompetence probably involved in recurrence of ulcers [17]. Acute life-threatening mucosal damage related to NSAIDs is well known [18]; in *H. pylori*-related damage, we still have to learn more about its direct cytotoxic actions [19]. In clinical practice, the immense problem of NSAID-induced gastroduodenopathy has become even more complicated considering another powerful factor causing mucosal damage via different pathways; there is the possibility of a severe outcome of combined actions. Thus, the question of testing NSAID takers for *H. pylori* positivity should be considered and further courses

– after eradication – be carefully evaluated. Since new *H. pylori* infections are rather rare (at least in well-developed countries), antimicrobial therapy and immunization, both needed for the elimination of *H. pylori*-associated disease, might influence quite fundamentally the development and course of peptic ulcer, and also help to manage NSAID-induced gastroduodenopathy [20].

CONCLUSIONS

Patients treated with NSAIDs and who have *H. pylori* gastric infection more frequently develop severe upper gastrointestinal mucosal lesions than those without *H. pylori* infection. This includes particularly the occurrence of frank bleeding and the development of duodenal and prepyloric ulcers.

Anti-ulcer treatment in NSAID takers prior to the manifestation of mucosal damage is frequently not sufficient or even missing. Maintenance treatment prior to clinical manifestations seems to decrease the risk (both in *H. pylori*-positive and -negative cases).

Mucosal defence, lowered due to NSAIDs, is even more impaired by *H. pylori*. This appears to justify testing for *H. pylori* in NSAID patients and employing adequate management (eradication) in positive cases.

REFERENCES

1. Development Panel on Helicobacter pylori in Peptic Ulcer Disease. J Am Med Assoc. 1994;272(1):65–9.
2. Marshall BJ. Helicobacter pylori. Am J Gastroenterol. 1994;89(8):S116–28.
3. Marshall BJ, Barrett LJ, Prakasch C et al. Urea protects Helicobacter (Campylobacter) pylori from the bactericidal effects of acid. Gastroenterology. 1990;99:697–702.
4. Murakami M, Yod JK, Teramura S et al. Generation of ammonia and mucosal lesion formation following hydrolysis of urea by urease in the stomach. J Clin Gastroenterol. 1990;12:S104–9.
5. Goggin PM, Northfield TC, Spychal RT. Factors affecting gastric mucosal hydrophobicity in man. Scand J Gastroenterol. 1991;181(Suppl):65–73
6. Tummura MX, Cover TL, Blaser MJ. Cloning and expression of a high-molecular mass major antigen of Helicobacter pylori: Evidence of linkage to cytotoxin production. Infect Immun. 1993;61:1799–809.
7. Salim AS. The relationship between Helicobacter pylori and oxygen-derived free radicals in the mechanism of duodenal ulceration. Intern Med. 1993;32:359–64.
8. Xiang Z, Bugnoli M, Rappuoli R et al. Helicobacter pylori host responses in peptic ulceration. Lancet. 1993;341:900–1.
9. Hirschl AM, Brandstatter RG, Dragosics B et al. Kinetics of specific IgG antibodies for monitoring the effect of anti-Helicobacter pylori chemo-therapy. J Infect Dis. 1993;168:763–6.
10. Crabtree JE, Wyatt JH, Sobala GM et al. Systemic and mucosal humoral responses to Helicobacter pylori in gastric cancer. Gut. 1993;34(10):1339–43.
11. Sobala GM, Pignatelli B, Schorah CJ et al. Levels of nitrite, nitrate, N-nitrose compounds, ascorbic acid and total bile acids in gastric juice of patients with and without precancerous conditions of the stomach. Carcinogenesis. 1991;12:193–8.
12. Correa P. Human gastric carcinogenesis: A multistep and multifactorial process. Cancer Res. 1992;52:6735–40.
13. Sobola GM, Schorah GJ, Pilnatell B et al. High gastric juice ascorbic acid concentrations in members of a gastric cancer family. Carcinogenesis. 1993;14:291–2.

14. Langmann MJS, Brooks P, Hawkey F et al. Management of non-steroidal anti-inflammatory drug gastroduodenopathy: Epidemiology, causation and treatment. Working party reports, World Congress of Gastroenterology, Sydney. 1990:11–16.
15. Flemstroem G, Garner A, Nylander O et al. Surface epithelial bicarbonate transport by mammalian duodenum in vivo. Am J Physiol. 1982;243:G348–58.
16. Robert A, Nezamis J, Lancaster C et al. Cytoprotection by prostaglandin in rats. Prevention of gastric necrosis produced by alcohol, HCl, NaOH, hypertonic NaHCl and thermal injury. Gastroenterology. 1979;77:433–43.
17. Cullen DJE, Collins J, Christiansen HJ et al. Long term risk of peptic ulcer disease in people with Helicobacter pylori infection – a community based study. Abstr. Gastroenterology. 1993;104(Suppl 2):60.
18. Fries JF, Miller SR, Spitz FW et al. Towards an epidemiology of gastropathy associated with non-steroidal anti-inflammatory drug use. Gastroenterology. 1989;96:647–55.
19. Tytgat GNJ, Axon ATR, Dixon MF et al. Helicobacter pylori: causal agent in peptic ulcer disease? Working party reports of the World Congress of Gastroenterology, Sydney. 1990:36–45.
20. Adamek RJ, Wegeler M, Opferkuch W et al. Successful Helicobacter pylori eradication: A systemic effect of antibiotic? Am J Gastroenterol. 1993;88:792–3.

G Mózsik et al. Cell Injury and Cytoprotection in the GI Tract. 175–185.
© 1997 Kluwer Academic Publishers.

THE ROLE OF CYSTEINE AND SERINE PROTEASES IN GASTRIC CARCINOGENESIS AND THEIR PROGNOSTIC IMPACT IN GASTRIC CANCER

L. HERSZÉNYI[1*], F. FARINATI[2], M. PLEBANI[3], P. CARRARO[3], M. DE PAOLI[3], G. ROVERONI[3], R. NACCARATO[2] AND Z. TULASSAY[1]

[1]Second Department of Medicine, Semmelweis University Medical School, Budapest, Hungary; [2]Cattedra Malattie Apparato Digerente, Istituto di Medicina Interna; [3]Dipartimento di Medicina di Laboratorio, Laboratorio Centrale, Universitá di Padova, Italy
*Correspondence

ABSTRACT

Cysteine proteases (cathepsin B [CATB], cathepsin L [CATL], the serine protease urokinase-type plasminogen activator (UPA) and its inhibitor PAI-1 play an important part in cancer invasion. Little is known about their prognostic value in gastric cancer and no data are available on the possible relationship between these proteases and gastric precancerous changes.

Aims:

1. To determine CATB, CATL, UPA, PAI-1 in chronic atrophic gastritis with intestinal metaplasia and in gastric epithelial dysplasia – as precancerous changes – in gastric cancer and in cancer-free mucosa;

2. To evaluate their prognostic value with respect to survival in gastric cancer.

Samples of tumour and of normal mucosa were obtained from 25 patients undergoing gastrectomy. Biopsies were taken from 33 patients with chronic atrophic gastritis (12 with dysplasia) and from 47 control subjects. Antigen concentrations were measured using ELISA. Survival was analysed by Cox's model.
    CATB, CATL, UPA and PAI-1 were significantly higher in cancer vs. cancer-free tissue. Chronic atrophic gastritis showed intermediate values between cancer and non-cancerous tissue. CATB and UPA were significantly higher in chronic atrophic gastritis with vs. without dysplasia. Low UPA, PAI-1 and CATB were associated with better survival. These proteases and PAI-1 have a role, not only in cancer invasion, but also in the progression of precancerous changes into cancer and have a strong prognostic impact.

Keywords: protease, cathepsin, plasminogen activator, chronic atrophic gastritis, precancerous changes, prognosis

This paper was presented at the Symposium on 'Cell injury and protection in the gastrointestinal tract: from basic science to clinical perspectives', October 8–11, 1995, Pécs, Hungary.

INTRODUCTION

The proteolysis of the extracellular matrix is an essential step in cancer invasion [1]. It has been suggested that cathepsin B (CATB) and cathepsin L (CATL) – both of which form part of the cysteine protease family – may have an important role in this process [2–4]. Previous reports have claimed that cysteine proteases are involved in the development of several gastrointestinal tumours. For instance, Ohta et al. [5] demonstrated that CATB may be active in the process of pancreatic cancer invasion and Shuja et al. [6] reported significantly higher CATB and CATL activity in colorectal cancer than in normal tissue at a distance from the tumours.

Plasminogen activators (which belong to the serine protease family) are involved in many degrading processes, converting plasminogen into active plasmin. It is known that tissue-type plasminogen activator (TPA) is responsible mainly for thrombolysis, whereas urokinase-type plasminogen activator (UPA) appears to influence inflammation, tissue degradation and tumour invasion [7–11]. Plasminogen activators are controlled by plasminogen activator inhibitors (PAI-1 and PAI-2), which are members of the serine protease inhibitors (serpin) family [12].

Increased UPA and PAI-1 levels have been found in solid tumours, such as those of the breast [13,14], brain [15] and colorectum [16–20], strongly suggesting that not only UPA but also PAI-1 may have an important role in tumour invasion and metastasis.

Similar results have been obtained with gastric cancer [10,21–26], and we have previously reported data obtained studying cathepsins, UPA and PAI-1 simultaneously in gastric cancer patients [27]. Some of the above studies have also pointed to the possible prognostic role of tissue proteases. For instance, the importance of UPA and PAI-1 determination has been demonstrated in breast cancer patients [13,14] and also in completely resected gastric cancer patients [26]. However, to our knowledge, the prognostic relevance of cathepsins in gastric cancer has not been evaluated or compared with that of UPA and PAI-1.

As for precancerous changes, Shuja et al. [6] suggested that CATB may be a sensitive marker of the progression from premalignant colorectal adenoma to colorectal cancer, and De Bruin et al. [28] found that adenomatous polyps of the colon exhibit intermediate UPA levels between those of normal colonic mucosa and adenocarcinoma, concluding that measuring UPA expression may be a useful parameter for the early detection of colorectal cancer.

Since in our own and other authors' experience, other proteolytic enzymes, such as aspartic proteases pepsinogen A and pepsinogen C, also provide a valuable means for screening patients at risk for gastric cancer [29–32] and since no data are currently available on the possible relationship between cysteine–serine proteases, PAI-1 and gastric precancerous changes, we decided to evaluate:

1. The antigen levels of CATB, CATL (cysteine proteases), UPA (serine protease) and its inhibitor PAI-1 in chronic atrophic gastritis with intestinal metaplasia (CAG), in gastric cancer (cancer), and in normal tissue obtained from a tumour-free area (non-cancer);

2. Any relationship these proteases may have with CAG activity, grade, degree of intestinal metaplasia (IM), and the presence or absence of gastric epithelial dysplasia (GED);

3. The prognostic impact of these proteases and PAI-1 in gastric cancer patients.

PATIENTS AND METHODS

Our study involved 105 patients. Twenty-five were patients undergoing gastrectomy for gastric cancer (17 males, 8 females; mean age 62 years, range 31–84). Immediately after removal of the stomach, fresh samples of tumour (cancer) and tumour-free tissue (non-cancer) (taken more than 10 cm from the border of the tumour and in an area macroscopically free from any change) were obtained. After removing fat and muscle layers, the samples were frozen at $-70°C$ until needed. All patients had histologically confirmed advanced adenocarcinoma. From the macroscopic point of view, the gastric cancer could be classified according to Borrmann: 5 type I (exophytic), 11 type II (ulcer-expansive), 5 type III (ulcer-infiltrative), and 4 type IV (scirrhus-infiltrative). Pathological staging was obtained for the presence ($n = 13$) or absence ($n = 12$) of metastases; for differentiation (well-differentiated G1 $n = 4$, moderately-differentiated G2 $n = 14$, for poorly-differentiated G3 $n = 7$), and for histotype (intestinal type $n = 13$, or diffuse-type $n = 12$, according to Lauren).

Biopsy specimens were taken for histology from 33 patients followed up for chronic atrophic gastritis and intestinal metaplasia (13 males, 20 females; mean age 62 years, range 40–78; 12 of these patients also had confirmed mild GED). Forty-seven control subjects with upper gastrointestinal complaints but negative endoscopy with either negative ($n = 7$) or unspecific histology (mild superficial gastritis; $n = 40$); [CONTROL] were also included in the study (29 males, 18 females; mean age 49 years, range 25–79).

Endoscopy was carried out in the usual fashion. Before withdrawal, biopsy specimens were routinely taken from the antrum ($n = 2$), body ($n = 2$) and fundus ($n = 2$). Multiple biopsies were also obtained of any focal change observed (in cases of CAG), plus one biopsy at the antrum, about 5 cm from the pylorus, for biochemical determination. The mean weight of the biopsy specimen was approximately 5 mg.

Samples for biochemical determinations were snap-frozen at $-70°C$, while those for histology were fixed in 5% buffered formaldehyde, stained in H&E and a modified Giemsa, and then observed blindly by the same pathologist for the presence of:

- Superficial gastritis [33];

- Atrophy (CAG) [34];

- Disease activity, according to a semiquantitative score considering the extent of polymorphonuclear infiltration (+ = low activity ($n = 8$); ++ and +++ = high activity ($n = 25$) [35];

- CAG grade, according to the Sydney system [35] (semiquantitatively scored considering the extent of atrophic changes and the severity of glandular loss replacement by metaplastic cells (low grade $n = 13$, high grade $n = 20$);

- Presence of GED (12 patients, always multifocal and of mild degree) according to Morson et al. [36] and Riddel et al. [37];

- Presence and degree of IM [low grade (+) ($n = 5$), consisting of a few tubules to one third of the total area biopsied; high grade (++/+++), consisting of one third to more than two thirds of the total area biopsied ($n = 28$).

Informed consent was obtained from all patients.

Extracts of resected tissues were prepared from 50–100 mg wet weight tissue sampling. Essentially, the specimens were homogenized in melting ice in 1 ml (vol/vol) Tris Tween buffer (0.1 mol/L, 0.1% Tween 80, pH 7.5) per 60 mg wet tissue. Biopsy tissue extracts were prepared similarly, except for the wet tissue concentration at homogenization, which was 25 mg. After centrifugation for 10 min at 10 000g at 4°C, the supernatants were stored at –70°C before assay. Protein concentrations of the supernatants were determined by the Bradford method [38] (Bio-Radd, München, Germany). The antigen levels were measured using the ELISA method as follows.

Assay for cathepsin B and cathepsin L

Briefly, the cathepsin immunoassay was a solid-phase enzyme-linked immunosorbent assay (ELISA) based on the sandwich principle (BioAss, Diesen, Germany). One hundred ml of tissue extract was added to a polyclonal immunoselected anti-human-cathepsin antibody and incubated. A second anti-cathepsin antibody labelled with horseradish peroxidase (conjugate) was added. Absolute quantities of CATB, CATL antigens on the samples were calculated from a 7-point standard curve of CATB/CATL (0–250 ng/ml). The lowest detectable levels of CATB and CATL is estimated to be 10 ng/ml.

Assay for urokinase-type plasminogen activator (UPA)

Antigen quantification was performed using the TintElize UPA-ELISA (Biopool, Umea, Sweden). A mouse monoclonal anti-UPA was used as a catching antibody. After incubation with the tissue homogenates, a second goat anti-human UPA, conjugated with horseradish peroxidase, was used to form a 'sandwich' ELISA and ortho-phenylene diamine was added as a substrate. The amount of UPA antigen in the samples was calculated from a 6-point standard curve of UPA (0–4 ng/ml). The detection limit is about 0.1 ng/ml for UPA.

Assay for plasminogen-activator inhibitor type-1 (PAI-1)

PAI-1 antigen was determined using Asserachrom PAI-1-ELISA (Diagnostica Stago, Asnieres-sur-Seines, France) with mouse monoclonal anti-human PAI-1 as a catching antibody. A second mouse monoclonal anti-PAI-1 is coupled with peroxidase and binds to another antigenic determinant at a distance from the first, forming the 'sandwich'. The bound enzyme peroxidase is then revealed, in the same way as for UPA, in the presence of hydrogen peroxide. Absolute quantities of PAI-1 antigen on the samples were calculated from a 5-point standard curve of PAI-1 (0–20 ng/ml). The detection limit is about 0.5 ng/ml for PAI-1.

Antigen concentrations were expressed as ng of antigen per mg of protein. Results were given as mean values $\pm$ SD.

Differences betweeng groups were statistically tested using Student's t-test, the Mann–Whitney U-test where applicable, ANOVA one-way and Kruskall–Wallis analysis of variance.

Differences were considered as significant with $2p < 0.05$. The ROC (receiver operating characteristics) curve was used to determine the optimal cut-off values (with the Youden J-test for overall accuracy).

To determine the prognostic value of proteases by comparison with histomorphological prognostic factors, survival was analysed according to Cox's proportional hazard model for: CATB, CATL, UPA, PAI-1, T stage, N stage, grade, Borrmann classification and Lauren classification. Twelve patients (48%) died of tumour recurrence during the follow-up study. Their median survival time was 8 months (range 4–17 months). At the end of the follow-up period, 13 patients (52%) were still alive; their median follow-up is 18 months (range 8–27 months). The median survival time, calculated over all patients, is 12.3 months. Finally, stepwise logistic regression analysis was used to evaluate the most significant independent prognostic variables.

RESULTS

The antigen concentrations for cysteine–serine proteases and PAI-1 in CAG, cancer, non-cancer and controls are shown in Table 1.

CATB, CATL, UPA, PAI-1 were significantly higher in cancer than in non-cancer tissues, CAG showed intermediate values between cancer and non-cancer (CATB, CATL, UPA, PAI-1). Cathepsins, UPA and PAI-1 were significantly higher in CAG than in non-cancer or control.

As shown in Table 2, CATB and UPA were significantly higher in CAG with GED than in specimens without GED. PAI-1 levels were also higher in CAG with GED than in CAG without GED, though not significantly so. No significant differences were observed with respect to degree of IM (high-degree IM (++/+++) vs. low-degree (+)), even though patients with a more extensive IM showed a trend towards higher antigen levels (Table 2).

No significant correlation was found with either CAG disease activity (high activity (++/+++) vs. low activity (+)), or CAG grade (high grade vs. low grade) (Table 3).

TABLE 1
Cathepsin B, cathepsin L, urokinase-type plasminogen activator and its inhibitor type-1 in gastric cancer, chronic atrophic gastritis and in control subjects, expressed as ng/mg protein (mean ± SD)

	CATB	CATL	UPA	PAI-1
Cancer (n = 25)	325.88 ± 427.08	43.63 ± 24.47	1.85 ± 1.05	2.35 ± 2.69
CAG (n = 33)	229.50 ± 115.02	35.27 ± 12.67	1.45 ± 0.83	1.11 ± 1.02
Non-cancer (n = 25)	155.02 ± 180.48	27.55 ± 19.34	0.45 ± 0.37	0.50 ± 0.30
Control (n = 47)	130.87 ± 43.54	27.02 ± 8.35	0.49 ± 0.48	0.48 ± 0.23
Statistics (t-test):				
Cancer vs. non-cancer and control	$p < 0.05$	$p < 0.005$	$p < 0.000001$	$p < 0.005$
CAG vs. non-cancer and control	$p < 0.001$	$p < 0.005$	$p < 0.000001$	$p < 0.005$

CATB, cathepsin B; CATL, cathepsin L; UPA, urokinase-type plasminogen activator; PAI-1, plasminogen activator type-1; cancer, gastric cancer; non-cancer, cancer-free tissue; CAG, chronic atrophic gastritis; control, control subjects

TABLE 2
Cathepsin B, cathepsin L, urokinase-type plasminogen activator and its inhibitor type-1 in chronic atrophic gastritis in the presence or absence of gastric epithelial dysplasia and in relation to the degree of intestinal metaplasia, expressed as ng/mg protein (mean ± SD)

	CATB	CATL	UPA	PAI-1
CAG with GED (n = 12)	283.30 ± 149.21*	34.45 ± 7.46	1.89 ± 1.09*	1.40 ± 1.53
CAG without GED (n = 21)	198.75 ± 78.69	35.75 ± 15.02	1.21 ± 0.51	0.95 ± 0.55
High-grade IM (n = 28)	240.55 ± 119.10†	36.55 ± 12.28†	1.47 ± 0.89	1.15 ± 1.10
Low-grade IM (n = 5)	167.62 ± 66.62	28.16 ± 13.83	1.35 ± 0.28	0.91 ± 0.32

Statistics (t-test): *CAG with GED vs. CAG without GED (CATB, UPA: $p < 0.05$); †High-grade IM vs. low-grade IM (CATB, CATL: $0.1 > p > 0.05$)

CATB, cathepsin B; CATL, cathepsin L; UPA, urokinase-type plasminogen activator; PAI-1, plasminogen activator inhibitor type-1; CAG, chronic atropic gastritis; GED, gastric epithelial dysplasia; IM, intestinal metaplasia

TABLE 3
Correlation of cathepsin B, cathepsin L, urokinase-type plasminogen activator and its inhibitor type-1 with activity and grade of chronic atrophic gastritis, expressed as ng/mg protein (mean $\pm$ SD)

	CATB	CATL	UPA	PAI-1
High-activity CAG ($n = 25$)	243.70 ± 129.34	35.72 ± 12.45	1.56 ± 0.89	1.19 ± 1.15
Low-activity CAG ($n = 8$)	197.62 ± 96.46	33.87 ± 14.11	1.12 ± 0.46	0.85 ± 0.22
High-grade CAG ($n = 20$)	244.89 ± 118.00	34.58 ± 13.22	1.33 ± 0.59	1.22 ± 1.18
Low-grade CAG ($n = 13$)	205.83 ± 110.59	36.35 ± 12.22	1.64 ± 1.10	0.94 ± 0.73

CATB, cathepsin B; CATL, cathepsin L; UPA, urokinase-type plasminogen activator; PAI-1, plasminogen activator inhibitor type-1; CAG, chronic atrophic gastritis

With respect to control patients, no significant differences were found in protease and PAI-1 antigen levels between subgroups with normal histology ($n = 7$) and with mild superficial gastritis ($n = 40$) (data not shown).

The optimal cut-off value for CATB was 265 ng/mg protein (J = 0.63). This discriminated 15 patients (60%) below and 10 (40%) above the cut-off. As for CATL, a cut-off of 45 ng/mg protein (J = 0.39) was found, distinguishing 17 patients (68%) with CATL $\leqslant$ 45 ng/mg and 8 patients (32%) having CATL > 45 ng/mg.

The cut-off for UPA was placed at 1.25 ng/mg (J = 70), with 8 patients (32%) below and 17 patients (68%) above this level. For PAI-1, the selected value of 0.9 ng/mg (J = 0.66) distinguished between 6 patients (24%) below and 19% (76) above the cut-off. The Cox's survival analysis showed that the following parameters were significantly correlated with survival time (in order of significance): UPA ($p = 0.0001$), PAI-1 ($p = 0.0004$), CATB ($p = 0.002$), staging N ($p = 0.0022$), Borrmann classification ($p = 0.0024$), staging T ($p = 0.005$) and grade ($p = 0.02$). No significant correlation with survival was observed with respect to CATL ($p = 0.17$) or histotype according to Lauren. UPA was selected as the single independent variable by the stepwise logistic regression analysis (F-value = 12.624, $p = 0.0001$).

DISCUSSION

Cysteine and serine proteases have been suggested to play an important role in several gastrointestinal diseases, such as peptic ulcer disease, as well as in gastrointestinal cancers, with a number of studies having been published on gastric cancer [5,6,10,16–26,28,39].

To our knowledge, however, no data are available on the possible relationship between cathepsins, UPA, PAI-1 and gastric mucosal precancerous lesions and very little is known on the prognostic role of these proteases in gastric cancer.

We moved from the consideration that a number of parameters, which are modified in gastric cancer, such as the levels of aspartic proteases or oncofetal antigens, are also altered, though to a lesser extent, in stomachs harbouring precancerous changes, both in our own and in other authors' experience [29–32,40–42]. We therefore wondered whether cysteine–serine proteases and PAI-1 could also be associated with the progression of precancerous conditions and lesions into cancer as has been suggested for CATB [6] and for UPA [28] in colorectal adenomatous polyps.

The results regarding gastric cancer patients were in complete agreement with those already present in the literature. CATB, CATL, UPA, PAI-1 were indeed significantly higher in cancer tissues than in the tumour-free counterpart of the stomach or in control samples. Our results therefore confirm earlier studies reporting increased levels respectively of cathepsins [21–23], UPA [10,24–26] and PAI-1 [26] in gastric cancer.

The clearcut difference between cysteine–serine proteases and PAI-1 levels in cancer and non-cancerous tissue demonstrate that they are involved in the process of gastric cancer invasion and, at the same time, validates the results we obtained in patients with precancerous changes, which represent the novel feature of the study.

In our experience, UPA, PAI-1 and CATB levels were significant in the prediction of survival, and, to be more specific, they correlated better with survival than staging, tumour grading or the Borrmann classification. UPA proved the only and most significant independent predictor variable in stepwise logistic regression analysis. Our findings concerning gastric cancer appear to be supported by experience with other tumours: studies on breast carcinoma have shown that high UPA and PAI-1 levels in tissue extracts are associated with an aggressive tumour and a poor prognosis, and appear to be independent prognostic factors [13,14]. Our results now add the finding that, not only UPA and PAI-1 [26], but also CATB may serve as important prognostic factors for survival in gastric cancer patients.

In our experience, CAG patients had CATB, CATL, UPA and PAI-1 antigen concentrations definitely higher than those of control subjects, or in the tumour-free area of resected stomachs, and approaching levels demonstrated in cancer samples. This finding indicates that the mechanisms underlying protease synthesis/release in gastric cancer are activated after the appearance of precancerous changes.

Further, the appearance of more severe damage correlated with higher levels of proteases. Indeed, CATB and UPA levels were significantly higher in CAG with than without GED; interestingly enough, with respect to UPA, the levels detected in samples obtained in patients with GED were in the same range as those found in cancer samples. Finally, when subgrouping patients with CAG according to the presence or absence of severe metaplastic changes, a trend towards higher levels was observed in patients with CAG and high-grade IM than in patients with low-grade IM, particularly, with respect to CATB and CATL. Overall, the above suggests a progressive alteration of the pathophysiological mechanisms involved in cancer development and invasion and a gradual shift from normality to cancer in which CAG, severe IM and GED represent three consecutive and interrelated steps. This view is supported by the finding that other factors, such as disease activity or grade, did not show any significant correlation with cathepsins, UPA or PAI-1 antigen levels. CATB, CATL, UPA and PAI-1, therefore, apparently follow a different trend with respect to aspartic proteases, such as cathepsin D and E, which were not detected immunohisto-chemically, in incomplete IM and/or dysplastic tissue [43]. All of the above considera-tions fit very well with the multifactorial and multistep model of gastric carcinogenesis described by Correa [44,45], the main stages of which have been characterized as chronic gastritis, atrophy, metaplasia, dysplasia and cancer.

We know that CAG and IM have long been identified as intermediate events in the stepwise development of cancer [46]. Our group, like others, has been involved for some time in studying the role of GED as a morphological precursor of gastric cancer [47–53]. This progression is further confirmed by data regarding oncofetal antigens [40–42] and aspartic proteases [29–32] and by results regarding the genotypic events in the onset of stomach cancer [54,55]. What might be the role of these changes in cysteine–serine proteases and PAI-1 gastric carcinogenesis? While cathepsins and UPA have been shown to be involved in the process of cancer invasion [2–4,7–11], the exact functional role of PAI-1 in tumour biology is not well established. PAI-1 may represent a specific protein of transformed tissue, or may serve to protect the transformed tissue itself from proteolytic degradation, since increased PAI-1 may also be viewed as an attempt to restrict the damage caused by increased UPA levels. Another possible explanation is that the inhibitor might also have a role in angiogenesis, thus favouring tumour spread and metastasis [19,56,57]. A genotypically mutated cell could trigger a number of mechanisms designed to facilitate the final evolution into cancer, including the release of proteases that can disrupt the extracellular matrix and the epithelial base membrane, thus making way for neoplastic invasion. This mechanism might be of specific relevance with respect to GED, which could be viewed as an intraepithelial neoplastic change.

In conclusion, our results demonstrate that cysteine–serine proteases and PAI-1 may have a crucial role, not only in the invasive and metastatic process of gastric cancer, but also in the progression of precancerous conditions and lesions to gastric cancer. Considering the correlation between higher antigen levels of proteases and the presence of GED in CAG patients, measuring CATB and UPA in tissues obtained during follow-up biopsies could prove a useful tool in the identification of patients with gastric precancerous conditions and lesions at a high risk of developing gastric cancer, who could be subjected to a more strict follow-up protocol. Finally, given the capacity of these biological markers to predict patients' survival, measuring UPA, PAI-1 and CATB in gastric cancer tissue might prove of great value in identifying patients with a poor prognosis.

REFERENCES

1. Nigam AK, Pignatelli M, Boulos PB. Current concepts in metastasis. Gut, 1994;35:996–1000.
2. Mason RW, Johnson DA, Barrett AJ, Chapman HA. Elastinolytic activity of human cathepsin L. Biochem J. 1986;233:925–7.
3. Okoda Y, Yokota Y. Purification and properties of cathepsin B from sea urchin eggs. Comp Biochem Physiol. 1990;96:381–6.
4. Sloane BF. Cathepsin B and cystatins: evidence for a role in cancer progression. Semin Cancer Biol. 1990;1:137–52.

5. Ohta T, Terada T, Nagakawa T et al. Pancreatic trypsinogen and cathepsin B in human pancreatic carcinomas and associated metastatic lesions. Br J Cancer. 1994;69:152–6.
6. Shuja S, Sheahan K, Murnane MJ. Cysteine endopeptidase activity levels in normal human tissues, colorectal adenomas and carcinomas. Int J Cancer. 1991;49:341–6.
7. Dano K, Andreasen PA, Grondahl-Hansen J, Kristensen P, Nielsen LS, Skriver L. Plasminogen activators, tissue degradation and cancer. Adv Cancer Res. 1985;44:139–266.
8. Saksela O, Rifkin DB. Cell-associated plasminogen activation: regulation and physiological functions. Ann Rev Cell Biol. 1988;4:93–126.
9. Markus G. The relevance of plasminogen activators to neoplastic growth – a review of recent literature. Enzyme. 1988;40:158–72.
10. Nishino N, Aoki K, Tokura Y, Sakaguchi S, Takada Y, Takada A. The urokinase type of plasminogen activator in cancer of digestive tract. Thromb Res. 1988;50:527–35.
11. Hart IR, Saini A. Biology of tumor metastasis. Lancet. 1992;339:1453–7.
12. Sprengers ED, Kluft C. Plasminogen activator inhibitors. Blood. 1987;69:381–7.
13. Janicke F, Schmitt M, Pache L et al. Urokinase (uPA) and its inhibitor PAI-1 are strong and independent prognostic factors in node-negative breast cancer. Breast Cancer Res Treat. 1993;24:195–208.
14. Bouchet C, Spyratos F, Martin PM, Hacéne K, Gentile A, Oglobine J. Prognostic value of urokinase-type plasminogen activator (UPA) and plasminogen activator inhibitors PAI-1 and PAI-2 in breast carcinomas. Br J Cancer. 1994;69:398–405.
15. Landau BJ, Kwaan HC, Verrusio EN, Brem SS. Elevated levels of urokinase-type plasminogen activator and plasminogen activator inhibitor type 1 in malignant human brain tumors. Cancer Res. 1994;54:1105–8.
16. Sier CFM, Verspaget HW, Griffioen G et al. Inbalance of plasminogen activators and their inhibitors in human colorectal neoplasia. Implication of urokinase in colorectal carcinogenesis. Gastroenterology. 1991;101:1522–8.
17. Kirchheimer JC, Huber K, Wagner O, Binder BR. Pattern of fibrinolytic parameters in patients with gastrointestinal carcinomas. Br J Haematol. 1987;66:85–9.
18. Tanaka N, Fukao H, Ueshima S, Okada K, Yasutomi M, Matsuo O. Plasminogen activator inhibitor 1 in human carcinoma tissues. Int J Cancer. 1991;48:481–4.
19. Buo L, Lyberg T, Jorgensen L, Johansen HT, Aasen AO. Location of plasminogen activator (PA) and PA inhibitor in human colorectal adenocarcinomas. APMIS. 1993;101:235–41.
20. Sier CFM, Vloedgraven HJM, Ganesh S et al. Inactive urokinase and increased levels of its inhibitor type 1 in colorectal cancer liver metastasis. Gastroenterology. 1994;107:1449–56.
21. Vasishta A, Baker PR, Hopwood D, Holley PM, Cuschieri A. Proteinase-like peptidase activities in malignant and non-malignant gastric tissue. Br J Surg. 1985;72:386–8.
22. Watanbe M, Higashi T, Watanabe A et al. Cathepsin B and L activities in gastric cancer tissue: correlation with histological findings. Biochem Med Metab Biol. 1989;42:21–9.
23. Chung SM, Kawai K. Protease activities in gastric cancer tissues. Clin Chim Acta. 1990;189:205–10.
24. Takai S, Yamamura M, Tanaka K et al. Plasminogen activators in human gastric cancers: correlation with DNA ploidy and immunohistochemical staining. Int J Cancer. 1991;48:20–7.
25. Sier CFM, Verspaget HW, Griffioen G, Ganesh S, Vloedgraven HJM, Lamers CBHW. Plasminogen activators in normal tissue and carcinomas of the human oesophagus and stomach. Gut. 1993;34:80–5.
26. Nekarda H, Schmitt M, Ulm K et al. Prognostic impact of urokinase-type plasminogen activator and its inhibitor PAI-1 in completely resected gastric cancer. Cancer Res. 1994;54:2900–7.
27. Plebani M, Herszényi L, Cardin R et al. Cysteine and serine proteases in gastric cancer. Cancer. 1995;76:367–75.
28. De Bruin PAF, Griffioen G, Verspaget HW, Verheijen JH, Lamers CBHW. Plasminogen activators and tumor development in the human colon: activity levels in normal mucosa, adenomatous polyps and adenocarcinomas. Cancer Res. 1987;47:4654–7.
29. Farinati F, Plebani M, Di Mario F et al. Aspartic proteinases and gastrin in the diagnosis of gastric cancer and gastric precancerous changes. Eur J Gastroenterol Hepatol. 1993;5:707–12.
30. Samloff IM, Varis K, Ihamaki T, Siurala M, Rotter JI. Relationship among serum pepsinogen I, pepsinogen II, and gastric mucosal history. Gastroenterology. 1982;83:204–9.
31. Miki K, Ichinose M, Ishikawa KB et al. Clinical application of serum pepsinogen I and II levels for mass screening to detect gastric cancer. Jpn J Cancer Res. 1993;84:1086–90.
32. Matsukura N, Onda M, Tokunaga A et al. Significance of serum markers pepsinogen I and II for chronic atropic gastritis, peptic ulcer and gastric cancer. J Clin Gastroenterol. 1993;17:146–50.
33. Rugge M, Baffa R, Farinati F et al. Epithelial dysplasia in atrophic gastritis. Bioptical follow-up study. Ital J Gastroenterol. 1991;23:70–3.

34. Correa P. Chronic gastritis: a clinicopathologic classification. Am J Gastroenterol. 1988;83:504–9.
35. Price AB. The Sydney system. J Gastroenterol Hepatol. 1991;6:209–22.
36. Morson BC, Sobin LH, Grundmann E, Johansen A, Nagayo T, Serck-Hanssen A. Precancerous conditions and epithelial dysplasia in the stomach. J Clin Pathol. 1980;33:711–21.
37. Riddel RH, Goldman H, Ransohoff DF et al. Dysplasia in inflammatory bowel disease: standardized classification with provisional clinical application. Hum Pathol. 1983;14:9331–68.
38. Bradford MA. Rapid and sensitive method for the quantitation of microgram quantities of protein utilizing the principle of protein-dye binding. Anal Biochem. 1976;72:248–54.
39. Wodzinski MA, Bardhan KD, Reilly JT, Cooper P, Preston FE. Reduced tissue type plasminogen activator activity of the gastroduodenal mucosa in peptic ulcer disease. Gut. 1993;34:1310–4.
40. Nitti D, Farini R, Grassi F et al. Carcinoembryonic antigen in gastric cancer juice collected during endoscopy. Value in detecting high-risk patients and gastric cancer. Cancer. 1984;52:2334–7.
41. Farinati F, Nitti D, Cardin F et al. CA 19-9 determination in gastric juice: role in identifying cancer and high-risk patients. Eur J Cancer Clin Oncol. 1988;24:923–7.
42. Farinati F, Holmgren J, Di Mario F et al. CA 50 determination in body fluids: can we screen patients at risk for gastric cancer? Int J Cancer. 1991;47:7–11.
43. Saku T, Sakai H, Tsuda N, Okabe H, Kato Y, Yamamoto K. Cathepsin D and E in normal, metaplastic, dysplastic, and carcinomatous gastric tissue: an immunohistochemical study. Gut. 1990;31:1250–5.
44. Correa P. A human model of gastric carcinogenesis. Cancer Res. 1988;48:3554–60.
45. Correa P. Human gastric carcinogenesis: a multistep and multifactorial process – First American Cancer Society Award Lecture on cancer epidemiology and prevention. Cancer Res. 1992;52:6735–40.
46. Sipponen P, Kekki M, Siurala M. Atrophic chronic gastritis and intestinal metaplasia in gastric carcinoma. Cancer. 1983;52:1062–8.
47. Farinati F, Cardin F, Di Mario F et al. Follow-up in gastric dysplasia patients. Am J Surg Pathol. 1989;13:173–4.
48. Rugge M, Farinati F, Di Mario F, Baffa R, Valiante F, Cardin F. Gastric epithelial dysplasia: a prospective multicenter follow-up study from the Interdisciplinary Group on Gastric Epithelial Dysplasia. Hum Pathol. 1991;22:1002–8.
49. Farinati F, Rugge M, Di Mario F, Valiante F, Baffa R. Early and advanced gastric cancer in the follow-up of moderate and severe gastric dysplasia patients. A prospective study. Endoscopy. 1993;25:261–4.
50. Rugge M, Farinati F, Baffa R et al. Gastric epithelial dysplasia in the natural history of gastric cancer: a multicenter prospective follow-up study. Gastroenterology. 1994;107:1288–96.
51. Ming SC, Bajtai A, Correa P et al. Gastric dysplasia: significance and pathologic criteria. Cancer. 1984;54:1794–801.
52. Lansdown M, Quirke P, Dixon MF, Axon AT, Johnston D. High grade dysplasia of the gastric mucosa: a marker for gastric carcinoma. Gut. 1990;31:977–80.
53. De Dombal FT, Price AB, Thompson H et al. The British Society of Gastroenterology early gastric cancer/dysplasia survey: an interim report. Gut. 1990;31:115–20.
54. Shiao YH, Rugge M, Correa P, Lehmann HP, Scheer WD. p53 alteration in gastric precancerous lesions. Am J Pathol. 1994;144:511–17.
55. Correa P, Shiao Y. Phenotypic and genotypic events in gastric carcinogenesis. Cancer Res. 1994;54(Suppl):1941–3.
56. Reilly D, Christensen L, Duch M, Nolan N, Duff MJ, Andreasen PA. Type-1 plasminogen activator inhibitor in human breast carcinomas. Int J Cancer. 1992;50:208–14.
57. Kristensen P, Pyke C, Lund LR, Andreasen PA, Dano K. Plasminogen activator inhibitor type-1 in Lewis lung carcinoma. Histochemistry. 1990;93:559–66.

G Mószik et al. Cell Injury and Cytoprotection in the GI Tract. 187–195.
© 1997 Kluwer Academic Publishers.

INHIBITION OF RABBIT GASTRIC EPITHELIAL RESTORATION BY A WATER EXTRACT OF *HELICOBACTER PYLORI*: EVIDENCE USING A CULTURED CELL MODEL

N. SATO[1], S. WATANABE[1], X-E. WANG[1], M. HIROSE[1], H. OIDE[1],
T. KITAMURA[1], R. OHKURA[1], K. OTAKA[1], H. MIWA[1], A. MIYAZAKI[1],
M. AIHARA[2], A. AZUMA[2], K. IMAGAWA[2] AND M. KIKUCHI[2]

[1]Department of Gastroenterology, Juntendo University School of Medicine, 2-1-1 Hongo, Bunkyo-ku, Tokyo 113; [2]Microbiological Research Institute, Otsuka Pharmaceutical Co. Ltd., 463-10 Kagasuno, Kawauchi-cho, Tokushima 771-01, Japan

This paper was first published in: Inflammopharmacology. 1996;4:341–349.

ABSTRACT

The detailed mechanism of *H. pylori*-induced gastric damage is still unknown. In this study, we showed that a water extract of *H. pylori* retarded the epithelial restoration in a cultured rabbit gastric epithelial cell model with the inhibition of both cell migration and proliferation. Although this inhibitory substance has not yet been biochemically characterized, it is different from known *H. pylori* associate-cytotoxins and ammonia. From these results, we hypothesize that these bacteria directly play a role in disturbance of peptic ulcer healing in vivo.

Keywords: gastric epithelial cell, restoration, restitution, *Helicobacter pylori*, cytotoxin, peptic ulcer

INTRODUCTION

It has been shown that damage to the gastric surface epithelium is followed by rapid epithelial cell migration called 'restitution' after removal of the injurious agents. Silen and his colleagues described early mucosal restitution and showed its importance in the whole process of gastric wound repair [1,3]. In order to investigate the precise process of wound repair in gastric ulcer diseases, a new restoration model was designed using primary monolayer cultured rabbit gastric mucosal cell sheets [4]. This model allows the assessment of the cellular capacity for mucosal restoration without the effects of systemic factors. Our series of experiments clearly shows that growth factors, extracellular matrix and the cytoskeleton play an important role in mucosal repair in this model [4–8].

Accumulating evidence clearly shows that *Helicobacter pylori* induce severe inflammation in the gastric mucosa and play an important role in the pathogenesis of active chronic gastritis, peptic ulcers and even in gastric carcinoma [9–13]. The detailed mechanism by which *H. pylori* contribute to the pathogenesis is still unclear. *H. pylori*

This paper was presented at the Symposium on 'Cell injury and protection in the gastrointestinal tract: from basic science to clinical perspectives', October 8–11, 1995, Pécs, Hungary.

have been reported to injure gastric epithelial cells by producing ammonia [14], cytotoxins called CagA (cytotoxin-associated gene A) gene product [15] and Vac A gene product (vacuolating cytotoxin) [16]. It has also been reported that *H. pylori* produce and release chemotactic substances that activate neutrophils and macrophages; the activated cells then cause gastric mucosal injury through the production of cytokines [17–19]. Recent studies showed that a water extract of *H. pylori* exhibited chemotactic activity for inflammatory cells and caused microvascular dysfunction [20,21]. However, the detailed mechanism of effects of *H. pylori* on peptic ulcer healing is entirely unknown.

In this study, we describe the effects of a water extract of *H. pylori* on gastric epithelial restoration using a recently developed gastric wound repair model with primary cultured rabbit gastric epithelial cells [4]. This model allows the quantitative assessment of epithelial restoration which includes cell migration and proliferation after artificial wounding in the confluent cell sheet.

MATERIALS AND METHODS

Helicobacter pylori

H. pylori used in this study were obtained from ATCC (strain ATCC 43504, American Type Culture Collection, Rockville, MD) and Otsuka Pharmaceutical Co. Ltd. (strain 0002, clinically isolated strain from chronic gastritis patients, Otsuka Pharmaceutical Company, Tokushima, Japan). A water extract of *H. pylori* was prepared according to the method reported by Yoshida et al. [21]. Briefly, *H. pylori* were grown in a brucella broth with 7% fetal bovine serum for 3 days. *H. pylori* were harvested with sterile cotton swabs into sterile distilled water, using 1 ml per plate (10^{11}–10^{12} *H. pylori*) and were kept at room temperature for 20 min. Then the *H. pylori* suspension was centrifuged at 17 000g for 15 min at 4°C. The resultant supernatant is the initial water extract of *H. pylori* and was stored at –20°C until use. Before use, an *H. pylori* water extract was re-centrifuged at 38 000g for 20 min. The extract was used at a final protein concentration of 50 µg/ml or 100 µg/ml and was added to the culture medium just after wounding, according to our previously described methods [4].

Detection of CagA gene

The CagA gene of *H. pylori* used in this study was detected using the primer reported by Tummuru et al., and all the procedures for polymerized chain reaction were carried out according to their report [22].

Cell culture and wound repair assay

Gastric epithelial cells were isolated from male Japanese white rabbits weighing 2.0 kg according to the methods described previously [4]. Briefly, the gastric mucosa was separated, minced, and incubated in a medium containing 0.07% collagenase (type I, Sigma Chemicals, St Louis, MO) for 15 min at 37°C. After the incubation, the tissue was washed with Ca^{2+}- and Mg^{2+}-free Hanks' balanced salt solution with 1 mmol/L EDTA. These procedures were repeated three times before the tissue was filtered through metal mesh (diameter 300 μm). Isolated cells were inoculated onto collagen-type-I-coated plastic culture dishes (diameter 60 mm, Corning Glass Works, Corning, NY) at a concentration of 5×10^6 cells per dish and cultured in a Coon's modified Ham's F-12 medium supplemented with inactivated 10% fetal bovine serum, 100 U/ml penicillin, 100 μg/ml streptomycin and 0.25 μg/ml amphotericin. Cells were kept in a 5% CO_2 incubator at 37°C.

The effects of a water extract of *H. pylori* on gastric epithelial cell restoration were assessed by the methods reported previously [4]. Forty-eight hours after the inoculation, gastric epithelial cells formed a complete monolayer cell sheet in which the majority (more than 90%) of cells were periodic acid–Schiff (PAS) staining-positive mucous cells [4]. A round shaped artificial wound with a cell-free area of constant size (2 mm^2) was made in the centre of the cell sheet without damaging the dish surface [4]. The process of epithelial restoration was monitored using an inverted phase-contrast microscope (Nikon TMD, Nikon, Tokyo) equipped with a time-lapse laser videodisc recorder (LVR-3000N, Sony, Tokyo) and the change in the cell-free area during restoration was quantitatively analysed by an image analyser (IBAS II, Carl Zeiss Japan, Tokyo).

DNA synthesizing cells were sequentially detected using indirect immunohistochemical methods with monoclonal anti-bromodeoxyuridine (BrdU, Sigma Chemicals) antibody during the process of restoration every 12 h and the BrdU labelling index (LI) around the wound was calculated according to the previous report [5]. Briefly, in the first group, BrdU (10 μg/ml) was added to the medium immediately after wounding and then incubated for 12 h; then the cells were processed for the immunostaining. In the second group, BrdU was added 12 h after wounding and the incubation was continued for an additional 12 h. In the third group, BrdU was added 24 h after wounding, and, in the fourth group, it was added 36 h after wounding. After staining, microscopic pictures were taken and BrdU-positive cells were calculated over a unit area (0.05 mm^2).

The effects of a water extract of *H. pylori* were assessed by adding it to the medium just after wounding at a protein concentration of 50 μg/ml and 100 μg/ml.

All the experiments were performed in triplicate from five separate cell preparations ($n = 5$); the results were expressed as means $\pm$ standard deviation and statistical analysis was performed using analysis of variance and non-paired Student's *t*-test.

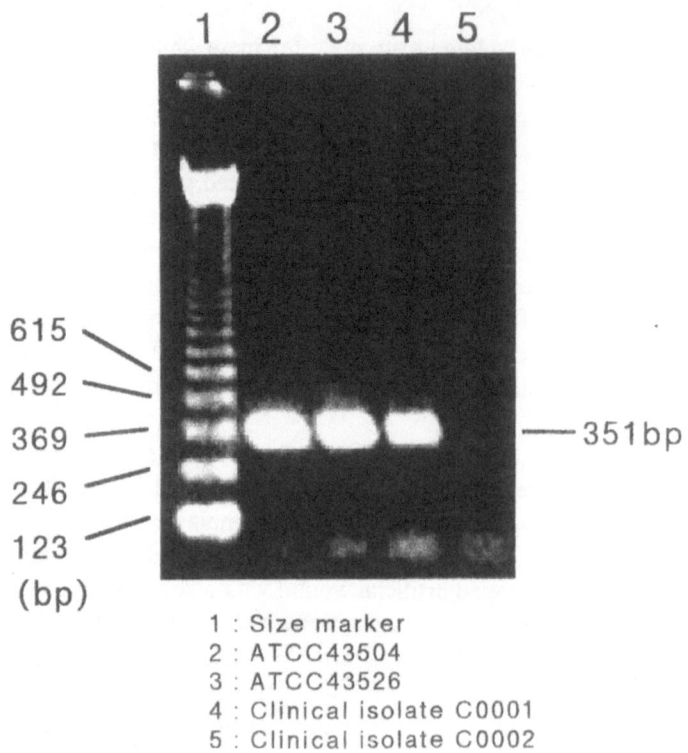

Figure 1. Polymerase chain reaction for the CagA gene. ATCC 43504 is a CagA-gene-positive strain and C-0002 is a CagA-gene-negative strain

RESULTS

Polymerase chain reaction of CagA gene revealed that ATCC 43504 is a CagA-gene-positive strain and C-0002 is a CagA-negative strain (Figure 1).

In controls, just after wounding, cells on the edge of the wound began to form pseudopodia-like structures (lamellipodia) that started ruffling and moving towards the centre of the cell-free area to repopulate; lamellipodia disappeared after complete restoration. This cell migration occurred with a form of sheet migration (Figure 1). The cell-free area was repopulated in a time-dependent manner (Figure 2).

In the groups treated with extracts of both ATCC 43504 and C-0002, the speed of epithelial restoration was much slower than controls. The cell-free area was not repaired completely even 48 h after wounding in both ATCC 43504 and C-0002 groups (Table 1; Figure 2), the suppressive effect being concentration-dependent.

In addition, the extracts of ATCC 43504 caused a dramatic morphological change in the epithelial cells. Several hours after addition of the extract, small vacuoles began to form in the cell cytoplasm. The vacuoles fused together and then increased in size.

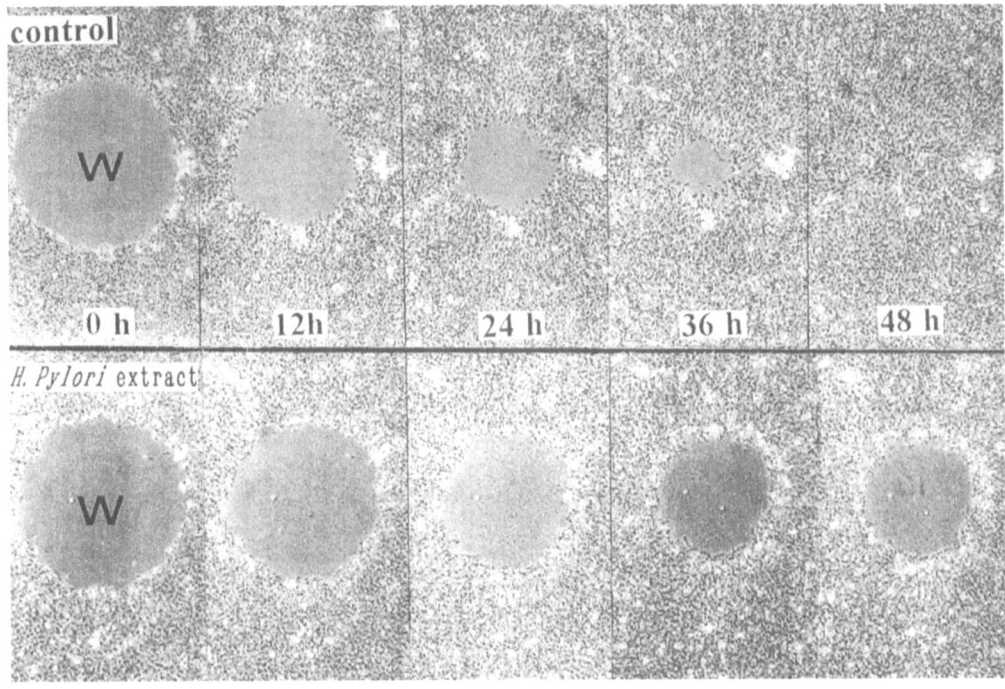

Figure 2. Phase-contrast micrographs showing the process of gastric epithelial restoration. In the control, restoration was complete within 48 h. A water extract of C-0002 inhibited the restoration process. W: artificial wound; original magnification × 40

TABLE 1
Quantitative analysis of wound repair: cell-free area in mm^2

	Wounding	12 h	24 h	36 h	48 h
Control	2.0 ±0.06	1.0 ±0.06	0.46±0.10	0.14±0.04	0±0
ATCC 43504					
50 µg/ml	2.02±0.07	0.98±0.07	0.56±0.10	0.32±0.11**	0.06±0.04*
100 µg/ml	2.0 ±0.06	1.24±0.04**	0.88±0.07**	0.64±0.10**	0.5 ±0.06**
C-0002					
50 µg/ml	2.02±0.04	0.98±0.07	0.54±0.08	0.34±0.08**	0.12±0.11
100 µg/ml	2.02±0.07	1.12±0.11	0.74±0.10**	0.64±0.12**	0.48±0.07**

All results are mean±SEM. Significantly different (Student's *t*-test) from control group: *$p<0.05$, **$p<0.01$, $n=5$

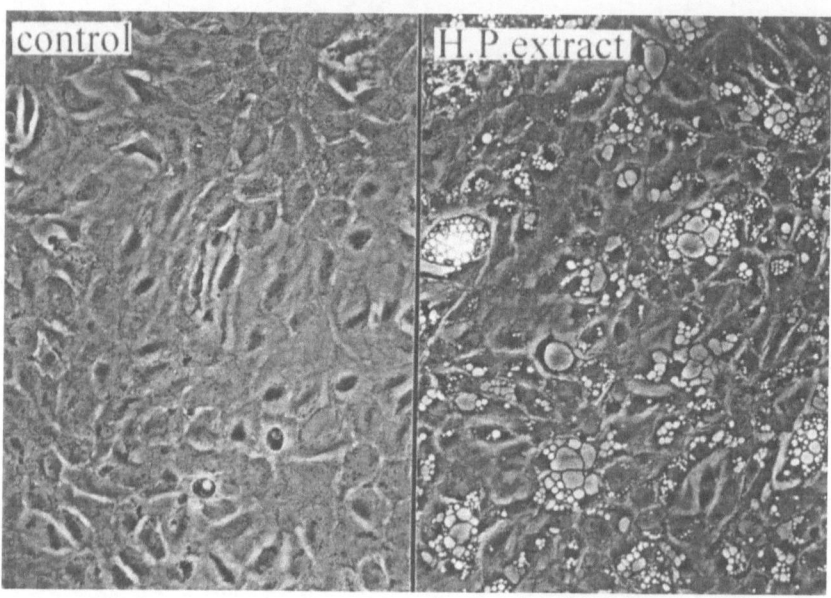

Figure 3. Phase-contrast micrographs showing vacuole formation in gastric epithelial cells. A water extract of ATCC 43504 caused vacuolization. × 150

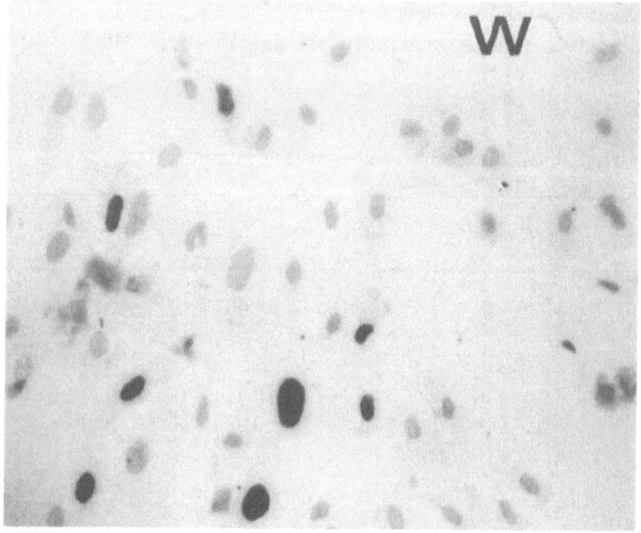

Figure 4. Cell proliferation during the process of restoration. Proliferating cells were detected around the wound by BrdU staining methods. W: wound. × 200

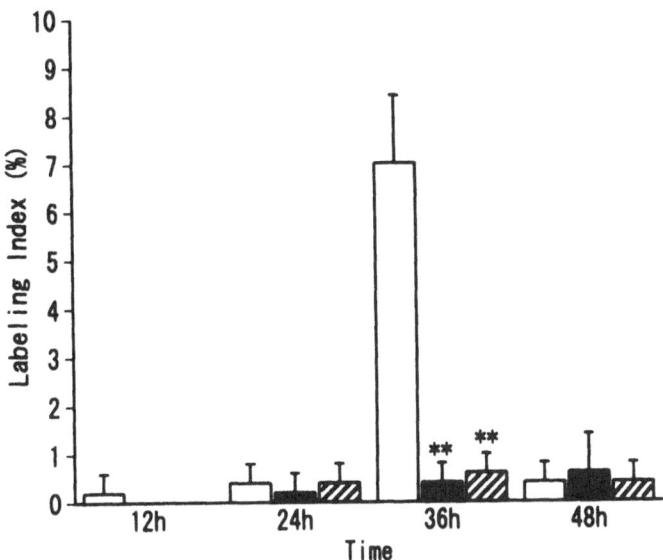

Figure 5. The sequential change of labelling index during the process of restoration. In controls (□), the number of BrdU-positive cells reached a peak level in the 36-h group. Water extracts of both ATCC 43504 (■) and C-0002 (□) had an inhibitory effect on cell proliferation. **$p < 0.05$, $n = 5$

Although no cells had vacuoles in the cytoplasm before addition of the extract, vacuoles were detected in $51.6 \pm 5.8\%$ of cells 24 h, and $90.2 \pm 4.1\%$ of cells 48 h, after addition of the extract (100 μg/ml; Figure 3). This vacuolization was dose-dependent and reversible. In contrast, the extract of C-0002 did not cause vacuolization in cultured epithelial cells.

All BrdU-positive cells were detected only around the cell-free area (Figure 4). Sequential staining of controls revealed that BrdU-positive cells were rarely detected in either 12-h (LI 0.2%) and 24-h (LI 0.4%) groups after wounding. The number of BrdU-positive cells reached peak levels in the 36-h group (LI 7.0%) and were rarely detected after complete repair at 48 h (LI 0.4%). The appearance of BrdU-positive cells was significantly suppressed in groups treated with extracts of both ATCC 43504 and C-0002. The labelling index was negligible throughout the experiment in the water-extract group (Figure 5).

DISCUSSION

The results of the polymerase chain reaction indicate that ATCC 43504 contains the CagA gene whereas C-0002 does not. Moreover, bioassay using cultured gastric epithelial cells showed that ATCC 43504 has a vacuolating cytotoxin, unlike C-0002.

These cytotoxins have been reported to produce vacuoles in the eukaryotic cells [16] and were believed to play a central role in the pathogenesis of *H. pylori*-associated diseases. We detected vacuole formation in primary cultured gastric epithelial cells. In this study, we show clearly that water extracts of *H. pylori* from both the CagA-gene-positive vacuolating toxin-positive strain and the CagA-negative vacuolating cyto-toxin-negative strain inhibited gastric epithelial cell migration and proliferation. Thus, this inhibitory effect on epithelial restoration was not caused by CagA gene products or vacuolating cytotoxin. Another major candidate for the inhibitory effect of *H. pylori* is ammonia, which is produced by bacterial urease. However, in this culture system, urea, the source of ammonia, was not present in the medium. Therefore, we can eliminate the role of ammonia in this study.

Water extracts from *H. pylori* have been reported to contain substances that increase the adhesion glycoproteins on neutrophils [21], increase neutrophil chemotactic activity, elicit an oxidative burst response from neutrophils, and promote leukocyte adhesion, emigration and albumin leakage from the venules and activated macro-phages and monocytes [23–25]. The identity of the proinflammatory factors in *H. pylori* water extracts is not known. Yoshida et al. indicated that the main proinflammatory factor was different from bacterial urease, cytotoxin and lipopolysaccharide, and they suspected that the phenomenon could be attributed to unknown factors, with a molecular weight of 25 000 or less, which are identified only from *H. pylori* extracts [21]. In the present study, the causative factors for the inhibition of gastric epithelial cell migration and proliferation are unknown but the effects of these factors disappeared after heat treatment (100°C, 5 min) and a water extract of *E. coli* did not contain this inhibitory factor (data not shown). This is the first evidence to show the direct suppressive effects of *H. pylori* water extract on gastric mucosal repair. The goal of future studies will be to analyse and identify the causative factors.

REFERENCES

1. Ito S, Lacy ER, Rutten MJ, Critchow J, Silen W. Rapid repair of injured gastric mucosa. Scand J Gastroenterol. 1984;19(Suppl.101):87–95.
2. Svanes K, Takeuchi K, Ito S, Silen S. Restitution of the surface epithelium of the in vitro frog gastric mucosa after damage with hyperosmolar sodium chloride. Morphological and physiological character-istics. Gastroenterology. 1982;83:1409–26.
3. Silen W, Ito S. Mechanism for rapid reepithelization of the gastric mucosal surface. Annu Rev Physiol. 1985;47:217–19.
4. Watanabe S, Hirose M, Yasuda T, Sato N. Role of actin and calmodulin in migration and proliferation of rabbit gastric mucosal cells in culture. Gastroenterol Hepatol. 1994;9:325–33.
5. Watanabe S, Hirose M, Wang XE et al. Hepatocyte growth factor accelerated the wound repair of cultured gastric mucosal cells. Biochem Biophys Res Commun. 1994;199:1453–60.
6. Watanabe S, Wang XE, Hirose M, Sato N. Effect of myosin light chain kinase inhibitor wortmannin on the wound repair of cultured gastric mucosal cells. Biochem Biophys Res Commun. 1994;199:799–806.
7. Mikami H, Watanabe S, Hirose M, Sato N. Role of extracellular matrix in wound repair by cultured gastric mucosal cells. Biochem Biophys Res Commun. 1994;202:285–92.
8. Watanabe S, Wang XE, Hirose M et al. Platelet-derived growth factor accelerates gastric epithelial restoration in a rabbit cultured cell model. Gastroenterology. 1996;110:775–9.
9. Axon AH. *H. pylori* and gastroduodenal disease. Practitioner. 1991;235:733–6.

10. Blaser MJ. Hypothesis on the pathogenesis and natural history of *Helicobacter pylori*-induced inflammation. Gastroenterology. 1992;102:720–7.
11. Cover TL. *Helicobacter pylori* and gastroduodenal disease. Annu Rev Med. 1992;43:135–45.
12. Graham DY. *Helicobacter pylori*: its epidemiology and its role in duodenal ulcer disease. J Gastroenterol Hepatol. 1991;6:97–105.
13. Megraud F, Lamouliatte H. *Helicobacter pylori* and duodenal ulcer: evidence suggesting causation. Dig Dis Sci. 1992;37:769–72.
14. Megraud F, Neman-Simha V, Brugmann D. Further evidence of the toxic effect of ammonia produced by *Helicobacter*. Infect Immun. 1992;60:1858–63.
15. Covacci A, Censini S, Bugnoli M et al. Molecular characterization of the 128-kDa immunodominant antigen of *Helicobacter pylori* associated with cytotoxicity and duodenal ulcer. Proc Natl Acad Sci USA. 1993;90:5791–5.
16. Cover TL. Purification and characterization of vacuolating toxin from *Helicobacter pylori*. J Biol Chem. 1992;267:10570–5.
17. Craig PM, Territo MC, Karnes WE, Walsh JH. *Helicobacter pylori* secretes a chemotactic factor for monocytes and neutrophils. Gut. 1992;33:1020–3.
18. Graham DY. Pathogenic mechanisms leading to *Helicobacter pylori*-induced inflammation. Eur J Gastroenterol Hepatol. 1992;4:S9–S16.
19. Wallace JL. Possible mechanisms and mediators of gastritis associated with *Helicobacter pylori* infection. Scand J Gastroenterol. 1991;26(Suppl.187):65–70.
20. Kurose I, Granger DN, Evans DJ Jr et al. *Helicobacter pylori*-induced microvascular protein leakage in rats: Role of neutrophils, mast cells, and platelets. Gastroenterology. 1994;107:70–9.
21. Yoshida N, Granger DN, Evans DJ Jr et al. Mechanisms involved in *Helicobacter pylori*-induced inflammation. Gastroenterology. 1993;105:1431–40.
22. Tummuru MR, Cover TL, Blaser MJ. Cloning and expression of a high-molecular-mass major antigen of *Helicobacter pylori*: Evidence of linkage to cytotoxin production. Infect Immun. 1993;61:1799–809.
23. Mai UEH, Perez-Perez GI, Wahl LM, Wahl SM, Blaser MJ, Smith PD. Soluble surface proteins from *Helicobacter pylori* activate monocytes/macrophages by lipopolysaccharide-independent mechanism. J Clin Invest. 1991;87:894–900.
24. Mai UEH, Perez-Perez GI, Allen JB, Wahl SM, Blaser MJ, Smith PD. Surface proteins from *Helicobacter pylori* exhibit chemotactic activity for human leukocytes and are present in gastric mucosa. J Exp Med. 1992;175:517–25.
25. Neisen H, Andersen LP. Chemotactic activity of *Helicobacter pylori* sonicate for human polymorphonuclear leucocytes and monocytes. Gut. 1992;33:738–42.

Section III

CELL INJURY AND PROTECTION IN SMALL INTESTINE AND IN THE LARGE BOWEL

G Mózsik et al. Cell Injury and Cytoprotection in the GI Tract. 199–206.
© 1997 Kluwer Academic Publishers.

ZINC SULPHATE HEALING EFFECTS ON CYSTEAMINE-INDUCED DUODENAL ULCER IN THE RAT

B. TROSKOT[1*], V.N. SIMICEVIC[2], M. DODIG[1], I. ROTKVIC[1], D. IVANKOVIC[3] AND M. DUVNJAK[1]

[1]Department of Gastroenterology, University Hospital "Sestre Milosrdnice", Medical School, University of Zagreb, Zagreb, Croatia; [2]PLIVA Pharmaceutical Company, Research Institute, Biomedical Department, Zagreb, Croatia; [3]Department of Statistics, Epidemiology and Informatics, School of Public Health Andrija Stampar, Medical School, University of Zagreb, Zagreb, Croatia
*Correspondence

ABSTRACT

Since zinc is an important requirement for the growth and repair of epithelial tissue, the aim of this study was to focus on the healing influence of $ZnSO_4$ on cysteamine-induced duodenal ulcer in the rat. Prior to the healing study, a separate study was carried out to determine the rate of spontaneous healing. Animals were sacrificed 7, 14, 21 and 28 days following cysteamine application and zinc concentrations in serum and tissue samples were determined using atomic absorption spectro-photometry. Animals used in the healing study received daily treatment with $ZnSO_4$ at a dose of 80 mg/kg body weight given orally starting 24 h after cysteamine application and were sacrificed 7, 14 and 21 days following cysteamine application. The serum and tissue levels of zinc as well as its antiulcerogenic effect were determined. To assess the absorption of $ZnSO_4$ a single dose of the substance (80 mg/kg body weight) was administered intragastrically to ten animals that did not receive cysteamine. The results of our study indicate that duodenal lesions induced with cysteamine spontaneously heal four weeks following its application. Spontaneous healing of the ulcer lesion was associated with positive shifts in zinc metabolism which returned to normal values upon ulcer healing. Daily treatment with $ZnSO_4$ progressively accelerated ulcer healing, and ulcers completely healed within one week of treatment. Shifts in zinc serum and tissue in this group were similar to shifts in the spontaneously healed group. A single intragastric treatment of zinc sulphate did not modify the normal aspect of the duodenal mucosa or serum and tissue concentrations.

Keywords: zinc sulphate, cysteamine, duodenum, ulcer healing, rat

INTRODUCTION

Zinc is an essential element for most organisms. Compared with most other trace elements, it is relatively non-toxic in vivo [1] and has been shown to be a functionally essential component of more than 200 enzymes encompassing all known classes of them as oxydoreductases, transferases, hydrolases, lyases, isomerases and lygases. Zinc ions are also important for the biosynthesis and catabolism of proteins. The synthesis of DNA and RNA is controlled by this element [2].

This paper was presented at the Symposium on 'Cell injury and protection in the gastrointestinal tract: from basic science to clinical perspectives', October 8–11, 1995, Pécs, Hungary.

The protective effect of zinc on the organism led to investigations of its influence on experimental stress lesions of the gastric mucosa. Oral administration of zinc salts have been shown to enhance the rate of healing in human gastric ulcers and to protect against experimental ulcers in different animal models including gastric ulceration induced by ethanol, cold-restraint stress, electric vagal stimulation, reserpine and acetic acid administration [2–4]. Previous reports have suggested that the antiulcerative effects of zinc could be due to several mechanisms, such as inhibition of histamine release from mast cells within the gastric mucosa [5], improvement of gastric microcirculation [6], an increase in the production of gastric mucus [7], stimulation of prostaglandin biosynthesis [8] and stabilization of biological membrane integrity including those of lysosomes [9].

However, little is known about zinc activity in duodenal ulcer disease. The aim of this study was, therefore, to focus on the influence of the healing effects of $ZnSO_4$ on duodenal ulcers in the rat. Duodenal ulcers were induced with cysteamine since this model has a similar pathomorphological history to that of human ulcers [10].

MATERIALS AND METHODS

Female Wistar rats, randomly assigned, ten rats to each group, 180–250 g body weight, were used in the experiment. They were housed in a temperature- ($22 \pm 1°C$) and humidity- (65–70%) controlled room. The animals were given food and tap water ad libitum throughout the entire study. Immediately after the experiment, the animals were sacrificed by decapitation.

Duodenal ulcers were induced by an already established noxious regimen. Cysteamine (cysteamine–HCl obtained from Aldrich Chemical Co.) was dissolved in distilled water and administered subcutaneously at a dose of 400 mg/kg [10].

Prior to the healing study, a separate study was carried out to determine the rate of spontaneous healing. Animal groups were sacrificed 7, 14, 21 and 28 days following cysteamine application and zinc concentrations in the serum and tissue samples were determined using atomic absorption spectrophotometry (AAS) [11]. Animals used in the healing study received daily treatment with $ZnSO_4$ at a dose of 80 mg/kg body weight [12, personal unpublished results] given orally starting 24 h after cysteamine and were sacrificed 7, 14 and 21 days following cysteamine application. The serum and tissue levels of zinc, as well as its antiulcerogenic effect were determined.

Duodenal lesions were assessed in the following manner. The degree of ulceration was assessed by averaging the haemorrhagic lesion sizes measured across their largest diameters. In the case of petechiae, five such lesions were taken as the equivalent of a 1-mm lesion [12]. The total lesion length in each group of rats divided by the number of the animals was expressed as the ulcer index.

Blood samples for the assessment of zinc concentration were taken from the carotid arteries into specially prepared test tubes. Following the assessment of duodenal lesions, duodenal tissue samples were also taken. Serum zinc concentrations (µg/ml) were determined using AAS [13]. Tissue samples were mineralized by the ashing procedure [14] and zinc concentrations (µg/g) were also determined by AAS. Quality control was achieved by comparison with references for blood and tissue, respectively (Seronorm Batch No. 116, Nycomed Pharma AS, Norway; SRM 1577, National Bureau of Standards, USA).

Ten unstressed animals served as a healthy control group.

To assess the absorption of $ZnSO_4$, a single dose of the substance (80 mg/kg body weight) was administered intragastrically to ten animals that did not receive cysteamine.

Results are expressed as mean $\pm$ SEM. The differences between means was compared using analysis of variance (ANOVA) followed by Dunnett's test. Differences were considered significant at a level of $p \leqslant 0.05$.

RESULTS

The results of our study confirm that, when applied subcutaneously, cysteamine induces duodenal lesions in rats. These lesions can vary in size and intensity ranging from petechiae to perforating ulcers and achieve their maximum diameter 24 h following cysteamine application. These lesions show a tendency to heal spontaneously within a period of four weeks with the most rapid healing rate being in the first week (Figure 1).

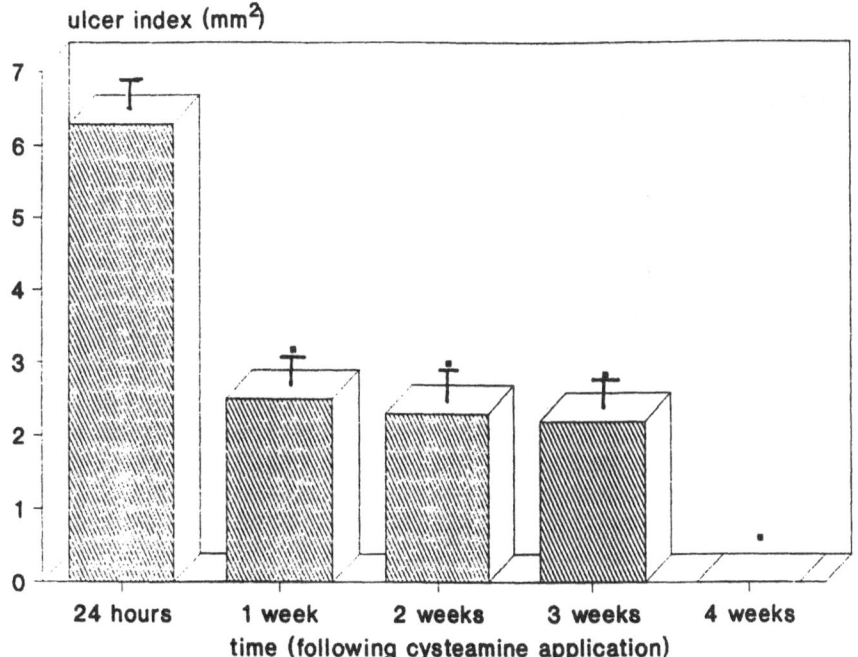

Figure 1. Spontaneous healing of duodenal ulcers induced with cysteamine. Ulcer index (mm^2) expressed as mean $\pm$ SEM; $n = 10$ animals per group; ■ $= p < 0.05$ vs. 24-h cysteamine

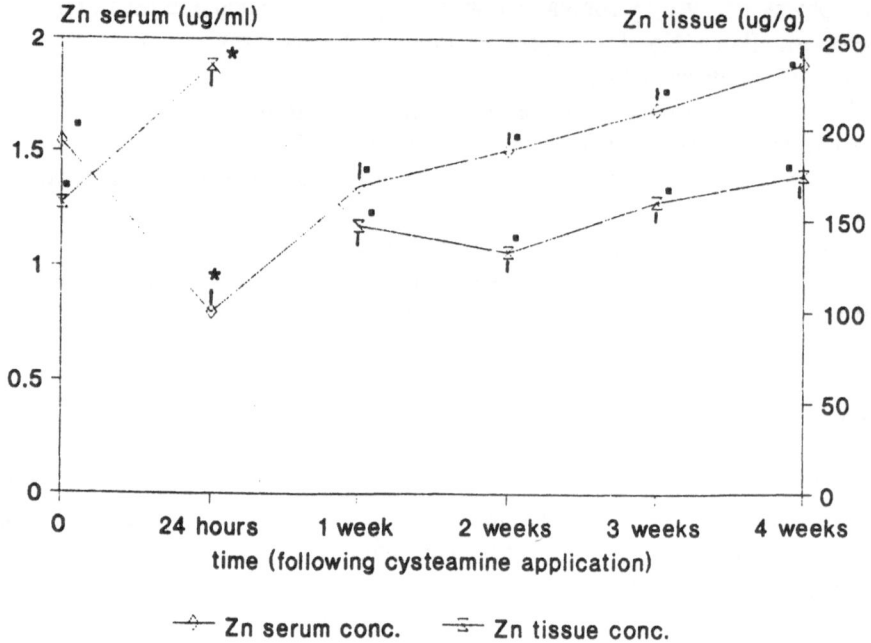

Figure 2. Dynamics of zinc serum (μg/ml) and tissue (μg/g) concentrations during the onset and spontaneous healing of duodenal ulcers. $n = 10$ animals per group; $*p < 0.05$ vs. healthy controls (time 0), ■ $= p < 0.05$ vs. 24-h cysteamine

The spontaneous healing of ulcer lesions was associated with certain shifts in zinc serum and tissue concentrations which could also be noted in the period of the onset and development of the lesions (report in preparation). With the onset of duodenal lesions, zinc serum concentrations significantly decreased, while there was a significant increase in duodenal tissue concentrations, when compared with the healthy control group. Tissue concentrations decreased and returned to starting values within the first week. This decrease in zinc tissue concentration corresponded to the healing rate of the duodenal ulcers (Figure 1). Serum zinc concentrations also returned to starting values within the first week (Figure 2). Aside from significant differences in zinc serum and tissue concentrations in the 24-h group, no difference was noted when groups were analysed among themselves (Table 1).

Daily oral administration of zinc sulphate at a dose of 80 mg/kg body weight, starting 24 h after cysteamine application, significantly accelerated ulcer healing and ulcers completely healed during the first week of treatment (Table 1). Shifts in zinc serum and tissue concentrations in this group (Figure 3) were similar to those of zinc concentrations in the spontaneous healing group (Figure 2). The comparison of zinc tissue concentrations between the spontaneous healing group and the zinc sulphate-treated group showed a statistically significant difference only at the first week time period and a significance in zinc serum concentrations in the second week (Table 1).

TABLE 1
The mean values of serum zinc and tissue concentrations and ulcer index in the investigated groups

Group	Serum Zn concentration (µg/ml)	Tissue Zn concentration (µg/g)	Ulcer index (mm²)
Healthy control (time 0)	1.5400[b]	158.6674[b]	0[b]
Cysteamine alone			
24 h	0.8000[a]	235.3613[a]	6.3[a]
1 week	1.3500[b]	147.3138[bc]	2.5[a,b]
2 weeks	1.5100[b,c]	133.2125[b]	2.3[a,b]
3 weeks	1.6900[b]	160.6775[b]	2.2[a,b]
4 weeks	1.8850[b]	174.5250[b]	0[b]
Cysteamine + ZnSO$_4$			
1 week	1.2825[a,b]	133.4875[b,c]	0[b]
2 weeks	1.1637[a,b,c,d]	138.9125[b]	0[b]
3 weeks	1.4100[b,d]	·145.9125[b]	0[b]
ZnSO$_4$ alone	1.5713[b]	138.4625[b]	0[b]

[a] $= p < 0.05$ vs. healthy control; [b] $= p < 0.05$ vs. 24-h cysteamine; [c] $= p < 0.05$ vs. corresponding time period among groups; [d] $= p < 0.05$ values within the same group

A single intragastric administration of zinc sulphate did not modify the normal aspect of the duodenal mucosa or the zinc serum and tissue concentrations ($p > 0.05$ vs. healthy animals; Table 1).

DISCUSSION

Studies that have been described over the years mainly focused on the protective effects of various zinc compounds on the prevention of acute gastric lesions [2–9,12,15–21]. Since little is known about the activity of zinc in the duodenal mucosa, we investigated the healing effects of zinc sulphate on cysteamine-induced duodenal ulcers in rats.

Our study demonstrated that oral administration of zinc exerted a dramatic healing activity in cysteamine-induced duodenal ulcers. This finding was also backed by the fact that it was possible to measure an increase in the zinc concentrations of the target tissue damaged by the noxious procedure. The increase of zinc tissue concentrations in stress have already been confirmed in the heart, kidney and muscles [22]. Our results confirm that zinc accumulates in the damaged duodenal tissue. A balance also exists between serum zinc concentration and the zinc content in the target tissue damaged by the noxious procedure.

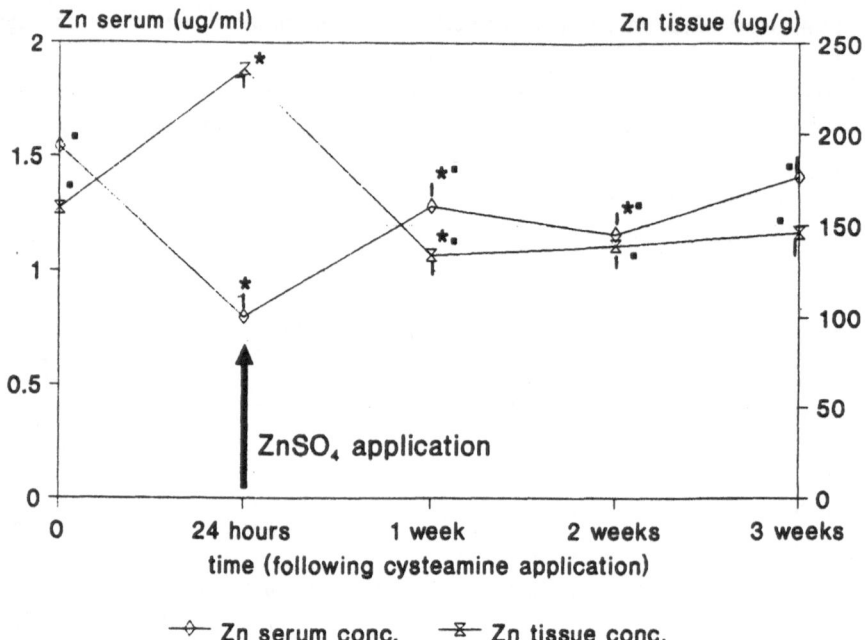

Figure 3. Dynamics of zinc serum (μg/ml) and tissue (μg/g) concentrations during the healing of ulcers in animals treated with ZnSO4. $n = 10$ animals per group; *$p < 0.05$ vs. healthy control (time 0), ■ = $p < 0.05$ vs. 24-h cysteamine

Despite the correlation between the changes in zinc concentrations and gastric ulcer healing, the healing pathway is not fully understood. However, several theories have been postulated. It has been suggested that zinc stablizes biological membranes by binding to sulphohydryl groups and forming mercapto-peptides [18]. Since zinc is an essential component of the superoxide dismutase enzyme [23], it protects against free radicals [19]. Additionally, the element is crucial for the synthesis of proteins as well as DNA and RNA [2].

Zinc compounds have been proved to preserve defence mechanisms which could contribute to increased resistance to ulceration and, in addition to this, have been shown to reduce gastric acid secretion when given in a pretreatment regimen [12,21,24]. This defence is very convincing in duodenal ulcer healing. The same protective role of zinc against cysteamine-induced duodenal ulcers could also be observed in pretreatment trials (report in preparation). This protection is dose and route-dependent. Only the per-os route exerted a protective action. On the basis of these experiments we focused on the healing effects of zinc.

In our study, the largest duodenal lesions (ulcer index 6.3) were observed 24 h following cysteamine application. At the same time, a dramatic decrease in the zinc serum concentration was noted as well as an obvious increase in duodenal tissue concentration. Both values were statistically significant when compared with healthy controls animals. In the groups of animals treated with zinc sulphate, all duodenal lesions healed within one week which corresponded to data of other authors who investigated the healing properties of zinc in gastric lesions [3,6–8,12,16,20,21,25]. A significantly higher zinc tissue concentration in the spontaneous healing group (ulcer index 2.5) vs. the $ZnSO_4$-treated group (ulcer index 0) in the first week of our experiment is most probably due to the fact that duodenal lesions still exist in the untreated group.

Taking together all these data, the positive influence of zinc in the protection and healing of gastroduodenal lesions in obvious, both in experimental conditions as well as in human disease [26], although further studies to determine the precise mechanism of these effects must be undertaken.

ACKNOWLEDGEMENTS

The authors wish to express their thanks to Dr Maja Blanusa PhD, and Durda Breski of the Institute for Medical Research and Occupational Health, Zagreb, Croatia for their contribution to this work.

REFERENCES

1. Borovansky J, Riley PA. Cytotoxicity of zinc in vitro. Chem–Biol Interact. 1989;69:279–91.
2. Cho CH. Current views of zinc as a gastrohepatic protective agent. Drug Devel Res. 1989;17:185–97.
3. Wong SH, Cho CH, Ogle CW. Protection by zinc sulphate against ethanol-induced ulceration: preservation of the gastric mucosal barrier. Pharmacology. 1986;33:94–102.
4. Cho CH, Ogle CW, Dai S. Acute gastric ulcer formation in response to electrical vagal stimulation in rats. Eur J Pharmacol. 1976;35:215–19.
5. Ogle CW, Lau HK. Disodium cromoglycate: its influence on gastric ulcers produced by stress in rats. IRCS Med Sci. 1979;7:393–4.
6. Lloris JM, Esplugues JV, Sarria B et al. Effects of zinc sulphate on gastric mucosal blood flow and gastric emptying in the rat. J Pharm Pharmacol. 1988;40:60–1.
7. Esplugues JV, Bulbena O, Escolar G, Marti-Bonmati E, Esplugues J. Effects of zinc acexamate on gastric mucosal resistance factors. Eur J Pharmacol. 1985;109:145–51.
8. Navarro C, Escolar G, Banos JE, Casanovas LI, Bulbena O. Effect of zinc acexamate on gastric mucosal production of prostaglandin E2 in normal and stressed rats. Prostagl Leucotrienes Essential Fatty Acids. 1988;33:75–80.
9. Pfeiffer CJ, Bulbena O, Esplugues JV, Escolar G, Navarro C, Esplugues J. Antiulcer and membrane stabilizing actions of zinc acexamate. Arch Inter Pharmacodyn. 1987;285:148–57.
10. Seyle H, Szabo S. Experimental model for production of perforating duodenal ulcers by cysteamine in the rat. Nature. 1973;244:458–9.
11. International Atomic Energy Agency. Elemental analysis of biological materials: current problems and techniques with special reference to trace elements. Technical report series No. 197. Vienna; 1980.
12. Cho CH, Ogle CW. A correlative study of the antiulcer effects of zinc sulphate in stressed rats. Eur J Pharmacol. 1978;48:97–105.
13. Momcilovic B, Belonje B, Shah BG. Effect of the matrix of the standard on results of atomic absorption spectrophotometry of zinc in serum. Clin Chem. 1975;21:588–90.
14. Blanusa M, Breski D. Comparison of dry and wet ashing procedure for cadmium and iron determination in biological material by atomic absorption spectrophotometry. Talanta. 1981;28:681–4.
15. Kong ML. Effect of zinc sulphate on acetic acid-induced gastric ulceration in rats. J Pharm Pharmacol. 1990;42:657–9.

16. Escolar G, Camarasa J, Navarro C, Vernetta C, Bulbena O. Antiulcerogenic activity of zinc acexamate in different experimental models. Meth Find Exp Clin Pharmacol. 1987;9:423–7.
17. Navarro C, Ramis A, Sendros S, Bulbena O, Ferrer LL, Escolar G. Relationship between gastric levels and antiulcerogenic activity of zinc. Arch Int Pharmacodyn. 1990;307:119–29.
18. Cho CH, Luk CT, Ogle CW. The membrane-stabilizing action of zinc carnosine in stress-induced gastric ulceration in rats. Life Sci. 1991;49:PL189–94.
19. Cho CH, Hui WM, Chen BW, Luk CT, Lam SK. The cytoprotective effect of zinc L-carnosine on ethanol-induced gastric gland damage in rabbits. J Pharm Pharmacol. 1992;44:364–5.
20. Cho CH, Chen BW, Poon YK et al. Dual effects of zinc sulphate on ethanol-induced gastric injury in rats: possibly mediated by an action on mucosal blood flow. J Pharm Pharmacol. 1989;41:685–9.
21. Oner G, Bor NM, Onug E, Oner ZN. The role of zinc ion in the development of gastric ulcers in rats. Eur J Pharmacol. 1981;70:241–3.
22. Cordova A. Zinc content in selected tissues in streptozotocin-diabetic rats after maximal exercise. Biol Trace Elem Res. 1994;42:209–16.
23. Carrico RJ, Deutsch HF. The presence of zinc in human cytocuperein and some properties of the apoprotein. J Biol Chem. 1970;245:723–7.
24. Abou-Mohamed G, El-Kashef H, Salem H, Elmazar MM. Effect of zinc on the anti-inflammatory and ulcerogenic activities of indomethacin and diclofenac. Pharmacology. 1995;50:266–72.
25. Rainsford KD. Protective effects of the slow-release zinc complex, zinc monoglycerolate, on the gastrointestinal mucosae of rodents. Exp Clin Gastroenterol. 1992;1:349–60.
26. Frommer DJ. The healing of gastric ulcer by zinc sulphate. Med J Aust. 1975;2:793–6.

G Mózsik et al. Cell Injury and Cytoprotection in the GI Tract. 207–213.

ENDOGENOUS VASOPRESSIN DAMAGES DUODENAL MUCOSA DURING HAEMORRHAGIC SHOCK IN RATS

F. LÁSZLÓ[1]*, Z. SZEPES[1], G. KARÁCSONY[1], C.S. VARGA[2] and F.A. LÁSZLÓ[2]
[1]First Department of Medicine, Albert Szent-Györgyi Medical University;
[2]Department of Comparative Physiology, Attila József University of Sciences, Szeged, Hungary
*Correspondence

This paper was first published in: Inflammopharmacology. 1996;4:379–385.

ABSTRACT

The role of endogenous vasopressin was studied in the development of mucosal erosions induced by haemorrhagic shock in the duodenum of the rat. Ischaemia–reperfusion provoked duodenal haemorrhagic lesions and elevated circulating and intramucosal vasopressin level. This mucosal injury was significantly attenuated by a vasopressin pressor receptor antagonist. Moreover, in the vasopressin-deficient Brattleboro homozygous rat, mucosal injury induced by haemorrhagic shock was also reduced. By contrast, when the vasopressin agonist, lysin–vasopressin, was administered, significant aggravation of ischaemia–reperfusion-induced duodenal mucosal injury was seen. These findings indicate the aggressive role of endogenous vasopressin, via its pressor receptors, in the generation of duodenal mucosal stress erosions in haemorrhagic shock.

Keywords: vasopressin, haemorrhagic shock, duodenal mucosa, vasopressin antagonist, Brattleboro rat

INTRODUCTION

Gastrointestinal stress erosions commonly occur among seriously ill patients, mostly in intensive care units, e.g. following severe trauma and burns, in septic, haemorrhagic, cardiogenic shock or after central nervous system injury [1]. Once the bleeding from these erosions becomes manifest, the severity of the condition is reflected in the mortality rate, which approaches 50% [1]. The prevention of stress erosions has a high impact, but this problem is not solved [2]. Stress ulcers have a complex aetiology, to which several factors contribute, including lowered intramucosal pH, impaired natural defence mechanisms, acid hypersecretion, mucosal energy deficit and hypoxia [1].

Vasopressin (VP) is a potent pituitary nonapeptide, released by stress, hypovolaemia and hyperosmosis. The presence of VP receptors in the mesenteric vascular beds [3], in the gastric intramucosal blood vessels [4] and on platelets [5,6] suggests its importance in the regulation of gastrointestinal microcirculation. VP acts on two different types of receptors [7], namely V_1 (pressor) and V_2 (antidiuretic), and, in the last decade, selective V_1 and V_2 receptor antagonists have been developed and used for receptor characterization in animal and in human studies [8,9].

This paper was presented at the Symposium on 'Cell injury and protection in the gastrointestinal tract: from basic science to clinical perspectives', October 8–11, 1995, Pécs, Hungary.

Endogenous VP has been recently shown to have an aggressive action, via its V_1 receptors, against the rat gastric mucosa following challenge with various ulcerogenic stimuli [4] and in the intestinal mucosa following the administration of endotoxin [10]. Therefore, using a V_1-receptor antagonist and vasopressin-deficient Brattleboro homozygous rats [11], in the present study, the possible role of endogenous VP in the acute damage in the duodenum induced by haemorrhagic shock has been evaluated in the rat.

METHODS

Experimental protocol

Female Wistar and Brattleboro homozygous rats, weighing 200–220 g, were fasted for 24 h, but received water ad libitum. The animals were anaesthetized with Nembutal (40 mg/kg ip) and duodenal lesions were produced by the same method as described by Leung et al. [12]. Briefly, blood was withdrawn from the right carotid artery, then reinjected 20 min later. Autopsy was performed 40 min after blood withdrawal. The duodenal lumen was perfused by 0.1 mol/L HCl (0.1 ml/min). Blood pressure during the shock period was 35–40 mmHg (measured from the left femoral artery by a cannula connected to an Elcomatic blood pressure transducer and a Grass Polygraph). The V_1-receptor antagonist ([Mca^1,Tyr,Me^2]AVP, 0.01–1 µg/kg, iv) and the VP agonist, lysin–vasopressin (LVP, 0.1 µg/kg, iv, into the left jugular vein) was injected 10 min before blood withdrawal. Controls and Brattleboro homozygous rats received the solvent (0.9%) at the same time and in the same volume as the V_1-receptor antagonist-treated groups.

Gross evaluation of lesions

Animals were killed by cervical dislocation, the duodenum was removed, stretched out on cork and photographed. The extent of lesions and total mucosa was examined planimetrically on enlarged (8–10 ×) pictures, and the ratio of the two was expressed as a percentage by an investigator unaware of the nature of the experiment.

Histology

The most extensively damaged site in the duodenum, on gross inspection, was taken, then fixed in formalin and embedded in paraffin. Haematoxylin–eosin staining was used. All sections were assessed according to the following scale: 0 = no damage; I = luminal surface damage; II = superficial lesions, swelling of superficial cells, with oedematous lamina propria, or superficial lesions due to the disruption of damaged cells; III = superficial lesions involving the upper half of the mucosa, surrounded by dilated vessels; IV = severe necrosis of the whole mucosa with an inflammatory cell reaction in the submucosa.

Measurement of plasma and intramucosal vasopressin contents

Blood was collected from the abdominal aorta before and after blood withdrawal (at 0 and 20 min, respectively) and when the autopsy for the gross evaluation was regularly performed (at 40 min). The duodenum was also removed and inspected grossly for the incidence of lesions, then the whole mucosa was immediately scraped off for tissue samples and stored at $-20°C$. In control studies, the plasma and intramucosal VP contents were measured in intact animals, fasted for 24 h.

Plasma and intramucosal VP was determined with a specific RIA system as described previously [4].

Statistics

The results were analysed with the Bonferroni test. Differences were taken as significant when the probability was $< 5\%$.

RESULTS

Gross evaluation of lesions

Haemorrhagic shock generated duodenal lesions in normal (Wistar) rats, involving $14.5 \pm 1.9\%$ of the total mucosal area.

The V_1-receptor antagonist caused a dose-dependent reduction in duodenal lesions induced by haemorrhagic shock (by a maximum reduction of $69 \pm 3\%$). In the duodenum of Brattleboro homozygous rats, the degree of such mucosal injury was found to be significantly attenuated by $65 \pm 2\%$. Additionally, in normal Wistar rats, exogenous VP aggravated duodenal mucosal damage by $97 \pm 15\%$ (Figure 1).

Histopathological analysis

The V_1-receptor antagonist protected the deeper layer of the duodenal mucosa (Table 1).

Plasma and intramucosal vasopressin levels in relation to the development of mucosal injury

Haemorrhagic shock caused a maximum of 45-fold increase in circulating VP level and a maximum of 4.5-fold elevation of intramucosal VP content (Table 2).

Plasma and intramucosal VP content were significantly elevated before and after blood withdrawal (at 0 and 20 min, respectively) and when the autopsy for the gross evaluation was regularly performed (at 40 min) as shown in Table 2. The incidences of duodenal lesions were $0/6$, $1/6$ and $6/6$ at 0, 20 and 40 min, respectively.

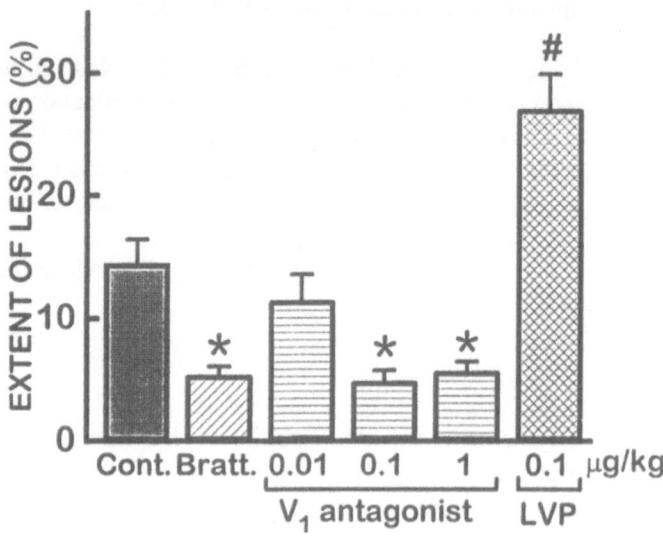

Figure 1. Inhibition and potentiation of duodenal erosions, induced by haemorrhagic shock, in the endogenous vasopressin-deficient Brattleboro homozygous rat (Bratt.), in normal rats treated with a V_1-receptor antagonist and in normal rats treated with the vasopressin agonist lysine–vasopressin (LVP). Data are expressed as the extent of macroscopic lesions in %, $n = 6$; means $\pm$ SEM, $*p < 0.05$ represents significant inhibition and $\#p < 0.05$ shows significant potentiation vs. controls (Cont., which received saline)

TABLE 1

Histopathology of haemorrhagic-shock-induced duodenal erosions in normal (Wistar) rats, and protection by a vasopressin V_1-receptor antagonist

Treatment	Histopathological distribution (%)				
	0	I	II	III	IV
Control	0.0	7.1	26.3	51.5	15.1
V_1 antagonist	0.0	12.8	30.8	57.1	0.0

$n = 6$; 0–IV: histopathological severity scale; controls received saline

TABLE 2
Intramucosal and plasma vasopressin levels during the generation of haemorrhagic shock-induced duodenal erosions in the rat

	Time (min)	Incidence of lesions	Mucosal vasopressin	Plasma vasopressin
Control		0/6	6.5 ± 0.5	$2.9 \pm 0.5^*$
Haemorrhagic shock	0	0/6	$16.1 \pm 0.7^*$	$54.8 \pm 8.4^*$
	20	1/6	$31.2 \pm 1.1^*\dagger$	$141.2 \pm 7.5^*\dagger$
	40	6/6	$27.8 \pm 3.2^*$	$97.4 \pm 12.8^*$

Means $\pm$ SEM; $^*p < 0.05$ vs. control; $\dagger p < 0.05$ vs. the values before and after blood withdrawal (0 and 20 min); the control value is the intramucosal vasopressin content (pg/mg protein) or plasma vasopressin level (pg/ml) of intact rats after fasting for 24 h

DISCUSSION

The action of endogenous VP in the formation of haemorrhagic-shock-induced duodenal mucosal injury was investigated in the rat. Brattleboro homozygous rats have a congenital deficiency of vasopressin synthesis, and consequently they have diabetes insipidus [11]. In these animals, the generation of lesions during haemorrhagic shock is decreased. Furthermore, in normal rats, the VP pressor receptor antagonist was shown to attenuate the extent of mucosal injury and to protect the deeper layer of the mucosa (assessed by histology). Moreover, in normal animals, exogenous VP aggravated duodenal lesions provoked by haemorrhagic shock. All these findings, in conjunction with the observation that plasma and intramucosal VP content was shown to be elevated, suggest that endogenous VP, via its V_1 receptors, plays a role in the formation of mucosal lesions provoked by haemorrhagic shock in the duodenum.

Surgical intervention [13,14], anaesthetics such as nembutal [13,14] and haemorrhagic shock [13,15,16] elevate plasma VP level. Plasma VP level was shown in our study to be increased at 0 min, i.e. before blood withdrawal but in surgically manipulated rats, which confirms these previous observations and, additionally, also demonstrates the simultaneous increase in intramucosal VP content. The low incidence of duodenal lesions in the earlier phase of the experiment (0/6 and 1/6 at 0 and 20 min, respectively) should be mentioned here, because it is in contrast with the role of endogenous VP in this model, since, in this period, elevated intramucosal and plasma VP contents were found. These results suggest that endogenous VP is not the only factor to be involved in the generation of duodenal ulceration. The lesions started to occur when acid perfusion was initiated (from 0 min) and became complete when the reperfusion ended (at 40 min). This finding indicates that gastric acid is needed for VP-mediated duodenal injury in haemorrhagic shock.

In relation to the pathomechanism(s) by which VP, released endogenously or injected exogenously, may have a pathological importance in the development of mucosal injury in haemorrhagic shock, several direct or indirect pathways may be contributed. VP is a potent vasoconstrictor in intestinal macro- and microcirculation [17–21]. Moreover, VP, via its V_1 receptors, can aggregate platelets, which can cause microthrombi and vascular occlusion [5,6]. Additionally, VP may provoke intestinal vasocongestion, vasoconstriction or microvascular damage through a thromboxane-dependent mechanism, since VP can release thromboxanes from vascular tissue and from platelets [22,23]. Other investigators have found that the vascular permeability of the mucosa is increased during haemorrhagic shock [12] and VP also can increase vascular permeability [24,25]. These microcirculatory processes possibly lead to duodenal hypoxia, and consequently the generation of lesions. Further studies are needed to evaluate the microcirculatory effects of VP in this model.

Our current results thus suggest that VP released endogenously injures the duodenal mucosa by a V_1-receptor-mediated pathway during haemorrhagic shock. Taken together with other recent observations that V_1-receptor antagonists have a protective action against various ulcerogenic stimuli in the stomach [4,26], V_1-receptor antagonists, as prophylactic agents, may have potential therapeutic benefits in the prevention of gastrointestinal stress erosions.

ACKNOWLEDGEMENTS

This work was supported by the Hungarian Research Foundation (No. OTKA T 1404) and by the Hungarian Academy of Sciences (No. AKA 88-0-556).

REFERENCES

1. Robert A, Kauffman GL. Stress ulcers, erosions, and gastric mucosal injury. In: Sleisenger MH, Fordtran JS, eds. Gastrointestinal Disease. Pathophysiology, Diagnosis, Management. Philadelphia: Saunders; 1989:772–92.
2. Ben-Manachem T, Fogel R, Patel RV. Profilaxis for stress-related gastric hemorrhage in the medical intensive care unit. Ann Intern Med. 1994;121:568–75.
3. St-Louis J, Schiffrin EL. Biological actions and binding sites for vasopressin on the mesenteric artery from normal and sodium depleted rats. Life Sci. 1984;35:1489–95.
4. Laszio F, Karacsony G, Pavo I, Varga CS, Rojik I, Laszio FA. Aggressive role of vasopressin in development of different gastric lesions in rats. Eur J Pharmacol. 1994;258:15–22.
5. Hourani SMO, Cusack NJ. Pharmacological receptors on blood platelets. Pharmacol Rev. 1991;43:243–98.
6. Siess W, Stiefel M, Binder H, Weber PC. Activation of V_1-receptors by vasopressin stimulated inositol phospholipid hydrolysis and arachidonate metabolism in human platelets. Biochem J. 1986;233:83–91.
7. Michell RH, Kirk CJ, Billah MM. Hormonal stimulation of phosphatidyl–inositol breakdown, with particular reference to the hepatic effect of vasopressin. Biochem Soc Trans. 1979;7:861–5.
8. Laszlo FA, Laszlo F, de Wied D. Pharmacology and clinical perspectives of vasopressin antagonists. Pharmacol Rev. 1991;43:73–108.
9. Manning M, Sawyer WH. Synthesis and receptor specificities of vasopressin antagonists. J Cardiovasc Pharmacol. 1986;Suppl 7:S29–35.
10. Laszlo F, Whittle BJR. Constitutive nitric oxide modulates the injurious actions of vasopressin on rat intestinal microcirculation in acute endotoxaemia. Eur J Pharmacol. 1994;260:265–8.

11. Sokol HW, Valtin H, eds. The Brattleboro rat. Ann NY Acad Sci. 1982;394:1–828.
12. Leung FW, Itoh H, Hirabayashi K, Guth PH. Role of blood flow in gastric and duodenal mucosal injury in the rat. Gastroenterology. 1985;88:281–9.
13. Reichlin S. Neuroendocrinology. In: William RH, ed., Textbook of Endocrinology. Philadelphia: Saunders; 1985:492–511.
14. Melville RJ, Forsling ML, Frizis HI, LeQuesne LP. Stimulus of vasopressin release during elective intra-abdominal operations. Br J Surg. 1985;72:929–35.
15. Robertson GL. Posterior pituitary. In Baxter JD, ed., Endocrinology and Metabolism. New York: McGraw-Hill; 1987:335–56.
16. Share L. Role of vasopressin in cardiovascular regulation. Physiol Rev. 1988;68:1248–84.
17. Liard JF, Deriaz P, Schelling P, Thibonnier M. Cardiac output distribution during vasopressin infusion or dehydration in conscious dogs. Am J Physiol. 1982;243:H663–9.
18. Baker CH, Sutton ET, Zhou Z, Deitz JR. Microvascular vasopressin effects during endotoxin shock in the rat. Circ Shock. 1990;30:81–95.
19. Vanner S, Jiang M-M, Brooks VL, Surprenant A. Characterization of vasopressin actions in isolated submucosal arterioles of the intestinal microcirculation. Circ Res. 1990;67:1017–26.
20. McNeill JR, Stark RD, Greenway CV. Intestinal vasoconstriction after hemorrhage: role of vasopressin and angiotensin. Am J Physiol. 1970;219:1342–7.
21. Stark RD, McNeill JR, Greenway CV. Sympathetic and hypophyseal roles in the splenic response to hemorrhage. Am J Physiol. 1970;220:837–40.
22. Filep J, Rosenkrantz B. Mechanism of vasopressin-induced platelet aggregation. Thromb Res. 1987;45:7–16.
23. Nadasy GL, Szekacs B, Juhasz I, Monos E. Pharmacological modulation of prostacyclin and thromboxane production of rat and cat venous tissue slices. Prostaglandins. 1992;44:339–55.
24. Rosenbar GA, Kyner WT, Fenstermacher JD, Patlak CS. Effect of vasopressin on ependymal and capillary permeability to tritiated water in cat. Am J Physiol. 1986;251:F485–9.
25. Doczi T, Szerdahelyi P, Gulya K, Kiss J. Brain water accumulation after the central administration of vasopressin. Neurosurgery. 1982;11:402–6.
26. Laszlo F, Karacsony G, Szabo E, Lang J, Balaspiri L, Laszlo FA. The role of vasopressin in the pathogenesis of ethanol-induced gastric hemorrhagic erosions in rats. Gastroenterology. 1991;101: 1242–8.

G Mózsik et al. Cell Injury and Cytoprotection in the GI Tract. 215–222.

THE VASCULAR EVENT AS A TARGET IN CHANGES OF INDOMETHACIN-INDUCED GASTROINTESTINAL MUCOSAL DAMAGE AFTER ACUTE SURGICAL AND 'CHEMICAL' VAGOTOMY IN RATS

O. KARÁDI, B. BÓDIS AND Gy. MÓZSIK*

First Department of Medicine, Medical University of Pécs, Pécs, Hungary
*Correspondence

ABSTRACT

The key role of the vagal nerve in gastrointestinal (GI) organoprotection has already been proved but the possible role of the different fibres of the vagal nerve has not been cleared in this mechanism.

Aim: The aim of our study was to make a comparison between the effects of acute surgical vagotomy (ASV) and cholinergic blockade (as 'chemical vagotomy' (CV) produced by atropine) on indomethacin (IND)-induced GI mucosal damage and changes of vascular permeability.

Materials and methods: The mucosal damage was produced by subcutaneous administration of IND at 20 mg/kg 24 h prior to killing the rats at the same time with ASV or CV. Atropine was given in three doses (0.1, 0.5 and 1.0 mg/kg ip) every five hours. Evans blue (1 mg/100 g) was employed to measure the serum protein extravasation and was given intravenously 15 min before sacrificing the rats. The number and severity of mucosal lesions and the Evans blue levels of mucosa and intraluminal contents were determined in the stomach, small intestine and colon.

Results: The results showed, that: (a) the IND-induced mucosal damage and increased the vascular permeability in the whole GI tract; and (b) the ASV increased while the CV dose-dependently and significantly decreased the IND-induced GI mucosal and vascular injury in the stomach, small intestine and proximal colon.

Conclusions: These different effects of ASV and CV show that there is a difference in the role of the different fibres of the vagal nerve on GI organoprotection and that vascular integrity is one of the targets of ASV and CV in changing the development of IND-induced GI mucosal damage.

Keywords: acute surgical vagotomy, atropine, indomethacin, gastrointestinal tract

INTRODUCTION

The essential role of the vagal nerve in gastrointestinal (GI) organoprotection against different aggressive agents, for example indomethacin (IND), has been demonstrated [1,2]. IND-induced GI mucosal lesions appear in the stomach 3–4 h after IND treatment [3]. However the greatest lesions appear in the small intestine 24–48 h after IND administration [4]. Significant erosions exist in both the stomach and the intestine 24 h after IND treatment [4].

This paper was presented at the Symposium on 'Cell injury and protection in the gastrointestinal tract: from basic science to clinical perspectives', October 8–11, 1995, Pécs, Hungary.

Acute surgical vagotomy (ASV) alone does not cause mucosal damage and changes in the vascular integrity after 24 or 48 h [2,5] but it increases mucosal lesions induced by different necrotizing agents in the vagal-nerve-innervated parts of the GI tract [1]. This aggravating effect of ASV is significant already 24 h after IND administration but the mucosal and vascular damage is significantly higher after 48 h than after 24 h in the stomach and small intestine [2]. ASV (after 24 and 48 h) clearly showed the effect of the lack of vagal innervation (afferent and efferent) because earlier studies suggested that at 10–14 days after surgical vagotomy different changes developed in the GI mucosa and in its function [5].

On the other hand, the atropine treatment ('chemical vagotomy', CV) decreases the aggressive-agent-induced mucosal and vascular lesions in the vagal-nerve-innervated regions of the GI tract [6]. The vagal nerve consists of different fibres – such as afferent sensory nerves, efferent cholinergic, catecholaminergic and other fibres – which have different effects on the GI tract, indicating that the effect of the vagal nerve on the GI tract is very complex [7,8]. The background to these various effects is not clear. The aim of our study was to make a comparison between the effects of ASV and CV on IND-induced GI mucosal damage and vascular permeability after 24 h in rats.

MATERIALS AND METHODS

The observations were performed on male Sprague–Dawley (LATI, Gödöllő, Hungary) rats weighing 180–210 g. The animals were fasted for 24 h before the experiments but they received tap water ad libitum.

The mucosal damage was produced by subcutaneous administration of IND (Indomethacinum, Chinoin, Hungary) 20 mg/kg given 24 h prior to killing the animals at the same time with ASV or CV. IND (20 mg/kg) was dissolved in 0.5 ml of 5% NaHCO$_3$ solution. Bilateral surgical vagotomy was performed after median laparotomy with ether anaesthesia. All fibres of the vagal nerve were cut around the cardia in the subdiaphragmatic location at the same time as IND application.

Atropine (Atropinum sulfuricum, EGIS, Hungary), dissolved in 0.5 ml of saline, was given intraperitoneally at three doses: 0.1 mg/kg (this dose being without any effect on gastric acid secretion), 0.5 and 1.0 mg/kg (antisecretory doses) every 5 h in order to produce a permanent 'chemical vagotomy' (anticholinergic effect). Control groups received IND (20 mg/kg sc) plus saline (0.5 ml ip) or atropine (1.0 mg/kg ip) plus saline (0.5 ml sc) or saline alone (0.5 ml ip and sc) at the same times.

The animals were sacrificed 24 h after IND administration and the stomach, small intestine and colon were removed. The large bowel was divided into three equal (proximal, middle and distal) parts. All parts of the GI tract were opened lengthways. The number of GI mucosal ulcerations was noted and the severity of mucosal damage was calculated on a semiquantitative scale for all parts [9].

The changes in vascular permeability were measured by the intravenous administration of Evans blue (1 mg/100 g) (Evans-kék, Chinoin, Hungary) 15 min before sacrifice [10]. The mucosa of the stomach, small intestine and the three equal parts of the large bowel were scraped, weighed and the intraluminal contents were collected and measured. The mucosa and the intraluminal content were digested in 32% (v/v) HCl for 1 h, when the Evans blue was extracted from the precipitatum with 4 ml formamide for 60 min [6]. The absorbance of Evans blue was measured from each sample spectrophotometrically (Hitachi 124 Spectrophotometer, Japan) at a wavelength of 620 nm and compared with standards of known concentrations of Evans blue. The albumin extravasation was calculated from the Evans blue concentration of the samples and the Evans-blue-bound protein concentration in blood. The concentration of infiltrated serum protein was expressed in µg/g of wet mucosa and µg in the intraluminal juice. Protein content was assayed by the method of Lowry et al. [11].

Statistical analysis

The results were calculated as means ± SEM. The non-paired Student's *t*-test was used for statistical analysis of data. The evaluation of semiquantitatively estimated mucosal lesions (severity) was carried out by the Mann–Whitney U test. Differences were considered significant when a $p \leqslant 0.05$ was obtained.

RESULTS

Single administration of IND caused mucosal ulcerations and increased Evans-blue-bound serum protein extravasation into the mucosa and intraluminal juice of the whole GI tract. The greatest mucosal damage was found in the small intestines of fasted rats after 24 h (Figures 1–4).

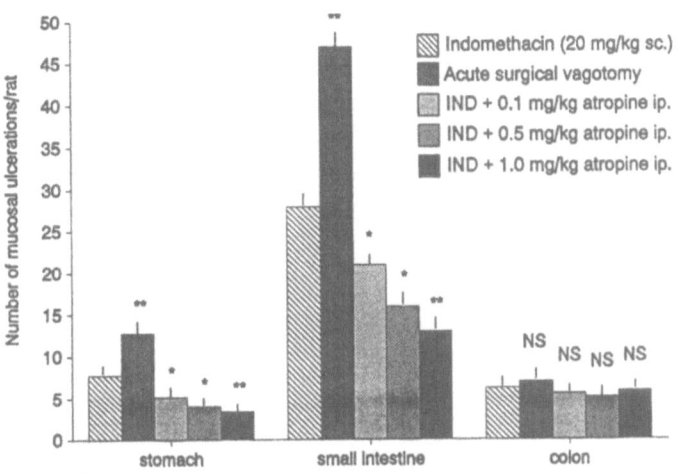

Figure 1. Effect of ASV and CV (different doses of atropine) on the number of IND-induced GI mucosal lesions after 24 h (means ± SEM; $n = 10$). NS, not significant; $*p < 0.05$; $**p < 0.01$

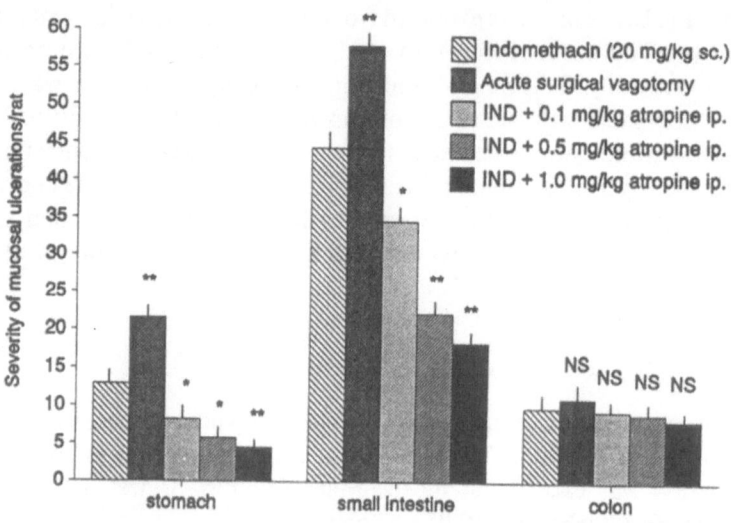

Figure 2. Effect of ASV and CV (different doses of atropine) on the severity of IND-induced GI mucosal lesions after 24 h (means ± SEM; $n = 10$). NS, not significant; *$p < 0.05$; **$p < 0.01$

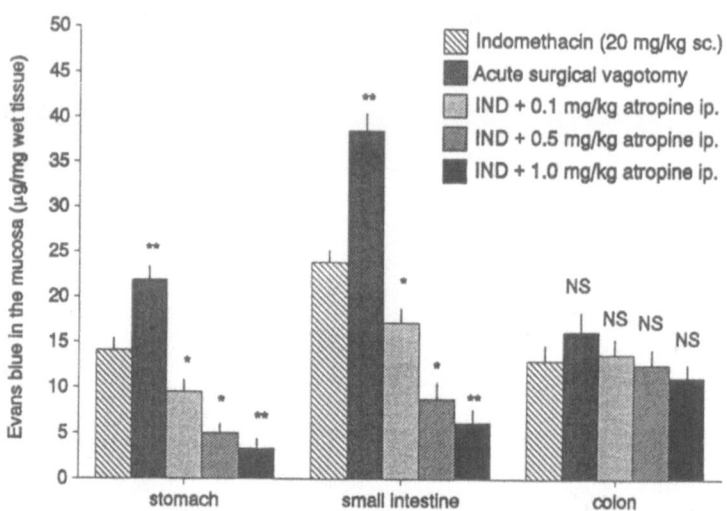

Figure 3. Effect of ASV and CV (different doses of atropine) on IND-increased Evans-blue-bound serum protein extravasation into the GI mucosa after 24 h (means ± SEM; $n = 10$). NS, not significant; *$p < 0.05$; **$p < 0.01$

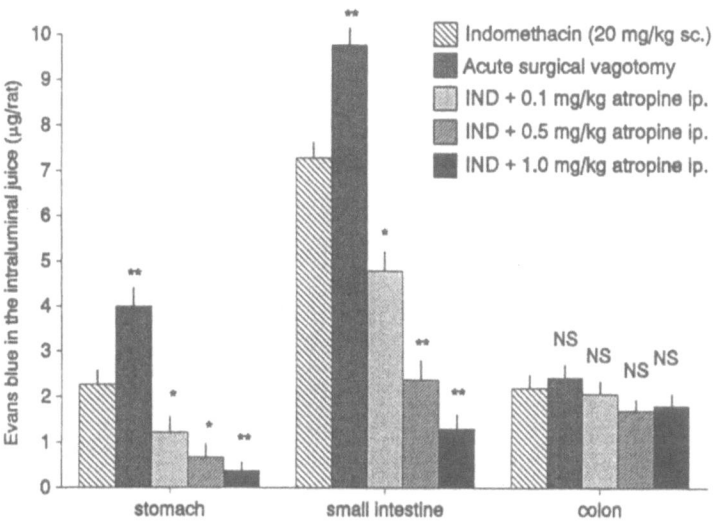

Figure 4. Effect of ASV and CV (different doses of atropine) on the IND-increased Evans-blue-bound serum protein extravasation into the GI lumen after 24 h ((means $\pm$ SEM; $n = 10$). NS, not significant; $*p < 0.05$; $**p < 0.01$

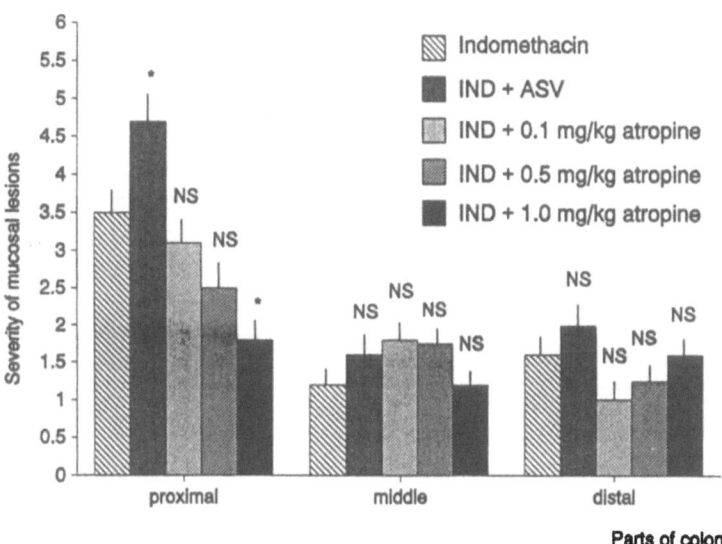

Figure 5. Effect of ASV and CV (different doses of atropine) on the severity of IND-induced mucosal lesions in the three equal parts of the colon after 24 h (means $\pm$ SEM; $n = 10$). NS, not significant; $*p < 0.05$; $**p < 0.01$

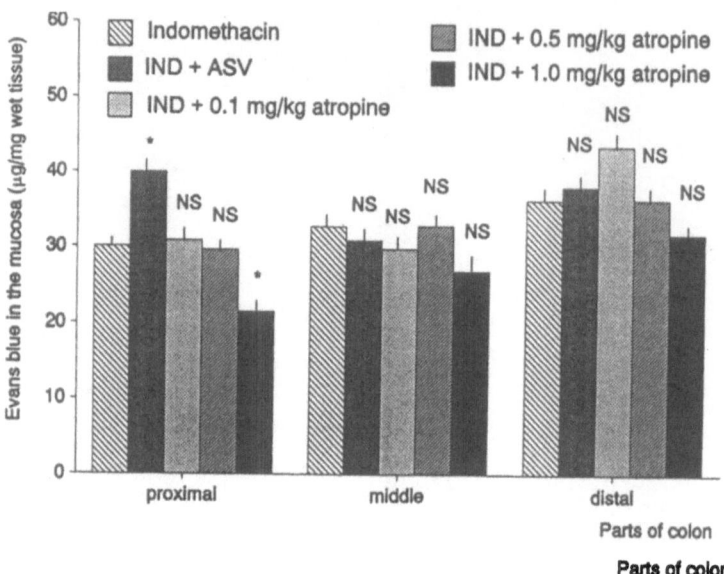

Figure 6. Effect of ASV and CV (different doses of atropine) on IND-increased Evans-blue-bound serum protein extravasation into the mucosa of the three equal parts of the colon after 24 h (means ± SEM; $n = 10$). NS, not significant; $*p < 0.05$; $**p < 0.01$

ASV significantly increased the number and severity of IND-induced GI mucosal lesions and the serum protein extravasation into the mucosa and intraluminal juice of the stomach, small intestine and proximal colony (Figures 1–6).

Atropine ('chemical vagotomy') dose-dependently and significantly decreased the number and severity of mucosal ulcerations and serum protein extravasation into the mucosa and lumen of the stomach, small intestine and proximal colon (Figures 1–6).

There were no significant changes in the extent of IND-induced mucosal erosions and serum protein extravasation in the middle and distal parts of the colon or considering the whole colon after ASV or atropine treatment (CV).

DISCUSSION

The effects of ASV and anticholinergic treatment with atropine (given to induce 'chemical vagotomy') on IND-induced GI mucosal damage and changes of vascular permeability were compared after 24 h.

The ASV significantly aggravated, while the CV dose-dependently and significantly decreased the extent of IND-induced GI mucosal injury and IND-increased vascular permeability in the vagal-nerve-innervated parts of the GI tract, namely the stomach, small intestine and proximal colon [7,8,12]. The ablation of vagal nerve (ASV) and the blocking of the cholinergic fibres only (CV) produced opposite effects on the GI organoprotection against IND. The vagal nerve contains different fibres, which have different roles in the development of GI mucosal protection against aggressive agents [7,8]. Some studies have shown that the afferent sensory fibres of vagal nerve have an important role in the mucosal defence mechanisms. Ablation of these fibres by high doses of capsaicin has been found to enhance IND-induced gastric mucosal lesions [13], while stimulation of these fibres by small doses of capsaicin protects the GI mucosa against IND [14]. A role of these fibres in GI organoprotection via the vago-vagal reflex has also been demonstrated [15].

However, the ulcerogenic effect on the GI mucosa of some peptides (TRH, VIP) injected in the brain occurs via the cholinergic fibres of vagal nerve [16]. Other studies have shown the role of the peripheral adrenergic and dopaminergic pathways in the GI protective effect of other peptides in the brain (e.g. neurotensin) [17].

ASV abolished all fibres of vagal nerve, while CV blocked only the cholinergic (muscarinergic). The different functions of the different fibres of the vagal nerve offer an explanation for the contrasting effects of ASV and CV on IND-induced mucosal lesions in the vagal-nerve-innervated parts of the GI tract.

Earlier studies have demonstrated that an increase in vascular permeability precedes the appearance of macroscopic mucosal ulceration after application of necrotizing agents [10]. Damage to the vascular integrity of the GI mucosa is also an important part of the ulcerogenic action of IND [2]. ASV increased serum protein exudation, while CV dose-dependently decreased it. The protective effects of atropine on vascular permeability are significantly greater than the protective effects of atropine on the development of IND-induced macroscopic mucosal ulcerations in the stomach, small intestine and proximal colon [6]. These results suggest that vascular integrity is one of the important targets of ASV and CV in changing the development of IND-induced GI mucosal lesions.

In summary, the cholinergic and the other fibres of vagal nerve have an important role in GI organoprotection. Vascular integrity is one of those protective mechanisms which develop via the vagal nerve.

ACKNOWLEDGEMENTS

This study was supported by a grant from The Hungarian National Research Fund (OTKA T-020098).

REFERENCES

1. Mózsik Gy, Kiŕly Á, Garamszegi M et al. Failure of prostacyclin, β-carotene, atropine and cimetidine to produce gastric cyto- and general mucosal protection in surgically vagotomized rats. Life Sci. 1991;49:1383–9.
2. Karádi O, Mózsik Gy, Király Á, Süto G, Vincze Á. Surgical vagotomy enhances the indomethacin-induced gastrointestinal mucosal damage in rats. Inflammopharmacology. 1994;2:389–9.
3. Djahanguiri B. The production of acute gastric ulceration by indomethacin in the rat. Scand J Gastroenterol. 1969;4:265–7.

4. Whittle BJR. Temporal relationship between cyclooxygenase inhibition, as measured by prostacyclin biosynthesis, and the gastrointestinal damage induced by indomethacin in the rat. Gastroenterology. 1981;80:94–8.
5. Király Á, Süto G, Vincze Á, Mózsik Gy. Acute and chronic surgical vagotomy and gastric mucosal vascular permeability in ethanol treated rats. Acta Physiol Hung. 1992;80:219–24.
6. Karádi O, Abdel-Salam OME, Bódis B, Mózsik Gy. Dose-dependent preventive effect of atropine on the indomethacin-induced gastrointestinal mucosal and vascular damage in rats. Pharmacology. 1996;52:46–55.
7. Grijalva CV, Novin D. The role of the hypothalamus and dorsal vagal complex in gastrointestinal function and pathophysiology. Ann NY Acad Sci. 1990;597:207–21.
8. Gabella G, Pease HL. Number of axons in the abnormal vagus of the rat. Brain Res. 1973;58:465–9.
9. Mózsik Gy, Móron F, Jávor T. Cellular mechanisms of the development of gastric mucosal damage and of gastrocytoprotection induced by prostacyclin in rats. A pharmacological study. Prostagl Leukotriene Med. 1982;9:71–84.
10. Szabó S, Trier JS, Brown A, Schnoor J. Early vascular injury and increased vascular permeability in gastric mucosal injury caused by ethanol in the rat. Gastroenterology. 1985;88:228–36.
11. Lowry OH, Rosebrough NJ, Farr AL, Randal RJ. Protein measurements with the Folin phenol reagent. J Biol Chem. 1951;193:265–75.
12. Berthoud HR, Neuhuber WL. Distribution and morphology of vagal afferents and efferents supplying the digestive system. In: Taché Y, Wingate DL, Burks TF, eds. Innervation of the Gut. Pathophysiological Implications. Boca Raton, Florida: CRC Press; 1994:39–61.
13. Holzer P, Sametz W. Gastric mucosal protection against ulcerogenic factors in the rat mediated by capsaicin-sensitive afferent neurons. Gastroenterology. 1986;91:975–81.
14. Gray JL, Bunnett NW, Orloff SL, Mulvihill SJ, Debas HT. Role for calcitonin gene-related peptide in protection against gastric ulceration. Ann Surg. 1994;219:58–64.
15. Yonei Y, Holzer P, Guth PH. Laparotomy-induced gastric protection against ethanol injury is mediated by capsaicin-sensitive sensory neurons. Gastroenterology. 1990;99:3–9.
16. Hernandez DE. The role of brain peptides in the pathogenesis of experimental stress gastric ulcers. Ann NY Acad Sci. 1990;597:28–35.
17. Hernandez DE, Nemeroff CB, Orlando RC, Prange AJ. The effect of intracisternally administered neuropeptides on the development of stress induced gastric ulcers in rats. J Neurosci Res. 1983;9:145–57.

G Mózsik et al. Cell Injury and Cytoprotection in the GI Tract. 223–235.
© 1997 Kluwer Academic Publishers.

INVOLVEMENT OF CORTICOTROPIN RELEASING FACTOR (CRF) AND VASOPRESSIN (AVP) IN STRESS-INDUCED EXACERBATION OF EXPERIMENTAL COLITIS IN RATS

M. GUÉ[1,2]*, C. DEL RIO-LACHEZE[1], J. FIORAMONTI[1], J. MORÉ[1],
J. LOUIS JUNIEN[2] AND L. BUÉNO[1]
[1]Department of Pharmacology, INRA, 180 chemin de Tournefeuille, BP3, 31931
Toulouse cedex; [2]Institut de Recherche Jouveinal, Fresnes, France
*Correspondence

ABSTRACT

Stress is supposed to be associated with exacerbation of inflammatory bowel diseases. Furthermore, stress-induced immune suppression is supposed to be mediated by activation of the hypothalamo–pituitary–adrenal (HPA) axis. This study was performed to evaluate the role of the key HPA modulator factors, corticotropin-releasing factor (CRF) and arginine vasopressin (AVP) in stress-induced exacerbation of colitis in rats chronically equipped with intracerebroventricular cannula.

Chronic partial restraint stress (PRS) was applied before colitis induced by trinitrobenzene sulphonic acid (TNB) in rats. In subsequent experiments, rats were centrally injected with α-helical CRF_{9-41} or AVP antagonist before each session of PRS. The colitis was assessed by macroscopic scoring, myeloperoxidase (MPO) activity, body weight and histological evaluation.

PRS, applied before TNB, increased the colitis and the leukocyte infiltration as reflected by MPO activity. Central α-helical CRF_{9-41} of AVP antagonist treatment before PRS, increased the severity of colitis, loss of weight and the MPO activity.

Stress may have a promoting effect on the development of colitis in rats but CRF and AVP can exert a protective effect in such a situation.

Keywords: colitis, corticotropin releasing factor, rats, vasopressin

INTRODUCTION

Ulcerative colitis and Crohn's disease are inflammatory bowel diseases (IBD) that exhibit an unpredictable clinical course usually characterized by successive exacerbations and remissions of variable intensity and duration. In patients with IBD, emotional stress may alter intestinal motility [1,2] and is clinically associated with exacerbation of IBD [3]. In rats, 4 h of cold restraint stress increases prostaglandin E_2 and LTC_4 synthesis in the proximal colon [4]; and McHugh et al. [5] observed that stress induced exacerbation of experimental colitis when stress was applied several weeks after induction of colitis.

Activated neutrophils [7] and macrophages [8–10] are major components of active lesions in both ulcerative colitis and Crohn's disease [6,11]. Large numbers of neutrophils and macrophages pass out of the circulation and enter the inflamed mucosa and submucosa of the bowel during acute inflammation [6,11]. In rats,

---

This paper was presented at the Symposium on 'Cell injury and protection in the gastrointestinal tract: from basic science to clinical perspectives', October 8–11, 1995, Pécs, Hungary.

intrarectal instillation of trinitrobenzenesulphonic acid (TNB) causes a profound colonic inflammation with histological changes and mediator release mimicking that found in human IBD [12].

Exposure to aversive stimuli or stressors modulates various aspects of immune function. For instance, prolonged restraint stress resulted in a decreased incidence and severity of experimental autoimmune encephalomyelitis when applied before but not after its induction [13]. Integrative physiological models initially proposed that stress-induced immune suppression was mediated by activation of the pituitary–adrenal axis with the release of glucocorticoids [14,15] but numerous reports failed to demonstrate that adrenal mechanisms fully accounted for stress-induced immune suppression [16]. Now there is no doubt that a counter-regulatory feedback loop exists between the immune system and CNS, in which immune or pro-inflammatory mediators stimulate corticotropin-releasing hormone (CRF) activation of the hypothalamic–pituitary–adrenal (HPA) axis [17–19]. The resultant increase in plasma glucocorticoids serves to restrain and limit the intensity of the inflammatory/immune response. Recently, we have shown that stress applied before TNB instillation increases colitis in terms of macroscopic aspect and myeloperoxidase activity [20].

Since CRF acts in synergy with arginine vasopressin (AVP) to regulate pituitary ACTH secretion and ultimately the activity of the pituitary–adrenal axis [21,22], we have examined the role of CRF and AVP in the modulation of colitis severity by stress.

METHODS

Animals

Eight groups of 6 male Wistar rats (Centre d'élevage R. Janvier, Le Genest Saint Isle, France) weighing 225–300 g were used for these experiments. Animals were housed individually in polypropylene cages ($37.5 \times 17 \times 15$ cm) and kept in a temperature-controlled room ($21 \pm 1°C$, $50 \pm 5\%$ relative humidity) on a 12-h light–dark cycle (light on at 8:00 am). The rats were fed standard laboratory chow and tap water ad libitum. All experimental procedures described in this report were performed in accordance with the guidelines of the local ethical committee for in-vivo animal studies (agreement No. 94.203 A).

Under general anaesthesia with ketamine (Imalgene 1000, Rhône Mérieux, Lyon, France, 100 mg/kg ip), four groups of rats were fitted with a small polyethylene catheter (ID 0.3 mm; OD 0.7 mm) inserted into a lateral ventricle of the brain using the following co-ordinates from bregma: anteroposterior –1.3 mm; lateral 1.8 mm; ventral 3.5 mm. Two screws were implanted in bone surface and dental cement secured the catheter.

Induction of colitis

Rats ($n = 6$ per group) were randomized into treatment groups. After an overnight fast and under general anaesthesia (ketamine, 100 mg/kg ip), colitis was induced by intracolonic administration of 0.25 ml of 50% ethanol (vol/vol) containing 15 mg of 2,4,6-trinitrobenzenesulphonic acid (TNB) as previously described [12].

Stress procedure

Partial restraint stress, a relatively mild, non-ulcerogenic model of restraint, was used in all stress sessions [23]. Animals were lighlty anaesthetized with di-ethyl-ether, and their foreshoulders, upper forelimbs and thoracic trunk were wrapped in a confining harness of paper tape to restrict, but not to prevent, body movements; then the animals were placed in their home cage for 2 h.

The stress protocol involved submitting rats to chronic PRS before either saline (non-inflamed group) or TNB instillation at 15 mg. Rats were killed on day 4 after TNB instillation for assessment of colitis.

Effect of CRF antagonist and AVP antagonist

In the last series of experiments, rats were intracerebroventricular (ICV) injected with saline alone (control group) or containing 5 µg of either α-helical CRF_{9-41} or [deamino-Pen^1,Val^4,D-Arg^8]vasopressin, a synthetic analogue of AVP with antagonist properties, 5 min before each PRS session. The animals were submitted to daily PRS over 4 consecutive days and were instilled with either TNB (15 mg) or saline as described above. The rats were killed on day 4 after induction of colitis. Doses of CRF antagonist and AVP antagonist were chosen in accordance with previous studies [24,25].

Assessment of colonic damage and inflammation

The severity of colitis was assessed in three ways: macroscopic scoring, histological evaluation and quantification of granulocyte infiltration through measurement of myeloperoxidase (MPO) activity. MPO is an enzyme found in cells of myeloid origin, especially neutrophils, and has been used as a quantitative marker of granulocyte infiltration into gastrointestinal tissues [12,26].

Rats of the randomized treated groups were weighed and killed by cervical dislocation, and the 10 cm of distal colon were removed. The colon was opened by a longitudinal incision, rinsed with saline, and pinned out on a wax block. The macroscopic scoring of colonic damage was performed using the criteria modified from Wallace and Keenan [27], which take into consideration the area of damage involvement and the presence or absence of ulcers. All scoring of damage and excision of tissue samples were performed by an observer unaware of the treatment group (C. Bonbonne and M. Gué).

One sample was taken from a region of grossly visible damage (5–6 cm proximal to the anus) and excised in the length in two pieces: one piece was immersed in neutral buffered formalin and was then processed by routine techniques before embedding in paraffin. Thin sections (5 μm) were mounted on glass slides and stained with haematoxylin and eosin to reveal structural features. Histological assessment was performed using coded slides to prevent observer (J. Moré) bias using criteria modified from Fabia et al. [28].

The other piece of tissue sample was excised, frozen on dry ice and stored at −80°C for subsequent measurement of MPO activity no more than 10 days later. MPO activity was measured using the modified technique of Bradley et al. [29]. Protein concentration was measured by the modified method of Lowry et al. [30] utilizing BIO-RAD DC test (BIO-RAD SA, Ivry-sur-Seine, France) and results were expressed as units myeloperoxidase assay per g of tissue protein.

Statistical analysis

Data are expressed as mean ± SEM. Groups of data were compared using one-way or multiple-way analysis of variance followed by a Dunnett's test; $p \leqslant 0.05$ was considered significant.

RESULTS

Induction of colitis in prestressed rats

Chronic PRS applied in healthy rats had no effect on the mean weight gain or on colitic aspect, since no change was detected macroscopically or histologically, even though chronic PRS reduced by 66% the MPO activity compared with control (not stressed) animals (35 ± 3 vs. 104 ± 8 U/g of protein; Figure 1). Four days after TNB administration, rats exhibit a drastic colitis characterized by severe hyperaemia and ulceration extending along the distal colon up to 2 cm. The colitic damage scores reached a value of 5.6 ± 0.8. Adhesions between the affected portion of the colon and other organs, usually the small intestine, were not frequently observed in TNB-treated rats. When they existed, adhesions were invariably located very close to a site of ulceration. Histological observations showed mucosal extended ulceration and moderate-to-severe mucin cell depletion, in addition to mucosal atrophy and oedema (10–30%), dilated vessels and inflammatory cell infiltration in the submucosa (Figure 2). MPO activity was increased by approximately three times for TNB-treated rats over that of saline controls (293 ± 31 vs. 104 ± 8 U/g of protein). Colitis observed in rats treated with TNB was paralleled by changes in body weight. Rats lost an average of 21 g in the TNB-treated group over a 4-day period.

With the chronic PRS for 4 consecutive days before induction of colitis, administration of TNB resulted in a significant increase in severity of colitis over that of non-stressed rats, assessed both macroscopically, with the areas of ulceration extended up to 5–6 cm instead of 2 cm, and by colonic damage score (9.6 ± 0.5 vs. 5.6 ± 0.8). Histological examination of tissues provided results complementary to the macroscopic data (Table 1). This consisted of mucosal ulcerations which did not exceed the

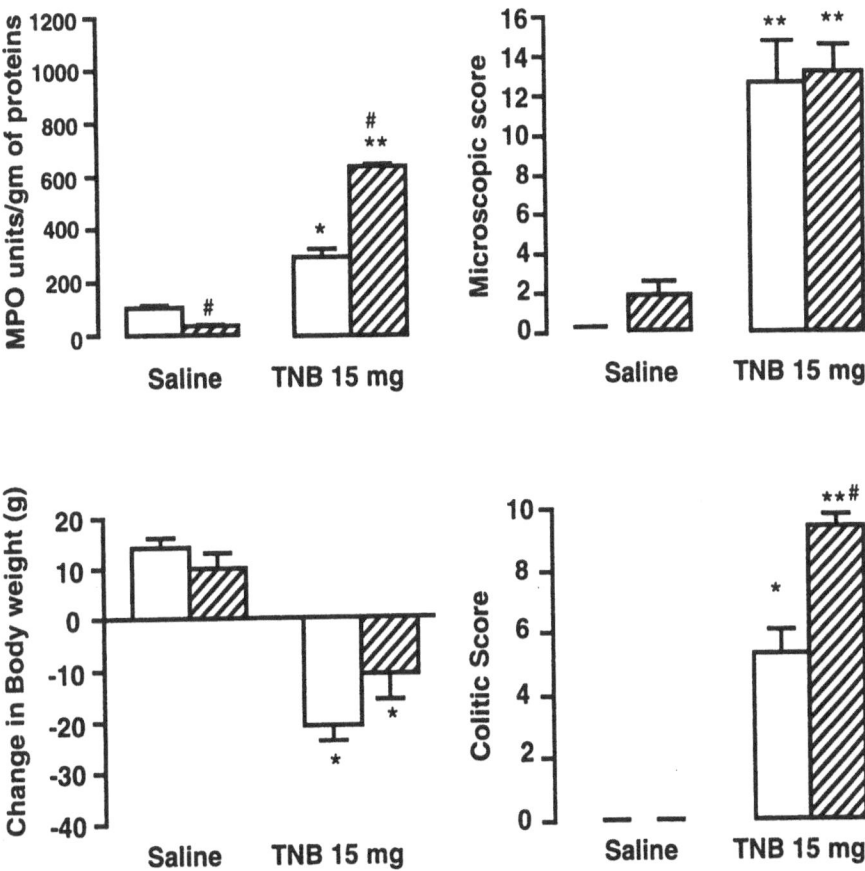

Figure 1. Body weight changes, myeloperoxidase (MPO) activity, colitic damage score in rats after intracolonic instillation of either saline or TNB (15 mg) in non-stressed (white columns) and chronic partial restraint stressed rats (hatched columns) *$p < 0.05$ significant difference from corresponding saline values, **$p < 0.01$ significant difference from corresponding saline values; #$p < 0.05$ significant difference from corresponding no-stress values; $n = 6$ rats per group

superior third of the lamina propria. The oedema was moderate and the mucosal atrophy about 50%. Mucus cell depletion was severe as well as the vascular dilatation (Figure 2). In all rats, there was marked inflammation in the colon even though there is no significant difference between non-stressed and prestressed rats submitted to colitis (Figure 1, Table 1). In contrast, the colonic tissues of these rats exhibit a significant increase, by 118%, in MPO activity compared with the TNB-treated group. However, chronic PRS had no effect on the change in body weight (Figure 2).

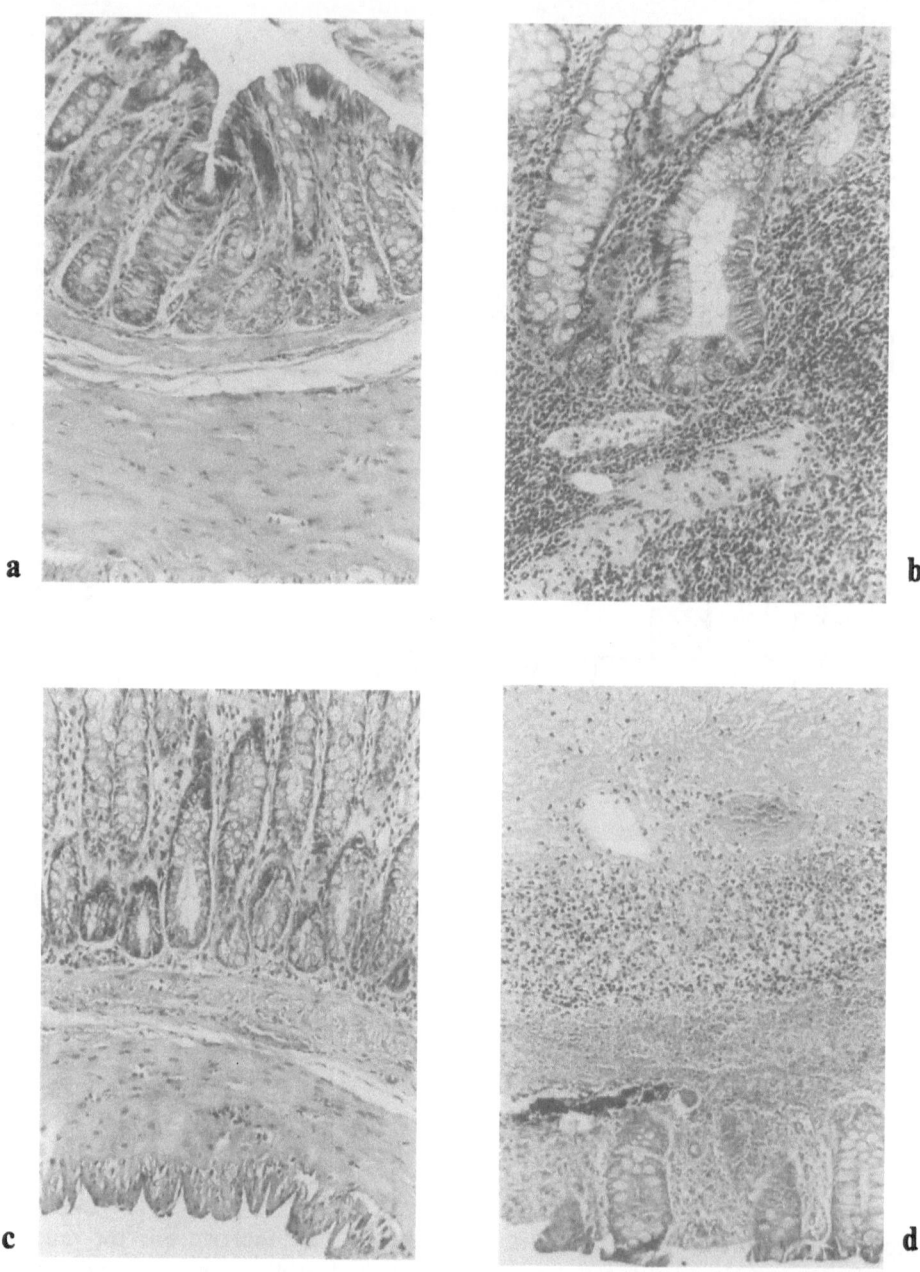

Figure 2. Light micrographs of colon of rat submitted or not to stress before induction of colitis with TNB (15 mg). Samples were taken 4 days after TNB instillation. Normal colon in (a) control rats; (b) stressed rats: observe the mild erosion of the surface epithelium. Inflammation and injury of colonic mucosa 4 days after intracolonic instillation of TNB (15 mg); (c) in non-stressed rats: note the infiltration of the mucosa and the submucosa by inflammatory cells; and (d) in stressed rat: the mucosa has shrunk and is partially necrotic

TABLE 1

Histologically assessed damage 4 days after intracolonic TNB instillation: effects of partial restraint stress (PRS) applied before induction of colitis with TNB

Treatment	Ulceration	Mucus cell depletion	Oedema	Mucosal atrophy	Inflammatory cell infiltration	Vascular dilatation
TNB (15 mg)	2.0 ± 1.1	1.8 ± 0.9	2.2 ± 0.7	1.7 ± 1.0	2.7 ± 0.8	1.8 ± 0.7
PRS + TNB	1.6 ± 0.4	$2.4 \pm 0.4*$	1.8 ± 0.4	2.4 ± 0.9	2.8 ± 0.4	$2.6 \pm 0.5*$

$*p < 0.05$ significantly different from corresponding no-stress value

Central injection of α-helical CRF$_{9-41}$ and AVP antagonist

Intracerebroventricular (ICV) injection of either α-helical CRF$_{9-41}$ or AVP antagonist, performed before each session of PRS, had no effect per se on MPO activity in saline rats or in rats receiving intrarectal insillation.

In rats previously injected with α-helical CRF$_{9-41}$ (5 µg ICV) before each session of PRS, the colitis was much more severe when measured 4 days after TNB (15 mg) instillation than in the PRS group (Figure 3). Indeed, MPO activity significantly ($p < 0.05$) increased compared with the PRS group (1429 ± 347 vs. 702 ± 31 U/g of protein). At the same time, rats lost an average of 45 ± 6 vs. 8 ± 3 g in PRD (Figure 3). In 1 of 6 animals, a cicatricial tissue was observed, while 5 or 6 rats presented ulcerations exceeding the submucosa, severe oedema and mucosal atrophy, inflammatory cell infiltration in the submucosa and severe dilatation of blood vessels (Figure 4). Similarly, AVP-antagonist (5 µg/kg) centrally injected before stress sessions, significantly increased the MPO activity and the loss of weight in rats treated with TNB and increased the severity of colitis, assessed macroscopically (Figure 3) and histologically (Figure 4).

DISCUSSION

Our findings show that partial restraint stress, applied over 4 consecutive days and considered as a chronic stress, does not alter immune reaction in the normal gut but increases the severity of experimental colitis in rats. These changes were expressed by an increase in colitis damage score, an aggravation of microscopic aspect and increase in granulocyte recruitment assessed by MPO activity. Our results reinforce the hypothesis that stress may cause an exacerbation of colitis in animals [5] and in humans [3].

Intrarectal administration of TNB in ethanol results in acute inflammation with ulcers that evolves into chronic inflammation of the distal colon in rats. When TNB,

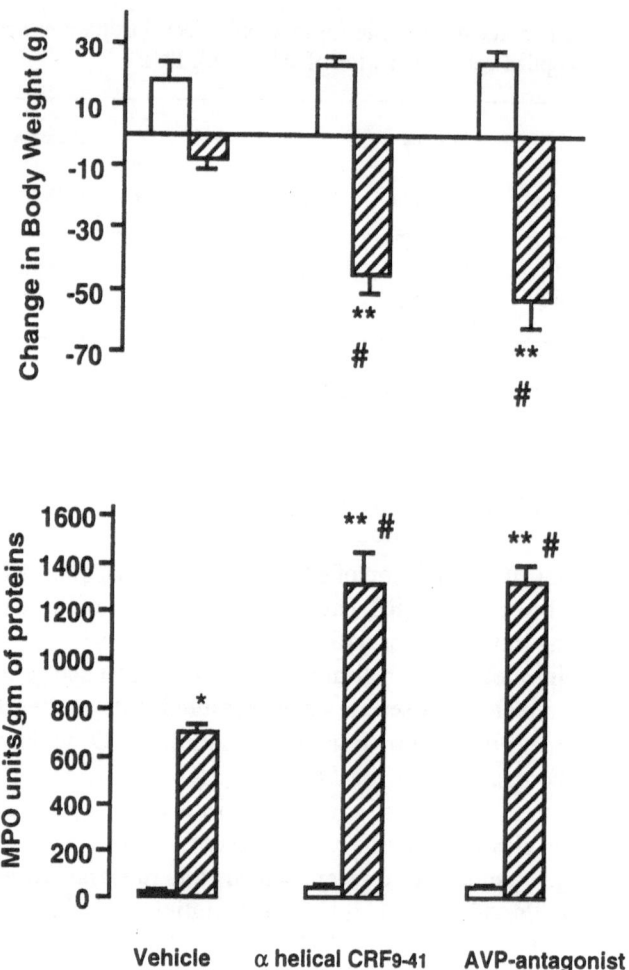

Figure 3. Effects of α-helical CRF$_{9-41}$ (5 μg ICV) and AVP antagonist (5 μg ICV) injected before each session of PRS on body weight and MPO activity 4 days after rectal instillation of saline (white columns) or TNB (15 mg) (hatched columns). *$p < 0.05$ significant difference from corresponding saline values, **$p < 0.01$ significant difference from corresponding saline values; #$p < 0.05$ significant difference from corresponding vehicle values; $n = 6$ rats per group

bound to tissue proteins, it elicits cell-mediated immune responses and induces an inflammation of the gut very similar to human Crohn's disease. In particular, the histologically observed infiltration of lymphocytes and histiocytes is exactly as described for the human disease [31]. Various inflammatory mediators such as PGE$_2$, TBA$_2$, prostacyclins, leukotrienes (LTB$_4$, LTC$_4$), platelet-activating factor (PAF) and interleukins (IL) may be involved in TNB colitis as in human IBD [27,32]. Among

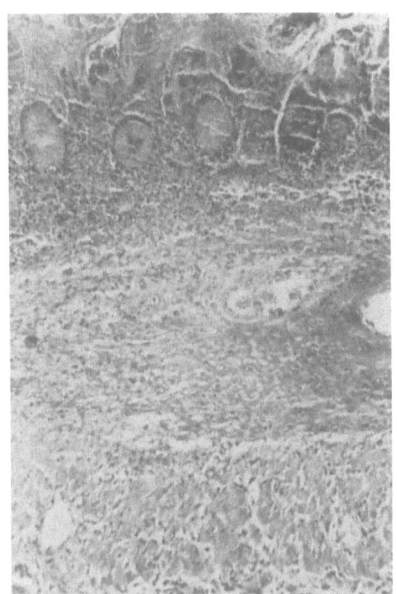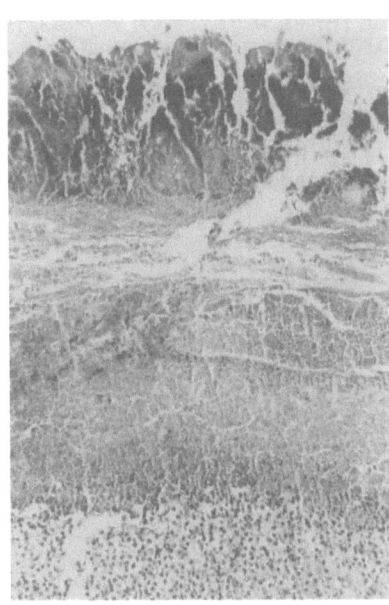

a   b

Figure 4. Histology of TNB colitis tissue obtained from α-helical CRF_{9-41} and AVP antagonist-pretreated rats. (a) Colonic mucosa 4 days after induction of colitis in the α-helical CRF_{9-41}-pretreated rat; (b) colonic mucosa 4 days after induction of colitis in the AVP antagonist-pretreated rat. Note, in both cases, the whole colonic wall is invaded by inflammatory cells and the necrosis of the mucosa

various inflammatory mediators in TNB-induced colitis, IL-1 is considered as a most significant indicator of mucosal inflammation because its level is correlated with MPO activity [33].

Peripherally generated inflammatory mediators and immune cytokines derived from various inflammatory and immune cells activate the HPA axis at some or all of its levels, which include hypothalamic CRF neurons, pituitary corticotrophs, and the adrenal cortex [17,18,20,33]. Among these substances are included mast-cell derived PAF, lymphocyte-derived γ-interferon, IL-2, IL-6, macrophage-derived IL-1 and tumour necrosis factor (TNF) and other interleukins. In addition, the central nervous system (CNS) contains neuronal pathways and receptors for cytokines such as IL-1, especially in the hypothalamus, an area of the brain that is important in the mediation of acute-phase response [34]. Whatever the mechanism of actions, IL-1 stimulates the HPA axis and then the release of glucocorticoids. Glucocorticoids are anti-inflammatory and block the production and action of several lymphokines such as IL-2, γ-interferon and also IL-1 production by macrophages. In fact, a feedback glucocorticoid-associated immunoregulatory system exists that may exert a continuous surveillance of the immunological state. However, when overstimulation of the pituitary–

adrenal axis by cytokines produced by immune-inflammatory cells occurs, it leads to pathological states. The massive and sustained release of IL-1, causing increased glucocorticoid blood levels may be one of the factors mediating immunosuppression of the acute phase following TNB instillation.

The principal effectors of the stress response include the CRF and locus coeruleus–norepinephrine systems in the central nervous system (CNS). CRF is widely distributed in many brain regions, including the paraventricular nucleus of the hypothalamus, the brain stem, the limbic system and the cortex. CRF was initially isolated as the principal hypothalamic stimulus to the pituitary–adrenal axis [36,37]. CRF is involved in behavioural and physiological responses to stress. These responses include HPA axis activation, sympathetic nervous system (SNS) activation, anorexia and changes in motor activity [34].

Increased levels of CRF have been implicated in the stress-induced suppression of immune function [38,39]. In the present study, we show that exposure to PRS for 4 consecutive days induces a decrease in MPO activity, in non-inflamed rats. Since MPO level is related to neutrophil infiltration [29], this result is in accordance with knowledge of a stress suppressive action on immune system [40], even though studies in adrenalectomized rats have shown that this response is independent of glucocorticoids [41]. Although the essential pathophysiology of stress-induced immunosuppression has not been determined, there is considerable evidence demonstrating that CRF is an essential agent in stress-induced impairment of immune function [38,41].

Our study shows the well-recognized stress-induced suppression of the immune system in intact rats but also provides evidence that chronic PRS has a pro-inflammatory effect in inflamed rats. Indeed, the MPO activity and the colitic damage score were higher in animals inflamed with TNB after chronic PRS. Cytokines appear to play a role in the response to stress and may mediate the release of hormones from the HPA axis. For instance, IL-6 which is not only produced by cells in immune tissues but also by cells in neuroendocrine and endocrine tissues, such as the hypothalamus [43,44], anterior pituitary [45,46] and adrenal cortex [47], is increased after tissue injury, infection and inflammation in which there is activation of the HPA axis. However, in rats exposed to a mild psychological stressor, blood IL-6 increased through a mechanism independent of endotoxaemia, tissue injury or inflammation [48]. Recently, Zhou et al. [49] reported that physical or psychological stressors elevated the plasma level of IL-6 in a manner that resembles that of corticosterone. The increase in IL-6 in response to stress may be under the regulation of the neural and endocrine system and may not come from immune tissues, since IL-6 production during stress was suppressed and because adrenalectomy reduced the elevation of plasma IL-6 due to stress [49]. Consequently, we can hypothesize that PRS stimulates the release of IL-6 which in turn increases the colitis in rats treated with TNB.

When animals received central administration of either CRF antagonist (α-helical CRF_{9-41}) or AVP antagonist before each PRS session applied before induction of colitis, these treatments enhanced the level of inflammation, already increased by stress. Indeed, the level of MPO was much higher than that observed in rats ICV injected with vehicle. The central injection of either α-helical CRF_{9-41} or AVP antagonist block the stress-induced stimulation of HPA axis and therefore the subsequent glucocorticoid release. Therefore, the colonic inflammation related to TNB is exacerbated as shown by increased MPO activity. These results provide evidence that, during a stress situation, CRF and AVP exert protective effects against inflammation and avoid over-inflammation.

Regarding body weight during colitis, we observed that stress applied before colitis had no effect on loss of body weight, although it did increase the inflammation state. Moreover, when stress was applied after induction of colitis, it reduced the loss of weight normally observed during colitis. In animals treated with α-helical CRF_{9-41} or AVP antagonist before stress sessions, the loss in body weight was greater, suggesting that CRF and AVP receptor antagonists prevent the inflammation-induced drastic weight loss. These observations reinforce the hypothesis that, during stress, CRF and AVP act to minimize the influence of general colitis through, at least, stimulation of the HPA axis. Indeed, the physiologically relevant ACTH secretagogues are CRF and AVP [22].

Several stress-induced alterations of GI functions such as intestinal [23] and colonic [28] motility are directly linked to the central release of either CRF [28] or AVP [29] but are not linked to the stimulation of the HPA axis [26,28]. Consequently, we could not reject the hypothesis that CRF and AVP may act on other pathways than the HPA axis to decrease the severity of colitis during stress.

ACKNOWLEDGEMENTS

The authors thank L. Ressayre for skillful technical assistance.

REFERENCES

1. Cann PA, Read NW, Cammack J. Psychological stress and the passage of a standard meal through the stomach and small intestine in man. Gut. 1983;24:236–40.
2. Narducci F, Snape WJ, Battle WM, London RL, Cohen S. Increased colonic motility during exposure to a stressful situation. Dig Dis Sci. 1985;30:40–4.
3. Collins SM. Is the irritable gut an inflamed gut? Scand J Gastroenterol. 1992;27(Suppl.192):102–5.
4. Stein TA, Keegan L, Auguste LJ, Bailey B, Wise L. Stress induced experimental colitis. Mediators Inflamm. 1993;2:253–6.
5. McHugh K, Weingarten HP, Khan I, Riddell R, Collins SM. Stress-induced exacerbation of experimental colitis (Abstract). Gastroenterology. 1993;104:A803.
6. MacDermott RP, Stenson WF. Inflammatory bowel disease. In: Targan SR, Shanahan F, eds. Immunology and Immunopathology of the Liver and Gastrointestinal Tract. New York, Tokyo: Igaku-Shoin; 190:459–86.
7. Hallgren R, Colombel JF, Dahl R et al. Neutrophil and eosinophil involvement of the small bowel in patients with celiac disease and Crohn's disease: studies on the secretion rate and immunohistochemical localization of granulocyte granule constituents. Am J Med. 1989;86:56–64.
8. Thyberg J, Graf W, Klingenstrom P. Intestinal fine structure in Crohn's disease; lysosomal inclusions in epithelial cells and macrophages. Virchows Arch (Pathol Anat.). 1981;39:141–52.
9. Tanner AR, Arthur MJP, Wright R. Macrophage activation, chronic inflammation and gastrointestinal disease. Gut. 1984;25:760–83.
10. Mahida YR, Wu KC, Jewell BC. Respiratory burst activity of intestinal macrophages in normal and inflammatory bowel disease. Gut. 1989;30:1362–70.

11. Herbay AJ, Gerbbers JO, Otto HF. Immunopathology of ulcerative colitis: a review. Hepatogastroenterology. 1990;37:99–107.
12. Morris GP, Beck PL, Herridge MS, Depew W, Szewczuk MR, Wallace JL. Hapten-induced model of chronic inflammation and ulceration in the rat colon. Gastroenterology. 1989;96:795–803.
13. Levine S, Strebel R, Wenk E, Harman P. Suppression of experimental allergic encephalomyelitis by stress. Proc Soc Exp Biol Med. 1962;109:294–8.
14. Riley V. Psychoneuroendocrine influences on immunocompetence and neoplasia. Science. 1981;212:1100–9.
15. Stein M, Schiavi RC, Camerino M. Influence of brain and behavior on the immune system. Science. 1976;191:435–40.
16. Keller SE, Weiss JM, Schleifer SJ, Miller NE, Stein M. Stress-induced suppression of immunity in adrenalectomized rats. Science. 1983;221:1301–4.
17. Berkenbosch F, van Oers J, del Rey A, Tilders F, Besedovsky H. Corticotropin-releasing factor-producing neurons in the rat activated by interleukin-1. Science. 1987;238:524–6.
18. Lumpkin MD. The regulation of ACTH secretion by IL-1. Science. 1987;238:452–4.
19. Sapolsky R, Rivier C, Yamamoto G, Plotsky P, Vale W. Interleukin-1 stimulates the secretion of hypothalamic corticotropin releasing factor. Science. 1987;238:522–4.
20. Gué M, Fioramonti J, Bonbonne C, Del Rio C, Junien JL, Buéno L. Chronic partial restraint stress (PRS) enhances trinitrobenzene sulfonic acid-induced colitis in rats. Gastroenterology. 1995;108:A828.
21. Axelrod J, Reisine TD. Stress hormones: their interaction and regulation. Science. 1984;224:452–9.
22. Rivier C, Vale W. Modulation of stress-induced ACTH release by corticotropin-releasing factor, catecholamines and vasopressin. Nature. 1983;305:325–7.
23. Williams CL, Villar RG, Peterson JM, Burks TF. Corticotropin releasing factor directly mediates colonic response to stress. Am J Physiol. 1987;253:G582–6.
24. Gué M, Junien JL, Buéno L. Mental stress in rats enhances colonic motility through the central release of corticotropin-releasing factor. Gastroenterology. 1991;100:964–70.
25. Buéno L, Gué M, Del Rio C. CNS vasopressin mediates emotional stress and CRH-induced colonic motor alterations in rats. Am J Physiol. 1992;262:G427–31.
26. Krawisz JE, Sharon P, Stenson WF. Quantitative assay for acute inflammation based on myeloperoxidase activity: assessment of inflammation in rat and hamster models. Gastroenterology. 1984;87:1344–50.
27. Wallace JL, Keenan CM. An orally active inhibitor of leukotriene synthesis accelerates healing in a rat model of colitis. Am J Physiol. 1990;258:G527–34.
28. Fabia R, Arrajab A, Johansson ML et al. The effect of exogenous administration of Lactobacillus reuteri R2LC and oat fiber on acetic acid-induced colitis in rats. Scand J Gastroenterol. 1993;28:155–62.
29. Bradley PP, Priebat DA, Christensen RD, Rothstein G. Measurement of cutaneous inflammation: estimation of neutrophil content with an enzyme marker. J Invest Dermatol. 1982;78:206–9.
30. Lowry OH, Rosebrough NJ, Farr AL, Randall RJ. Protein measurement with the folin phenol reagent. J Biol Chem. 1951;193:265–75.
31. Rabbins JL, Cotran RS. Pathologic basis of disease. Philadelphia: W.B. Saunders Co., 1979:958–87.
32. Sharon P, Stenson WF. Enhanced synthesis of leukotriene B4 by colonic mucosa in inflammatory bowel disease. Gastroenterology. 1984;86:453–60.
33. Rachmilewitz D, Simon PL, Schwartz LW, Griswold DE, Fondacaro JD, Wasserman MA. Inflammatory mediators of experimental colitis in rats. Gastroenterology. 1989;97:326–37.
34. Sternberg EM, Wilder RL, Chrousos GP, Gold PW. The stress response and the pathogenesis of arthritis. In: McCubbin JA, Kaufmann PG, Nemeroff CB, eds. Stress, Neuropeptides and systemic Disease. San Diego, California: Academic Press; 1991:287–300.
35. Breder CD, Dinarello CA, Saper CB. Interleukin-1 immunoreactive innervation of the human hypothalamus. Science. 1988;240:321–4.
36. Vale W, Spies J, Rivier C, Rivier J. Characterization of a 41-residue ovine hypothalamic peptide that stimulates secretion of corticotropin and beta-endorphin. Science. 1981;213:1394–7.
37. Sutton RE, Koob GF, Le Moal M, Rivier J, Vale W. Corticotropin releasing factor produces behavioral activation in rats. Nature. 1982;29:331–3.
38. Irwin M. Stress-induced immune suppression: role of brain corticotropin releasing hormone and autonomic nervous system mechanisms. Adv Neuroimmunol. 1994;4:29–47.
39. Jain R, Zwickler D, Hollander CS et al. Corticotropin releasing factor modulates the immune response to stress in the rat. Endocrinology. 1991;128:1329–36.
40. Keller SE, Weiss JM, Schleifer SJ, Miller NE, Stein M. Suppression of immunity by stress: effect of a graded series of stressors on lymphocyte stimulation in the rat. Science. 1981;213:1397–400.

41. Saperstein A, Brand H, Audhya T et al. Interleukin 1 b mediates stress-induced immunosuppression via corticotropin-releasing factor. Endocrinology. 1992;130:152–8.
42. Kort WJ. The effect of chronic stress on the immune response. Adv Neuroimmunol. 1994;4:1–11.
43. Schobitz B, Voorhuis DAM, De Kloet ER. Localization of interleukin 6 mRNA and interleukin 6 receptor mRNA in rat brain. Neurosci Lett. 1992;136:189–92.
44. Yamaguchi M, Yoshimoto Y, Komura H et al. Interleukin 1 b and tumour necrosis factor a stimulate the release of gonadotropin-releasing hormone and interleukin 6 by primary cultured rat hypothalamic cells. Acta Endocrinol. 1990;123:476–80.
45. Spangelo BL, MacLeod RM, Isakson PC. Production of interleukin 6 by anterior pituitary cells in vitro. Endocrinology. 1990;126:582–6.
46. Spangelo BL, Judd AM, Isakson PC, MacLeod RM. Interleukin-1 stimulates interleukin-6 release from rat anterior pituitary cells in vitro. Endocrinology. 1991;128:2685–92.
47. Judd AM, MacLeod RM. Adenocorticotropin increases interleukin-6 release from rat adrenal zona glomerulus cells. Endocrinology. 1992;130:1245–54.
48. LeMay LG, Vander AJ, Kluger MJ. The effects of psychological stress on plasma interleukin-6 activity in rats. Physiol Behav. 1990;47:957–61.
49. Zhou D, Kusnecov AW, Shurin MR, dePaoli M, Rabin BS. Exposure to physical and psychological stressors elevates plasma interleukin 6: relationship to the activation of hypothalamic–pituitary–adrenal axis. Endocrinology. 1993;133:2523–30.

G Mózsik et al. Cell Injury and Cytoprotection in the GI Tract. 237–248.
© 1997 Kluwer Academic Publishers.

PROTECTIVE EFFECT OF TRAPENCAINE IN ACETIC ACID-INDUCED COLITIS IN RATS

V. NOSÁLOVÁ AND V. BAUER

Institute of Experimental Pharmacology, Slovak Academy of Sciences, Bratislava, Slovak Republic

This paper was first published in: Inflammopharmacology. 1996;4:387–398.

ABSTRACT

Despite extensive research, the aetiology and pathogenesis of ulcerative colitis are still unknown and the therapeutic approach remains therefore empirical. Since trapencaine, a local anaesthetic, has been repeatedly demonstrated to protect the gastric mucosa from the injurious effects of a variety of noxious stimuli, its efficacy against acute inflammatory attack of the colonic mucosa was studied in a rat model of colitis induced by intracolonic administration of 4% acetic acid.

Vehicle or trapencaine in doses of 3, 10 and 30 mg/kg were given 30 min before acetic acid and the resulting injury was assessed after 48 h. Gross findings were ranked using the criteria of MacPherson and Pfeiffer. The length and wet/dry weight ratio of the colon were recorded, colonic fluid absorption was assessed and myeloperoxidase activity in colonic mucosal scrapings was determined. Contractility of colonic muscle strips was examined in vitro.

Trapencaine pretreatment was found to reduce the extent of the inflammatory colonic mucosal injury induced by acetic acid administration, as evidenced by the significant decrease in the rank of gross mucosal damage and in wet/dry colonic weight ratio, as well as by the attenuation of granulocyte infiltration. The increased responsiveness of colonic smooth muscle to acetylcholine and barium chloride associated with acute colitis was diminished by trapencaine pretreatment. The results indicate that trapencaine locally present in the colon seems to maintain the intregrity of colonic mucosa.

Keywords: acetic acid, colitis, rats, trapencaine

INTRODUCTION

The normal colonic mucosa provides an efficient barrier against a potentially harmful environment that normally exists in the intestinal lumen. This barrier is impaired in colitis. Ulcerative colitis is a chronically recurrent inflammatory bowel disease of unknown origin. A variety of aetiological and pathogenic mechanisms resulting in mucosal breakdown and subsequent inflammation have been proposed, e.g. biochemical, bacterial, immunoreactive, genetic, ischaemic and toxic factors [1–5].

Björck et al. [6,7] suggested a pathogenic role of hyper-reactive autonomic nerves in the disease based on the finding of hyperinnervation of the submucosa, the muscularis mucosae and the mucosa with adrenergic nerves and peptidergic nerves immunopositive for neuropeptide Y, substance P and VIP. They thought that an increased release of neurotransmitters from these nerves could possibly be related to some initial phenomena seen in ulcerative colitis. Noradrenaline and neuropeptide Y may reduce mucosal

This paper was presented at the Symposium on 'Cell injury and protection in the gastrointestinal tract: from basic science to clinical perspectives', October 8–11, 1995, Pécs, Hungary.

circulation, augment epithelial cell proliferation and enforce neuroimmune interactions. This would lead to vasoconstriction and congestion, cell loss and ulcer formation and to an inflammatory response. They proposed the use of a local anaesthetic to block these neural effects. In an open trial, patients with ulcerative proctitis and proctosigmoiditis were treated daily by intrarectally administered 2% lidocaine enemas. Symptomatic relief, improvement in histology and eventual healing were achieved in 83% of patients after lidocaine treatment for 6–34 weeks.

The use of local anaesthetics in ulcerative colitis is a new approach to mucosal inflammation. So far, their effect has not been fully elucidated. In the present study the effect of another local anaesthetic, trapencaine ($\pm$)-*trans*-2(1-pyrrolidinyl)cyclohexyl ester of 3(n)-pentyl-oxycarbanilic acid [8,9], an antiulcer and gastroprotective agent with some antisecretory activity, was examined in a rat model of colitis. This compound was found to prevent the development of gastric lesions induced by stress and non-steroidal anti-inflammatory drugs, to inhibit duodenal lesions induced by cysteamine and to protect the gastric mucosa against the necrotizing effect of absolute ethanol, concentrated HCl or NaCl [10,11]. To determine whether trapencaine could also protect the colonic mucosa against an acute inflammatory change, a model of acute acetic acid-induced colitis was used.

MATERIALS AND METHODS

Male Wistar rats weighing 200–280 g were housed in wire-mesh cages, given standard laboratory chow and tap water ad libitum and acclimatized for one week before experiments. The rats were randomly assigned to the experimental groups.

Induction of colitis

Rats were anaesthetized by 50 mg/kg pentobarbital ip and administered 1 ml either vehicle (0.9% saline) or trapencaine at doses of 3, 10 or 30 mg/kg intrarectally via a polyethylene cannula (fitted to a 1 ml syringe) with the tip inserted approximately 8 cm proximal to the anus. Following 30 min pretreatment, 1 ml of 4% acetic acid was introduced into the colon ir and, after exposure of 60 s, the excess fluid was withdrawn [12]. A similar treatment was given to the second group of rats by another mode of administration, i.e. injection into the ligated colon after laparatomy [13]. A reversible ligature at the junction of the caecum and the ascending colon was made, the colon was cleansed of its luminal contents with warm saline (37°C) and residual fluid was manually pressed out. Distal to the ligature, 2 ml of either vehicle or trapencaine at doses of 3, 10 or 30 mg/kg were injected. After 30 min, this pretreatment was followed by 30 s exposure to 2 ml of 4% acetic acid. The luminal content was then expelled by instillation of 10 ml air, the ligature was removed and the abdomen was sutured. Both groups of rats were allowed to recover with food and water and the resulting injury was assessed after 48 h.

Assessment of colonic damage

The rats were weighed, inspected for the presence of diarrhoea and sacrificed in diethyl ether. The colons were excised and opened longitudinally, rinsed with cold saline, pinned out and observed under a dissecting microscope. Colonic damage was scored on a 0–5 scale, using the scoring system of MacPherson and Pfeiffer [14]: 0 – normal appearance; 1 – hyperaemia; 2 – patchy petechial bleeding; 3 – diffuse petechial bleeding; 4 – partial exfoliated mucosa or single erosion or ulcer; 5 – diffuse exfoliated mucosa or multiple erosions or ulcers. The presence or absence of adhesions between the colon and the surrounding tissues was recorded. The scoring of the colonic damage was performed by an observer unaware of the treatment.

Wet weights of colons were recorded as well as their dry weights obtained after 48 h heating at 80°C and the colonic wet/dry weight ratio, considered an indirect index of inflammatory reaction, was calculated.

In-vivo colonic fluid absorption

Using the method of Fedorak et al. [15], colonic fluid absorption was measured 48 h after the induction of colitis. In anaesthetized rats (50 mg/kg sc pentobarbital), an occluding ligature was made at the caecal–ascending colon junction. The luminal contents were flushed out with warm saline and residual saline was emptied by manual expression. An intestinal loop of approximately 15 cm was created with ligatures, 2 ml of 154 mmol/L sodium chloride were instilled into the empty loop, the viscera were returned to the abdominal cavity and the incision was closed. After 60 min, the colon loop was removed and weighed, both full and emptied, to determine residual intraluminal volume.

Colonic myeloperoxidase activity

Myeloperoxidase (MPO) activity was determined in colonic mucosal scrapings 48 h after the induction of colitis by the modified method of Bradley et al. [16]. Tissue samples of approximately 50 mg were taken, weighed and homogenized three times for 30 s at 4°C in 1 ml ice-cold 0.5% hexadecyltrimethylammonium bromide in 50 mmol/L phosphate buffer (pH 6). The homogenate was subjected to three freeze/thaw cycles and centrifuged for 15 min at 40 000g. MPO activity was determined spectrophotometrically by the addition of 0.1 ml of the supernatant to 2.9 ml of 50 mmol/L phosphate buffer containing 0.167 mg/ml o-dianisidine dihydrochloride and 0.0005% w/v hydrogen peroxide. The change in absorbance at 460 nm over a 5-min period was measured at 25°C. The data are expressed as the mean absorbance $\pm$ SEM at 5 min/g wet weight [17].

Contractility of colonic longitudinal muscle

The contractile responses of isolated colonic segments to acetylcholine and barium chloride were studied in 3 groups of rats: control group (sham operated), a group of rats 48 h after induction of colitis with only vehicle pretreatment and a group of colitic rats pretreated in vivo with 30 mg/kg trapencaine. Segments of the proximal colon, approximately 4 cm from the caecum–ascendant colon junction, and of the distal colon, approximately 4 cm from the anus, were excised and the mucosa was removed, carefully avoiding damage to the underlying muscle. The muscular strips of long-itudinal orientation were suspended in a 20-ml organ bath containing oxygenated (95% O_2 and 5% CO_2) Krebs solution of the following composition (mmol/L): Na^+ 136.6, K^+ 5.9, Ca^{2+} 2.5, Mg^{2+} 1.2, Cl^- 133.3, HCO_3^- 15.4, $H_2PO_4^-$ 1.2 and glucose 11.5. Isometric contractions were recorded. The strips were allowed to equilibrate for 60 min prior to dosing and the resting tension was maintained at 10 mN. After equilibration, the cumulative concentration effect curves (CCEC) of acetylcholine in the concentra-tion range of 10^{-8} to 10^{-3} mol/L and of $BaCl_2$ in the concentration range of 0.15 to 13.5 mmol/L were obtained.

In separate experiments, the in-vitro effect of trapencaine on the isolated colonic smooth muscle from intact rats was studied. After recording the CCEC of the agonist (acetylcholine), the antagonistic effect of trapencaine was assessed using one or two of its concentrations on each preparation. The application of the agonist was repeated following a 15-min pretreatment period and in the presence of trapencaine in the bathing fluid.

The following drugs were used: acetylcholine chloride (Germed), barium chloride (Riedel–De Haenag), trapencaine hydrochloride was kindly supplied by L. Beneš (Faculty of Pharmacy, Comenius University), reagents used in the MPO assay (Sigma); other chemicals were of analytical grade.

Each experimental group consisted of at least six animals. Results are expressed as means $\pm$ SEM. Student's t-test was used for statistical analysis, $p < 0.05$ was considered significant. Non-parametric data were analysed with the Mann–Whitney U test. In studies on muscle contraction, the EC_{50} and pD_2 ($-\log EC_{50}$) were calculated by probit transformation of the data.

RESULTS

Intracolonic administration of 4% acetic acid induced diffuse hyperaemia and bleeding in the colon with focal erosions and ulcerations. As shown in Figure 1, trapencaine pretreatment reduced gross mucosal injury. The mean score of 4.1 in vehicle-treated colitic rats decreased to 1.2 after 3 mg/kg trapencaine, to 0.3 after 10 mg/kg and to 0.1 after 30 mg/kg trapencaine. The highest dose of trapencaine applied directly into the colon also reduced significantly the rank value of gross injury from 3.9 to 0.5 and the only visible sign of damage was hyperaemia. Increased mucus secretion was evident in the colon from trapencaine-treated rats.

Other indices of injury were also influenced by trapencaine (Table 1). The incidence of colon adhesions to the surrounding tissues and of diarrhoea was decreased after trapencaine pretreatment. Changes in body weight (typical weight loss on the 2nd postoperative day) were similar in non-treated rats and after 3, 10 and 30 mg/kg trapencaine (12.9 ± 0.7 g, 12.6 ± 0.9 g, 11.3 ± 1.1 g and 11.2 ± 1.4 g, respectively).

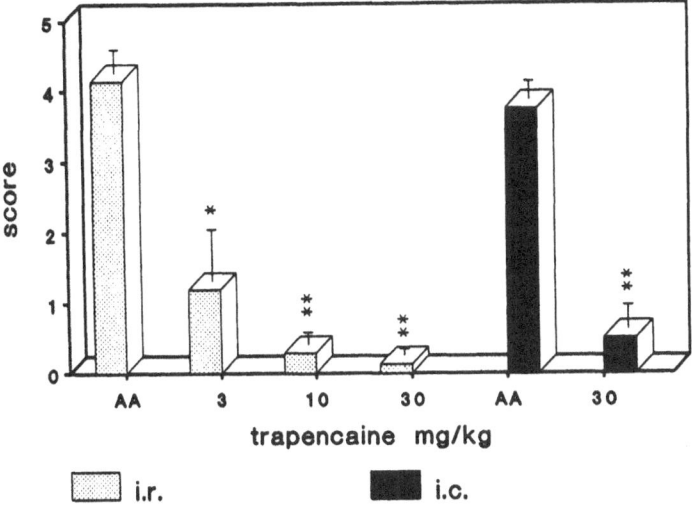

Figure 1. Effect of trapencaine on the score of gross mucosal injury 48 h after induction of colitis by intracolonic administration of 4% acetic acid (AA). Trapencaine was administered 30 min before acetic acid at doses of 3, 10 and 30 mg/kg intrarectally (ir) or injected at a dose of 30 mg/kg into the ligated colon after laparatomy (ic). Colonic damage was scored using the criteria of MacPherson and Pfeiffer by an observer unaware of the treatment. Values are means $\pm$ SEM, $n \geqslant 7$ animals per group, $*p < 0.05$, $**p < 0.01$ vs. acetic acid (vehicle-treated) group

TABLE 1
Effect of intracolonic trapencaine in rats with acetic acid-induced colitis

Feature	Colitis + vehicle	Colitis + trapencaine
Adhesions of colon to the surrounding tissues	+++	– (+)
Diarrhoea	+++	–
Body weight	Decrease by 6.6%	Decrease by 6.2%

As demonstrated in Table 2, colonic wet/dry weight ratio increased significantly in vehicle-treated colitic rats from 4.3 to 5.3. In the rats pretreated with trapencaine, the values did not differ from those of controls.

Colonic fluid absorption was measured 48 h after the induction of colitis. There was no significant change in residual volume in the colonic loop at this time interval (Figure 2).

Colonic MPO activity, which is almost exclusively located in neutrophils, was used to quantitate neutrophil infiltration. The results showed that, 48 h after the induction of

TABLE 2
Effect of trapencaine on colonic wet/dry weight ratio in acetic acid-induced colitis in rats

Treatment	Dose (mg/kg)	n	Wet/dry weight ratio
Intrarectal			
Sham operated		6	4.351
Acetic acid + vehicle		7	5.326*
Acetic acid + trapencaine	3	7	4.718
Acetic acid + trapencaine	10	7	4.713
Acetic acid + trapencaine	30	7	4.629
Intracolonic			
Sham operated		6	4.495
Acetic acid + vehicle		10	5.616*
Acetic acid + trapencaine	30	6	4.723

*$p < 0.05$ vs. control (sham-operated) rats

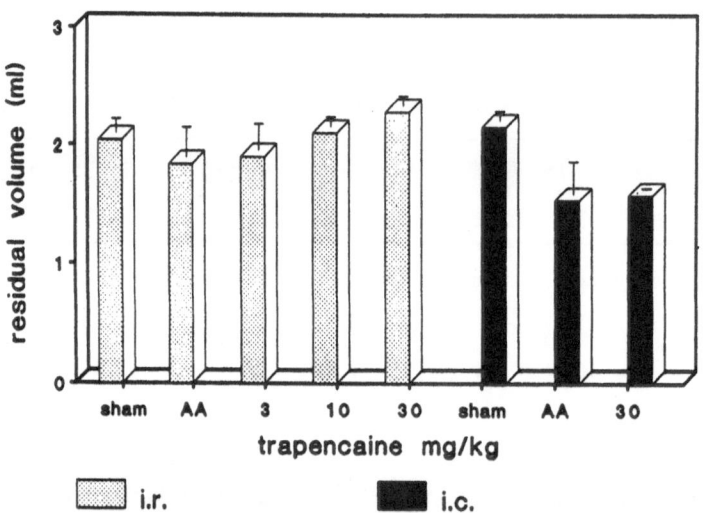

Figure 2. Effect of trapencaine on colonic fluid absorption measured in vivo 48 h after induction of colitis by intracolonic administration of 4% acetic acid. Trapencaine was administered 30 min before acetic acid in doses of 3, 10 and 30 mg/kg intrarectally (ir) or injected in a dose of 30 mg/kg into the ligated colon after laparatomy (ic). The acetic acid (AA) group was treated by vehicle and the control group was sham-operated (sham). Values are means $\pm$ SEM of at least 7 experiments, expressed as ml of residual volume

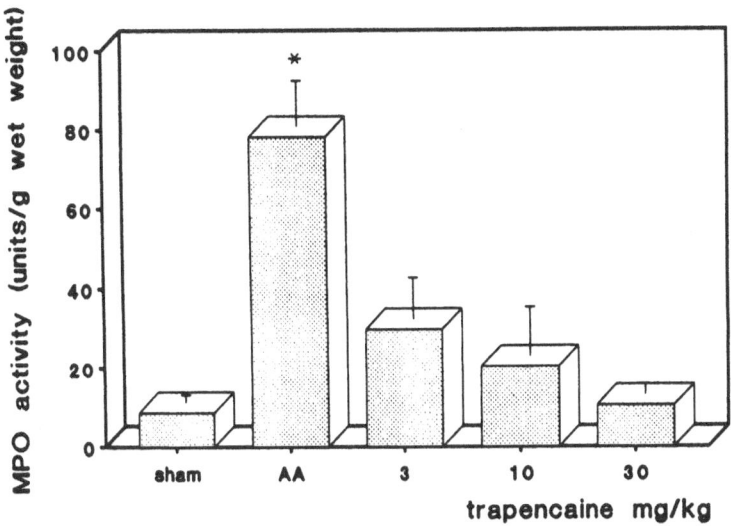

Figure 3. Effect of trapencaine on myeloperoxidase (MPO) activity measured in colonic mucosal scrapings 48 h after induction of colitis by intracolonic administration of 4% acetic acid. For further details of trapencaine pretreatment, see previous figures. Values are means $\pm$ SEM of at least 7 experiments, expressed as units MPO/g wet weight, *$p < 0.05$ vs. sham-operated rats

colitis, there was a significant increase in MPO activity which was dose-dependently diminished by trapencaine pretreatment (Figure 3).

Muscle preparations of colonic longitudinal strips showed spontaneous activity which was reduced by the removal of the mucosa. Trapencaine, at concentrations of 10^{-5} and 10^{-4} mol/L, reduced the basal tension by 3.43 ± 0.68 mN and 5.39 ± 0.67 mN, respectively, and attenuated the spontaneous smooth muscle activity. Cumulative administration of acetylcholine in a bath concentration range of 10^{-8} to 10^{-3} mol/L elicited contractions of the longitudinal colonic muscle strips. Trapencaine in the concentrations used shifted the CCEC to the right and reduced significantly the maximum of CCEC (Figure 4).

In control preparations, there was a difference between the proximal and distal colon in the response to the agonists used, with the proximal part being more responsive than the distal one. The contractions of muscle preparations from rats with colitis to acetylcholine had an increased amplitude in the longitudinal strips from the proximal colon compared with sham-operated rats (pD_2 values 6.7 and 5.4, respectively) and were unchanged in the distal colon (pD_2 values 5.8 for both groups). The responses of colonic preparations from colitic animals pretreated with 30 mg/kg trapencaine (pD_2 value 6.1) were not different in amplitude from those in controls (Figures 5 and 6). The same trend of changes was observed after the application of a musculotropic agent, $BaCl_2$ (Figure 7) with pD_2 values of 3.0 in sham-operated, 3.3 in colons with colitis and 2.8 in trapencaine-treated preparations.

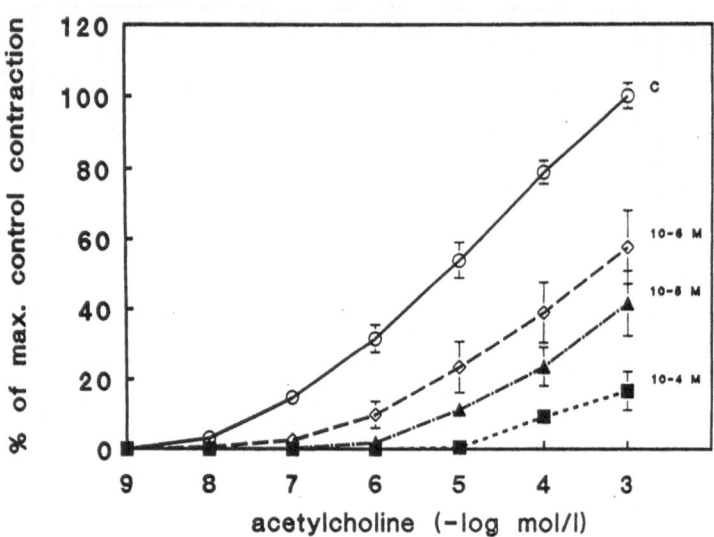

Figure 4. Effect of trapencaine on cumulative concentration–effect curves of acetylcholine in colonic longitudinal muscle strips from control rats. Values are means ± SEM, expressed as % of maximal control contraction. ○——○ control response, ◇- - -◇ trapencaine 10^{-6} mol/L, ▲-·--·-▲ 10^{-5} mol/L. ■- - - -■ 10^{-4} mol/L

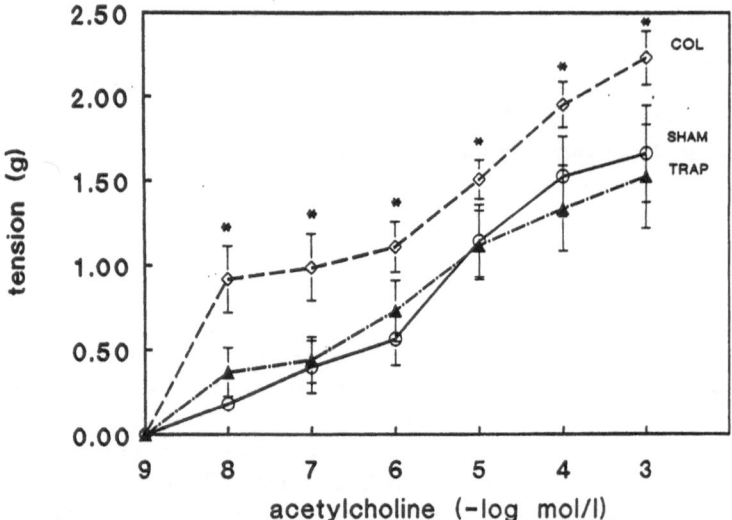

Figure 5. Isometric tension (g) induced by longitudinal muscle of the proximal colon from sham-operated control rats (SHAM, ○——○), rats with colitis induced by 4% acetic acid (COL, ◇- - -◇), and from colitis rats pretreated by 30 mg/kg trapencaine (TRAP, ▲-·--·-▲). Cumulative concentration–effect curve of acetylcholine applied in concentrations of 10^{-8}–10^{-3} mol/L. Values are means ± SEM from ≥ 6 experiments, *$p < 0.05$ vs. sham-operated group

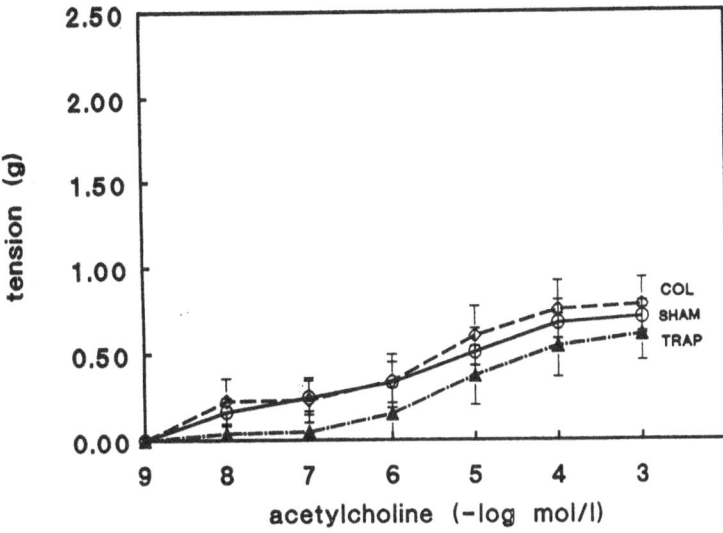

Figure 6. Isometric tension (g) induced by longitudinal muscle of the distal colon from sham-operated control rats (SHAM), rats with colitis induced by 4% acetic acid (COL), and colitis rats pretreated by 30 mg/kg trapencaine (TRAP). Cumulative concentration–effect curve of acetylcholine applied in concentrations of 10^{-8}–10^{-3} mol/L. Values are means $\pm$ SEM from at least 6 experiments

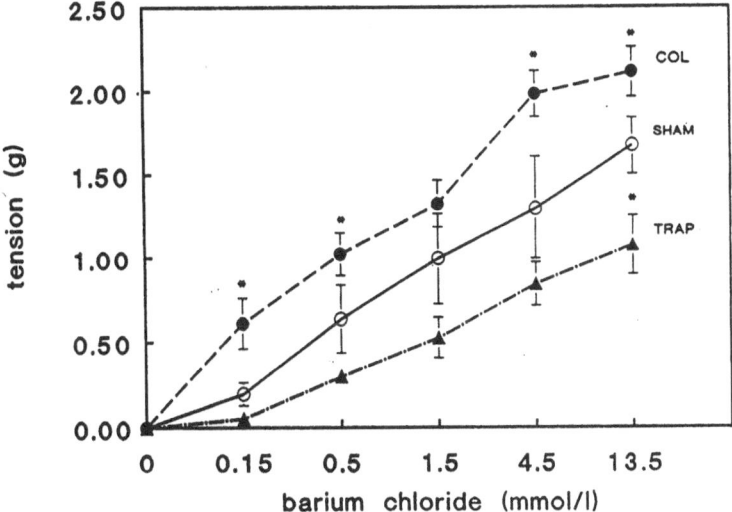

Figure 7. Isometric tension (g) induced by longitudinal muscle of the proximal colon from sham-operated control rats (SHAM), rats with colitis induced by 4% acetic acid (COL), and from colitis rats pretreated by 30 mg/kg trapencaine (TRAP). Cumulative concentration–effect curve of barium chloride applied in concentrations of 0.15–13.5 mmol/L. Values are means $\pm$ SEM from at least 6 experiments; $*p < 0.05$ vs. sham-operated rats

DISCUSSION

The use of local anaesthetics in ulcerative colitis is a new approach to mucosal inflammation. The possible mechanism of their action is through the blockade of certain neurally mediated effects, such as epithelial proliferation and congestion of the mucosal vasculature, with actions on cells of the immune system (subsets of T-lymphocytes). Local anaesthetics exert a variety of anti-inflammatory effects, independent of their action on neurons. Lidocaine was shown to suppress neutrophil secretion and superoxide production in vitro [18] and to inhibit granulocyte adherence and prevent granulocyte delivery to inflammatory sites [19]. Our results demonstrated that trapencaine could also protect the colonic mucosa against an inflammatory attack, as shown by the reduction of gross mucosal injury, inhibition of wet/dry weight ratio and by the attenuation of MPO activity. The protective effect of trapencaine against acetic acid-induced damage seems to require the presence of trapencaine in the colon since there was no protection observed after its subcutaneous administration (results not shown). Similarly, previous experiments on ethanol-induced gastric injury demonstrated a pronounced protection after orally administered trapencaine, yet a virtual lack of gastroprotective effect after parenteral administration [20].

Lidocaine was shown to have a similar protective effect in experimental colitis induced by trinitrobenzenesulphonic acid in rats [21]. If it is the local anaesthetic property that is mostly responsible for such a protection, then the use of trapencaine may prove very suitable since its local anaesthetic activity exceeds, by approximately one order of magnitude, that of lidocaine without having higher toxicity or undesirable side-effects.

Unlike the effect of most of the common local anaesthetics, the effect of trapencaine increases in low pH conditions, as shown in in-vitro experiments on action potential conduction [22]. This property would be of advantage with regard to the action of trapencaine in regions where pH is shifted toward acidity, e.g. in the stomach or at inflammatory sites.

A marked increase in mucosal permeability was observed by Yamada et al. [23] within one hour after the induction of colitis. This initial damage was followed by rapid repair of the mucosa over the following 48 h, as manifested by a fall in mucosal permeability. It is possible that the time interval of 48 h used in our experiments was too long for the assessment of colonic fluid absorption in vivo because the acute changes of permeability have already been returned to almost normal values.

Concerning the effect of trapencaine on colonic smooth muscle, its non-selective blockade of the cation influx might prevent membrane depolarization, resulting in reduced calcium influx and smooth muscle relaxation. Acetylcholine reacting with muscarinic receptors of the smooth muscle membrane enhances the influx of extracellular calcium. Barium chloride was shown to substitute for Ca^{2+} in the contractile process [24] and it may cause membrane depolarization due to suppression of potassium conductance independent of receptor activation [25]. The ability of trapencaine to antagonize the effect of both these spasmogens in vitro suggests that its action may be independent of a specific membrane receptor-mediated action. The shift of the acetylcholine CCEC to the right and the reduction of the maximum contraction are indicative of the non-competitive type of trapencaine action. A similar effect was described also for other local anaesthetics on different smooth muscles [26]. The non-specific action of trapencaine in the initial phase of colitis development might prevent influences elicited by hyperinnervation and local reflexes.

Studies on muscle contraction in colitis have yielded conflicting results. Experiments on nematode-infected rats indicated that acute inflammation was associated with an increase in tension generation by intestinal longitudinal muscle [27]. Cohen et al. [28] described a decrease in tension development by circular muscle from rabbits with immune complex colitis whereas Percy et al. reported unchanged responses [29]. Discrepancies could arise from species differences, from regional differences in the responses of the smooth muscle to inflammatory mediators, from differences in structural integrity or orientation of the preparations, or they may result from the diverse nature of the inflammatory responses in various experimental models [30].

We also observed difference in the responsiveness of longitudinal strips from the proximal and from the distal colon to acetylcholine and barium chloride in sham-operated rats, with the proximal part of the colon being more responsive than the distal one. In the inflamed colon, there was an increased responsiveness of the proximal longitudinal colonic muscle to acetylcholine and barium chloride compared with sham-operated rats which was restored to control values after trapencaine treatment, whereas, in the distal colon, the responses were unchanged. Similarly, in patients with colitis, the anorectal motor functions were not compromised after lidocaine topical treatment, yet some altered muscle function might have still been present.

The results indicate that the local anaesthetic, trapencaine, can protect the colonic mucosa during the early phase of the inflammatory response in acetic acid-induced colitis as documented by the reduction of gross mucosal injury and wet/dry weight ratio and by the inhibition of myeloperoxidase activity. The ability of trapencaine to restore the altered muscle function in colitis may contribute to its beneficial effect. The precise mechanisms of trapencaine action need to be further evaluated.

ACKNOWLEDGEMENTS

The authors are grateful to the Slovak Academy of Sciences for partially supporting this work (grant N 288).

REFERENCES

1. Roediger WEW, Nance S. Metabolic induction of experimental colitis by inhibition of fatty acid oxidation. Br J Exp Pathol. 1986;67:773–82.
2. Chester JF, Ross JS, Malt RA, Wietzman SA. Acute colitis produced by chemotactic peptides in rats and mice. Am J Pathol. 1985;121:284–90.
3. Grisham MB, Granger DN. Neutrophil-mediated mucosal injury. Dig Dis Sci. 1988;33(suppl):6S–15S.
4. Koo A, Leung FW. Microcirculation of the colon: macromolecular permeability and loss of the endothelial viability in experimental colitis in rats. Prog Appl Microcirc. 1990;17:90–100.
5. Sharon P, Stenson WF. Metabolism of arachidonic acid in acetic acid colitis in rats. Similarity to human inflammatory bowel disease. Gastroenterology. 1985;8:55–63.

6. Björck S, Dahlström A, Johansson L, Ahlman H. Treatment of the mucosa with local anaesthetics in ulcerative colitis. Agents Actions. 1992;Special Conference Issue:C60–72.
7. Björck S, Dahlström A, Ahlman H. Topical treatment of ulcerative proctitis with lidocaine. Scand J Gastroenterol. 1989;24:1061.
8. Beneš L, Borovanský A, Kopáčová L. Alkoxycarbanilic acid esters with high local anaesthetic activity. Arzneim.-Forsch (Drug Res). 1969;19:1902.
9. Beneš L. Trapencaine hydrochloride. Drugs Future. 1991;16:627–30.
10. Nosálová V, Babulová A, Beneš L. On gastric cytoprotective effect of pentacaine. Acta Pharmacol Toxicol. 1986;59(suppl):201.
11. Nosálová V, Babulová A, Jakubovský J, Beneš L. Experimental peptic ulcer: effect of pentacaine. In: Szabo S, Mozsik Gy, eds. New Pharmacology of Ulcer Disease. New York: Elsevier; 1987:505–16.
12. Eliakim R, Karmeli F, Okon E, Rachmilewitz D. Ketotifen effectively prevents mucosal damage in experimental colitis. Gut. 1992;33:1498–503.
13. Fedorak RN, Empey LR, MacArthur C, Jewell LD. Misoprostol provides a colonic mucosal protective effect during acetic acid-induced colitis in rats. Gastroenterology. 1990;98:615–25.
14. MacPherson BR, Pfeiffer CJ. Experimental production of diffuse colitis in rats. Digestion. 1978;17:135–50.
15. Fedorak RN, Empey LR, Walker K. Verapamil alters eicosanoid synthesis and accelerates healing during experimental colitis in rats. Gastroenterology. 1992;102:1229–35.
16. Bradley PP, Priebat DA, Christensen RD, Rothstein G. Measurement of cutaneous inflammation: estimation of neutrophil content with an enzyme marker. J Invest Dermatol. 1982;78:206–9.
17. Noronha-Blob L, Lowe VC, Muhlhauser RO, Burch RM. NPC 15669, an inhibitor of neutrophil recruitment, is efficacious in acetic acid-induced colitis in rats. Gastroenterology. 1993;104:1021–9.
18. Goldstein IM, Lind S, Hoffstein S, Weissman G. Influence of local anesthetics upon human polymorphonuclear leukocyte function in vitro: reduction of lysosomal enzyme release and superoxide anion production. J Exp Med. 1977;146:483–94.
19. MacGregor RR, Thorner RE, Wright DM. Lidocaine inhibits granulocyte adherence and prevents granulocyte delivery to inflammatory sites. Blood. 1980;56:203–9.
20. Nosálová V, Babulová A. Gastric antiulcer activity of pentacaine: possible mechanism of action. Physiol Res. 1994;43:181–6.
21. McCafferty D-M, Sharkey KA, Wallace JL. Beneficial effects of local or systemic lidocaine in experimental colitis. Am J Physiol. 1994;266:G560–7.
22. Štolc S, Stankovičová T. Effect of local anaesthetics and pH: new aspects. Drugs Exp Clin Res. 1986;12:753–60.
23. Yamada T, Specian RD, Granger DN, Gaginella TS, Grisham MB. Misoprostol attenuates acetic acid-induced increases in mucosal permeability and inflammation: role of blood flow. Am J Physiol. 1991;261:G332–9.
24. Ebashi S, Endo M. Calcium ion and muscle contraction. Progr Biophys Mol Biol. 1968;18:123–83.
25. Benham CD, Bolton TB, Lang RJ, Takewaki T. The mechanism of action of Ba^{2+} and TEA on single Ca^{2+}-activated K^+-channels in arterial and intestinal smooth muscle cell membranes. Pflugers Arch. 1985;403:120–7.
26. Feinstein MB, Paimre M. Pharmacological action of local anesthetics on excitation–contraction coupling in striated and smooth muscle. Fed Proc. 1969;28:1643–8.
27. Vermillion DL, Collins SM. Increased responsiveness of jejunal longitudinal muscle in Trichenella-infected rats. Am J Physiol. 1988;254:G124–9.
28. Cohen JD, Kao HW, Tan ST, Lechago J, Snape WJ Jr. Effect of acute experimental colitis on rabbit colonic smooth muscle. Am J Physiol. 1986;251:G538–45.
29. Percy WH, Burton MB, Jacobowitz Y, Burakof R. An investigation in vitro of the properties of the individual muscle layers of the rabbit colon in an induced colitis. In: Snape WJ, Collins SM, eds. Effect of immune cells and inflammation on smooth muscle and enteric nerves. Boca Raton: C.R.C.; 1991:95–108.
30. Grossi L, McHugh K, Collins SM. On the specificity of altered muscle function in experimental colitis in rats. Gastroenterology. 1993;104:1049–56.

G Mózsik et al. Cell Injury and Cytoprotection in the GI Tract. 249–258.
© 1997 Kluwer Academic Publishers.

PENTADECAPEPTIDE BPC 157 BENEFICIALLY INFLUENCES THE HEALING OF COLON–COLON ANASTOMOSES IN RATS

I. ZORICIC, P. SIKIRIC*, S. SEIWERTH, Z. GRABAREVIC, R. RUCMAN, M. PETEK, V. JAGIC, B. TURKOVIC, I. ROTKVIC, S. MISE, D. VUKUSIC, Z. PERKO AND P. KONJEVODA

Centre for Digestive Diseases, Medical and Veterinary Faculty, University of Zagreb, Zagreb, Croatia
*Correspondence

ABSTRACT

Protection of gastrointestinal tract and an evident anti-inflammatory effect have been shown by a pentadecapeptide BPC 157, a fragment of organoprotective gastric juice peptide (BPC) (ip/ig) in comparison with several reference standards in various ulcer models (pre-/co-/post-treatment). Since an effect on mucosal healing was also noted, the BPC 157 effect on healing of colon–colon anastomoses was further investigated.

Methods: Male Albino Wistar rats, 250 g body weight, were used for the experiments. Bursting pressure (mean ± SEM, mmHg) was measured on postoperative days 2, 5, 7 and 10 using a previously described method. The rats were treated with BPC 157 (10 μg or 10 ng/kg) given either (a) immediately after colon resection and colon–colon anastomosis, (i) ig, (ii) ip or (iii) locally, and sacrificed 2, 5, 7 or 10 days thereafter, or (b) with an additional (iv) ig or (v) ip application, 24 h after first medication (sacrifice on postoperative day 2). Controls received an equivolume of saline (5 ml/kg).

Results: After single administration of BPC 157, a dose-dependent increase in bursting pressure and maximal bowel wall tension relative to control values was evident after 2 days. When applied repeatedly, BPC resulted in a relative increase after 2 days at the lower BPC 157 dosage as well. Taken together, these data indicate that, in accordance with its strong protective effect on gastrointestinal tract, BPC 157 could beneficially influence healing of colon–colon anastomoses, and this was confirmed microscopically, and increase bursting strength, particularly in the early postoperative period. Whether this will have clinical implications remains to be seen.

Keywords: pentadecapeptide BPC 157, peptide BPC, colon–colon anastomosis, increased healing

INTRODUCTION

The physiological significance of the gut peptides is as yet not completely explored for possible therapeutic application. The discovery of novel peptides, their structure and actions, have received considerable attention [1,2]. We identified a new gastric juice peptide with mucosal protective properties and a huge range of organoprotective effects (MW 40 000 determined by gel chromatography) termed BPC [3–9]. Following these studies, a 15-amino-acid fragment (BPC 157), apparently with no sequence

---

This paper was presented at the Symposium on 'Cell injury and protection in the gastrointestinal tract: from basic science to clinical perspectives', October 8–11, 1995, Pécs, Hungary.

homology with known gut peptides, thought to be essential for activity of entire peptide, was synthesized and characterized [3–9]. This protective property was independently investigated and confirmed by others [10–14].

The protective effects of pentadecapeptide BPC 157 on gastrointestinal lesions were successfully evaluated in different experimental models in comparison with conventional agents and other gut peptides [3–14]. In this, the noted positive effects of BPC 157 and other gut peptides (secretin, glucagon and NPY) were in keeping with the suggested peptides' physiological significance and importance of BPC [3–15]. While having potent protection against liver lesions, a protective effect of BPC 157 was observed on different gastrointestinal lesion/ulcer models as well as acute anti-inflammatory and analgesic activity [3–15]. Consequently, it seemed possible that its activity could also be seen in intestinal wound healing.

Thus, the current study examines the effect of BPC 157 application on anastomosis healing in the intestine. Since resection and anastomosis of the colon is associated with a high incidence of anastomotic leakage and disruption [15], the colon anastomosis was used for this investigation.

METHODS

Preparation of BPC 157

The pentadecapeptide, BPC 157 (Gly Glu Pro Pro Pro Gly Lys Pro Ala Asp Asp Ala Gly Leu Val; MW 1419) is a part of the sequence of human gastric juice peptide BPC, freely soluble in water at pH 7.0 and in saline. It was prepared by solid phase peptide synthesis using t-BOC-Val loaded HYCRAM polymer carrier (ORPEGEN GmbH, Heidelberg). The t-BOC amino group was removed at each step with trifluoroacetic acid (50% in dichloromethane). The t-BOC amino acids were coupled in consecutive steps using diisopropylcarbodiimide/1-hydroxybenzetriazole reagent for activation. After sequence completion, the partially protected peptide was cleaved from the polymeric carrier by hydrogenation and purified on polymeric carrier and on a silica gel column. All protecting groups were removed with trifluoroacetic acid and the peptide finally purified by RP-HPLC. Peptide with 99% purity (1-des-Gly peptide as impurity) was used [3–9].

Experimental procedures

Animals

Wistar female albino rats randomly assigned, 10–16 rats per group (weighing 200–250 g) were used for all of these experiments.

General procedure: Immediately after preparation, a colon–colon anastomosis was performed, BPC 157 (10 µg or 10 ng/kg) or saline were given as a single application: (i) ig, (ii) ip (5.0 ml/kg), or (iii) locally as a 1-ml bath at the site of the anastomosis. Alternatively, in addition to the immediate intragastric or intraperitoneal application following anastomosis preparation, BPC or saline were given as a once-daily application, intragastrically or intraperitoneally, starting the next day, throughout the experiment. The final dose was given 24 h before sacrifice. The rats were sacrificed 2, 5, 7 and 10 days after surgery.

Anastomosis preparation: The colon was not prepared in any way preoperatively. Laparatomy was performed under ether anaesthesia through a lower abdominal midline incision. During operation, the abdomen was repeatedly moistened with small amounts of saline. The sigmoid colon was divided 2 cm above the lower peritoneal reflection, taking special care not to damage the mesenteric blood vessels. A colo-colostomy was made using 6.0 polyfilament (Synthophyl, B. Braun Melsungen AG, Germany) by a single layer of continuous inverting suture.

Measurement of bursting pressure of colon at the anastomotic site: The rats were anaesthetized by an intraperitoneal injection of sodium pentobarbital (60 mg/ml, 0.8 ml/kg), a midline abdominal incision was made and the abdominal cavity was filled with 0.9% NaCl. The intestinal segment was cleaned and connected to a pump on one side and a manometer on the other side. Subsequently, intraluminal pressure was increased by pumping oxygen at a rate of 1 ml/min into the segment. The bursting pressure (P; mmHg) was recorded, and appearance of bubbles in the abdominal cavity was taken to indicate leakage. The site of leakage was easily determined visually. A 3-cm segment containing the anastomosis was collected for further microscopic analysis.

The maximal bowel wall tension (BWT) was obtained according to Laplace's law as follows [15,16]:

$$BWT \ (dyn \times 10 \ cm^3/cm) = 1.330 \times P \ (mmHg) \times r \ (cm)$$

where r is the anastomotic radius, calculated from the circumference at the anastomtic site [15,16]. Healthy normal rats were used as an additional control group.

Statistical analysis

Kolmogorov–Smirnov test was performed for estimation of the normality of the data distribution. Further statistical analyses were performed by means of analysis of variance (ANOVA) and/or Kruskall–Wallis, Mann–Whitney U-, Student–Newman–Keuls, Dunn's and Dunnett's tests. Differences of $p < 0.05$ were considered to be statistically significant.

RESULTS

Bursting pressure, BWT measurement

Relative to the control data, increased values in the BPC 157 groups were noted in the earliest period following anastomosis preparation. Although BPC 157 seems to be effective after a single application (Figures 1 and 3), it is apparently increased when an additional application was given subsequently (Figures 2 and 4). In the groups of animals repeatedly treated with BPC and sacrificed at the earliest interval (48 h after surgery), a significant beneficial effect appeared in the rats treated with 10 ng/kg (Figures 1–4).

In the groups sacrificed at the later intervals, both the bursting pressure and BWT values in control rats markedly increased, and previously noted differences between BPC-treated groups could no longer be found (Figures 1 and 3).

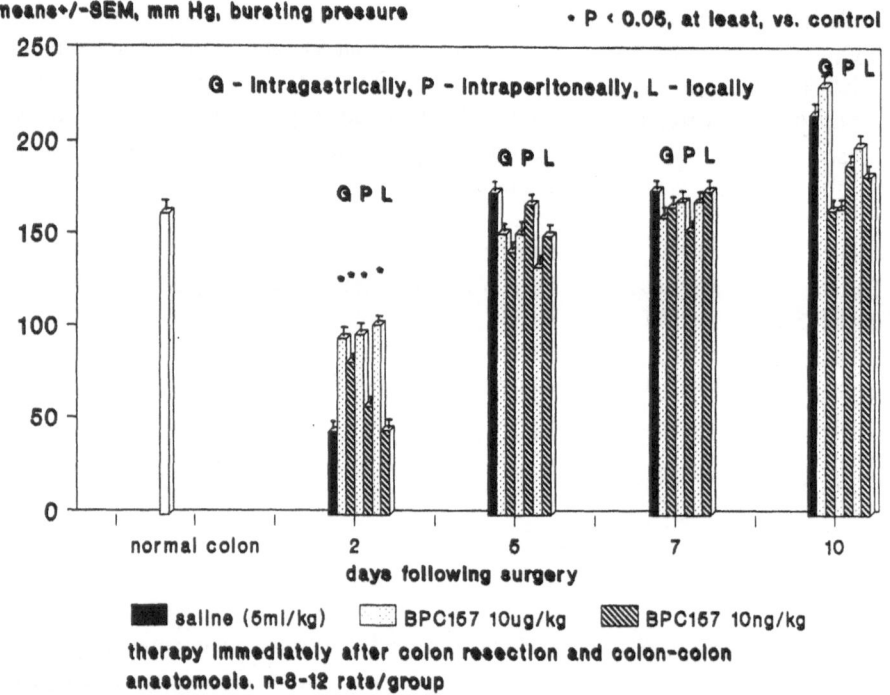

Figure 1. Bursting pressure measurement. Single application. Relative to the control data, the increased values in BPC groups were noted in the earliest period following anastomosis preparation

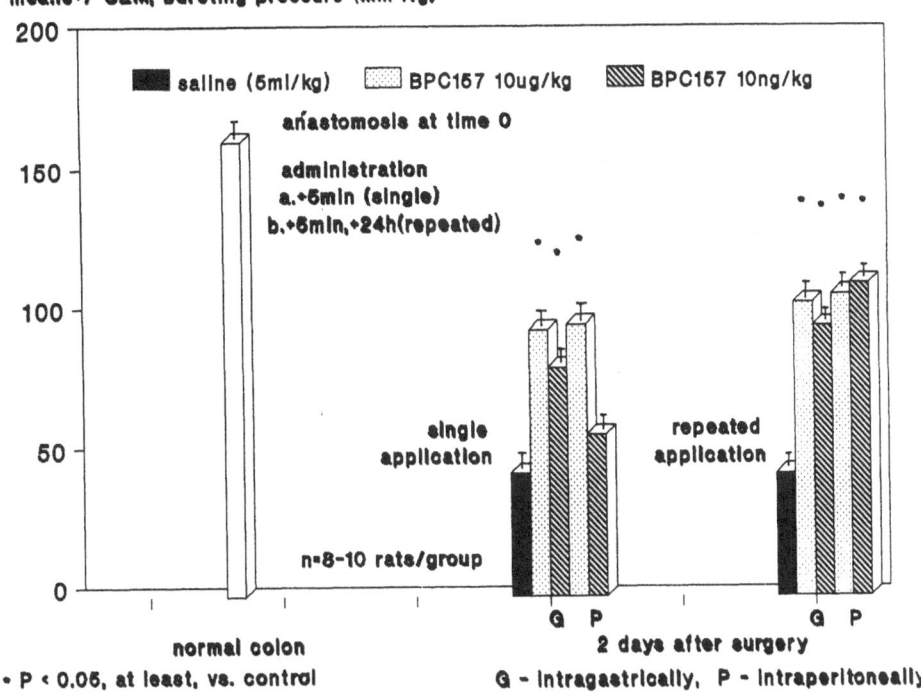

Figure 2. Bursting pressure measurement. Repeated application. Relative to the control data, the increased values in BPC groups were noted also in the groups treated with the lower dosage (ng/kg)

Pathohistological examination

In the control groups, the sequence of lesions was as follows:

1. Two days after surgery, at the site of anastomosis, submucosal oedema, perivascular and diffuse submucosal and epithelial infiltrate, with eosinophil predomination, lymphofollicular hyperplasia and microapostematous inflammation were found (Figure 5);

2. After five days, submucosal oedema was significantly decreased by lymphofollicular hyperplasia and eosinophilic infiltration was still noted;

3. Seven days after surgery, the predominant cells were monocytes and fibrocytes with obvious collagen deposition; lymphofollicular hyperplasia, predominantly in the submucosa, was also found. Similar findings were also noted ten days after anastomosis.

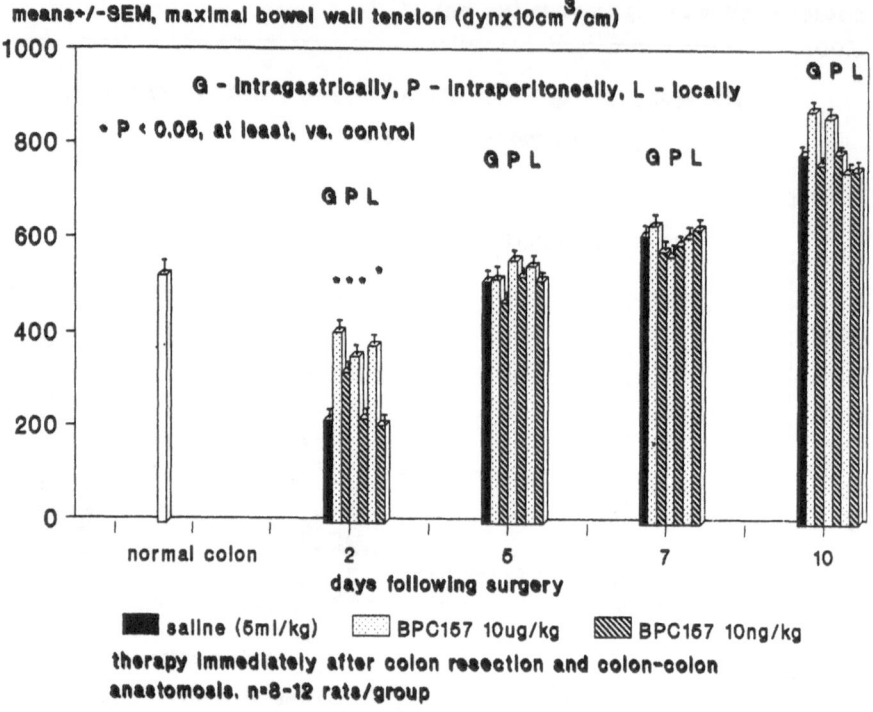

means+/-SEM, maximal bowel wall tension (dynx10cm³/cm)

G - Intragastrically, P - Intraperitoneally, L - locally

• P < 0.05, at least, vs. control

normal colon   2   6   7   10

days following surgery

■ saline (5ml/kg)   ▨ BPC157 10ug/kg   ▨ BPC157 10ng/kg

therapy immediately after colon resection and colon-colon
anastomosis, n=8-12 rats/group

Figure 3. BWT measurement. Single application. Relative to the control data, the increased
values in BPC groups were noted in the earliest period following anastomosis preparation

In the BPC-treated groups, the most striking difference, compared with controls,
was observed two days after surgery, particularly in the rats treated with the BPC 157
intragastrically at the dose of 10 µg/kg. An increased number of mononuclear cells
coincident with a decreased number of eosinophils and neutrophils was noted (Figure
6). Likewise, a less severe submucosal oedema and lymphofollicular hyperplasia was
also seen. However, the described difference was not present in the latter intervals.

DISCUSSION

It is generally known that anastomoses of the colon are more prone than most other
gastrointestinal anastomoses to leak and rupture, leading to a relatively high morbidity
and mortality [17-24]. Many factors may be involved in the leakage rate after colonic
surgery [17–24]. In the early course of colonic healing, a collagenolytic system is
inactivated, leading to breakdown of pre-existing collagen in the colonic wall, not only
in the immediate vicinity of the anastomosis but also for various distances away [22].
Infection further increases the collagenolytic activity [23]. The balance between
synthesis and breakdown of collagen is probably of great importance for successful
colonic healing [24].

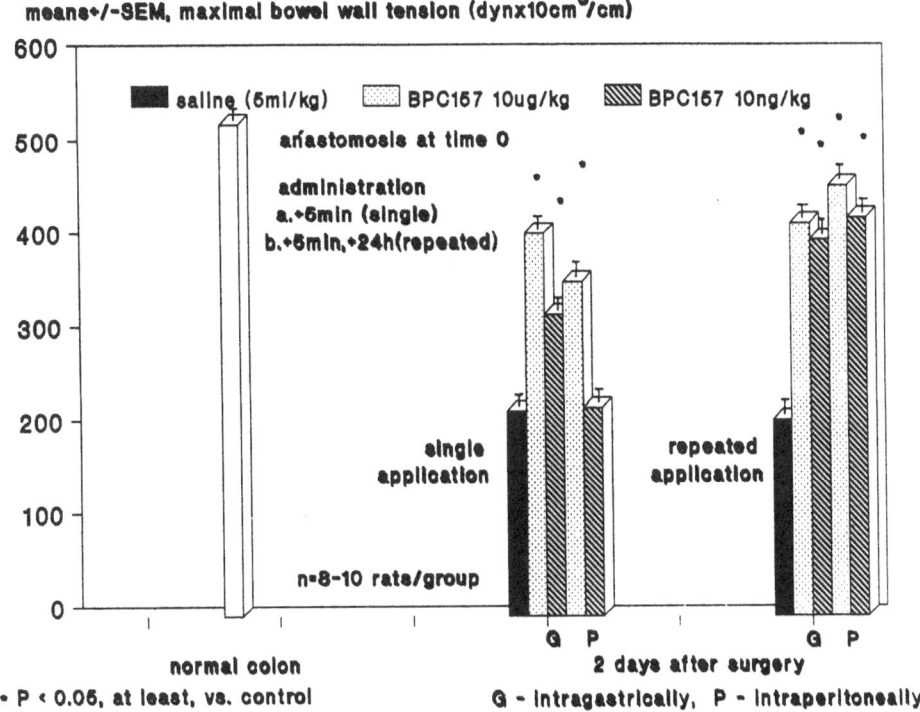

Figure 4. BWT measurement. Repeated application. Relative to the control data, the increased values in BPC groups were noted also in the groups treated with the lower dosage (ng/kg)

Thus, the evidence arising from our BWT measurements clearly emphasizes the significantly elevated BWT values noted in BPC groups. This suggests the involvement of BPC in the most critical early postwounding period and in the balance of the collagen system [17–24]. Accordingly, the raised BWT values were noted after just two postoperative days in the BPC-treated animals. This effect seems to be dose dependent. It was seen after only one single application of the higher µg-dosage, but it could be also observed in the lower ng-dosage when the dosage had been reapplied. This beneficial effect could be seen in either regimen with intragastric, intraperitoneal or local application. Thus, it seems likely that this effectiveness implies, besides systemic effects, a direct and potent local effect in the gastrointestinal tract, clearly seen also at the site of the injury [3–14]. This effect has to be rapid in onset consequently affecting the earliest events, but having a long-lasting positive influence.

Interestingly, BPC 157 has been shown to reduce MPO, LTB_4 and TXB_2 serum and inflamed tissue levels [12,13]. In support, BPC 157 appears to be a very stable protein. When incubated in human gastric juice or in water, this pentadecapeptide was not subject to any degradation over 24 h, unlike h-EGF and h-TGFα, stable in water, but degraded in human gastric juice after 15 min [25]. Likewise, acute toxicology shows a very high therapeutic index, since no death or pathological changes were observed despite the administration of a very high dosage (mg/g body weight) [5].

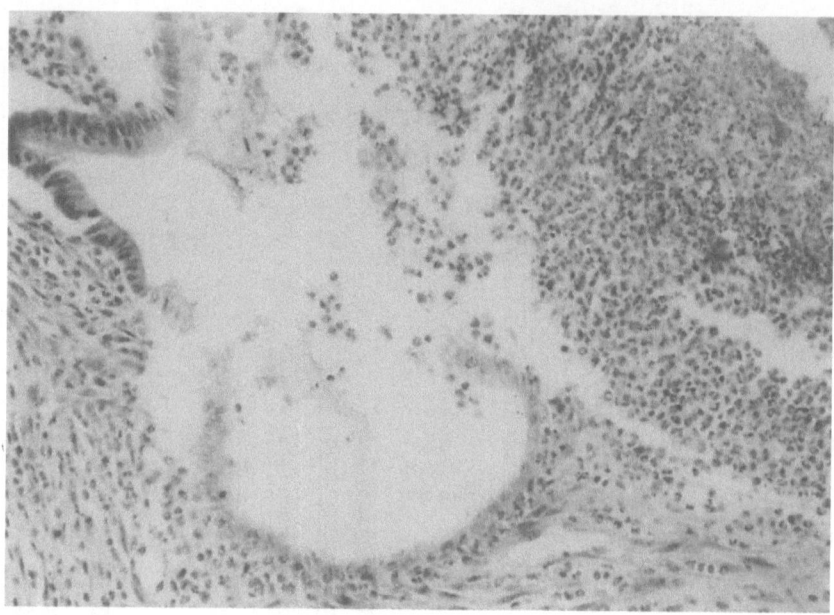

Figure 5. Control rat two days after surgery. Severe predominantly neutrophil infiltration at the location of anastomosis. HE, × 20

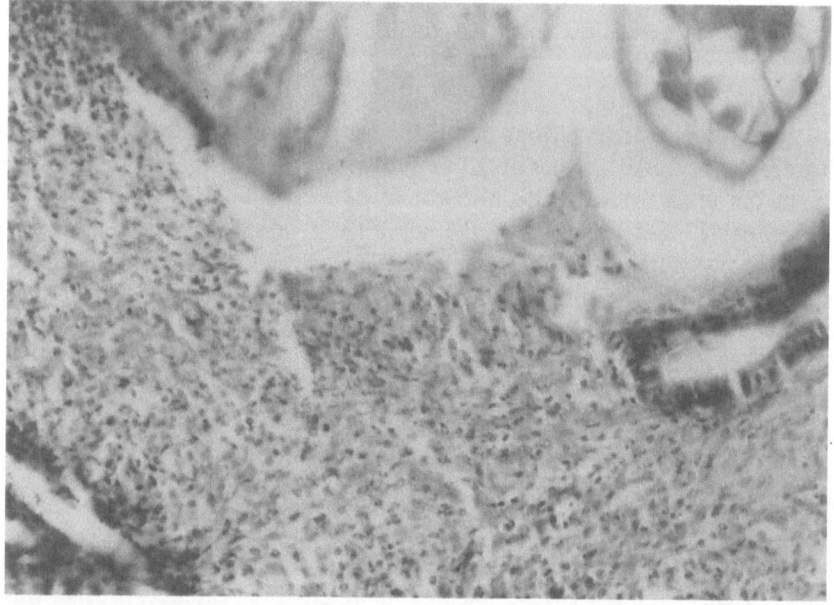

Figure 6. A rat treated with BPC 157. Predominantly mononuclear cell infiltration with sparse neutrophils in the colonic submucosa

ACKNOWLEDGEMENTS

This study was subsidized by grants from the Ministry of Science of the Republic of Croatia and Pliva, Zagreb, Croatia.

REFERENCES

1. Thompson JC, Greeley GH, Rayford PL, Townsend CM. Gastrointestinal Endocrinology. New York, St. Louis, San Francisco: McGraw-Hill Book Company; 1987.
2. Kriger TD. Brain peptides: what, where, and why? Science. 1983;222:975–85.
3. Sikiric P, Petek M, Rotkvic I et al. Hypothesis: stomach stress response, diagnostic and therapeutic value – a new approach in organoprotection. Exp Clin Gastroenterol. 1991;1:15–16.
4. Sikiric P, Petek M, Rucman R et al. The significance of the gastroprotective effect of body protection compound (BPC): modulation by different procedures. In: Mózsik Gy, Pár Á, Csomós G et al., eds. Cell Injury and Protection in the Gastrointestinal Tract: From Basic Science to Clinical Perspectives. Budapest: Akadémiai Kiadó; 1992:89–98.
5. Sikiric P, Petek M, Rucman R et al. A new gastric juice peptide, BPC – an overview of stomach/stress/ organoprotection hypothesis and BPC beneficial effects. J Physiol (Paris). 1993;87:313–27.
6. Sikiric P, Rotkvic I, Mise S et al. Dopamine agents efficacy in peptic ulcer healing and relapse prevention – a further indication for importance of stomach dopamine in the stress organoprotection concept. In: Szabo S, Taché Y, Glavin G, eds. Neuroendocrinology of Gastrointestinal Ulceration: Hans Selye Symposia on Neuroendocrinology and Stress. Vol 2. New York: Plenum Publishing Corporation; 1995:221–30.
7. Sikiric P, Seiwerth S, Grabarevic Z et al. Hepatoprotective effect of BPC 157, 15-aminoacid peptide, on liver lesions induced by either restraint stress or bile duct and hepatic artery ligation or CCl_4 administration. A comparative study with dopamine agonists and somatostatin. Life Sci. 1993;53:PL 291–6.
8. Sikiric P, Seiwerth S, Grabarevic Z et al. The beneficial effect of BPC 157, a 15 amino acid peptide BPC 157 fragment, on gastric and duodenal lesions induced by restraint stress, cysteamine and 96% ethanol in rats. A comparative study with H_2 receptor antagonists, dopamine promotors and gut peptides. Life Sci. 1994;54:PL63–8.
9. Sikiric P, Gyires K, Seiwerth S et al. The effect of pentadecapeptide BPC 157 on inflammatory, non-inflammatory, direct and indirect pain and capsaicin neurotoxicity. Inflammopharmacology. 1993;2:121–7.
10. Mózsik G, Sikiric P, Petek M. Preventing effect of body protective compound (BPC) on the development of ethanol and HCl-induced gastric mucosal injury. Exp Clin Gastroenterol. 1991;1:87–90.
11. Bosnjak ZJ, Graf BM, Sikiric P, Stowe DF. Protective effects of newly isolated gastric peptide following hypoxic and reoxygenation injury in the isolated guinea pig heart. FASEB J. 1994;8:A129.
12. Veljaca M, Pllana R, Lesch CA, Sanchez B, Chan K, Guglietta A. Protective effect of BPC 157 on a rat model of colitis. Gastroenterology. 1994;106:789.
13. Veljaca M, Lech CA, Pllana R, Sanchez B, Chan K, Guglietta A. BPC-15 reduces trinitrobenzene sulfonic acid-induced colonic damage in rats. J Pharmacol Exp Ther. 1994;272:417–22.
14. Paré W, Klucyznski JM. The effect of new gastric juice peptide BPC on classic stress triad in stress procedure. Exp Clin Gastroenterol. 1992;2:234–6.
15. Jiborn H, Ahonen J, Zederfeld B. Healing of experimental colonic anastomoses. Am J Surg. 1978;136:587–94.
16. Matsuse S, Walser M. Healing of intestinal anastomoses in adrenalectomized rats given corticosteroids. Am J Physiol. 1992;263:R164–8.
17. Rousselot LM, Slattery JR. Immediate complication of surgery of the large intestine. Surg Clin North Am. 1964;44:397.
18. Goligher JC, Graham NG, de Dombal FT. Anastomotic dehiscence after anterior resection of rectum and sigmoid. Br J Surg. 1970;57:109.
19. Dunphy JE. The cut gut. Am J Surg. 1970;119:1.
20. Morgenstern L, Yaamkawa T, Ben-Shoshan M, Lippman H. Anastomotic leakage after low colonic anastomosis. Am J Surg. 1972;123:104.

21. Dunphy JE. Preoperative preparation of the colon and other factors affecting anastomostic healing. Cancer. 1971;28:181.
22. Hawley PR, Faulk WP, Hunt TK, Dunphy JE. Collagenase activity in the gastrointestinal tract. Br J Surg. 1970;57:896.
23. Hawley PR, Hunt TK, Dunphy JE. Etiology of colonic leaks. Proc R Soc Med. 1970;(Suppl)63:28.
24. Hunt TK, Hawley PR. Surgical judgement and colonic anastomoses. Dis Colon Rectum. 1969;12:167.
25. Veljaca M, Chan K, Guglietta A. Digestion of h-EGF, h-TGF alfa, and BPC 15 in human gastric juice. Pharmacol Res. 1995;31:70.

G Mózsik et al. Cell Injury and Cytoprotection in the GI Tract. 259–269.
© 1997 Kluwer Academic Publishers.

CYSTEINE AND SERINE PROTEASES IN DUODENAL ULCER

L. HERSZÉNYI*[1], F. FARINATI[2], M. PLEBANI[3], P. CARRARO[3], M. DE PAOLI[3], F. DI MARIO[2], S. KUSSTATSCHER[2], R. NACCARATO[2] AND Z. TULASSAY[1]

[1]Second Department of Medicine, Semmelweis University Medical School, Budapest, Hungary; [2]Cattedra Malattie Apparato Digerente, Istituto di Medicina Interna; [3]Dipartimento di Medicina di Laboratorio, Laboratorio Centrale, Universitá di Padova, Italy
*Correspondence

ABSTRACT

Cysteine proteases (cathepsin B and L: CATB and CATL, respectively) are involved in gastric mucosal injury while urokinase- and tissue-type plasminogen activators (serine proteases; UPA, TPA) and their inhibitor PAI-1 may play a part in the pathogenesis of duodenal ulcer disease (DU).

The aim of this study was to determine CATB, CATL, UPA, TPA and PAI-1 levels in DU and in control patients.

Samples of duodenal mucosa were obtained from 26 patients with active DU, from 26 patients with healed DU and from 21 controls. Antigen concentrations were measured using ELISA methods.

Significantly higher cathepsins, UPA, PAI-1 and significantly lower TPA were found in active DU than in healed DU and controls.

Our results demonstrate that, in DU patients, impaired fibrinolysis (TPA), activation of intramucosal proteases (cathepsins) and, with respect to healing, tissue remodelling and angiogenesis (UPA, PAI-1) may play an important role.

Keywords: duodenal ulcer disease, cathepsin, plasminogen activator, protease

INTRODUCTION

The pathogenesis of peptic ulcer is a complex phenomenon in which several, only partly explained, factors are thought to be involved. In recent years, research has focused on the role of *Helicobacter pylori* infection and there is currently sound evidence that *H. pylori* causes non-autoimmune gastritis [1] and peptic ulcer [2–4]. With respect to the latter, it has been suggested that *H. pylori* may induce peptic ulceration also through the direct production of several proteases that could damage the gastroduodenal mucosa [1,5–7]. However, apart from any exogenous factors, the role of endogenous alterations must also be borne in mind when considering the pathogenesis of peptic ulcer. This is indeed the result of an imbalance between protective factors, such as the mucosal barrier, and aggressive factors, such as acid and *H. pylori*. In this respect, the role of proteases, as part of either of these groups, may be of considerable interest.

This paper was presented at the Symposium on 'Cell injury and protection in the gastrointestinal tract: from basic science to clinical perspectives', October 8–11, 1995, Pécs, Hungary.

For instance, cathepsin B and L (CATB, CATL), the most typical and best characterized cysteine proteases in lysosomes, that are widely distributed in gastroduodenal tissues [8–11], present a number of features which suggest a possible role for them in peptic ulcer disease because:

1. They are very efficient in their ability to degrade the extracellular matrix and have been implicated in processes of inflammation and cell growth [12–15];

2. They (and CATB in particular) contribute to the development of chemically induced gastric tissue damage in rats [16]; and

3. These proteases and their inhibitors have been shown to be involved in gastric mucosal injury and protection [17].

However, to our knowledge, the role of cathepsins in peptic ulcer has not been evaluated in clinical studies.

On the other hand, since mucosal blood flow is an important protective factor, vascular mechanisms (via alterations in oxygen supply and/or angiogenesis) may also be important in the pathogenesis of peptic ulcer, leading to necrosis and ulceration. The gastroduodenal mucosa certainly has a rich vascular supply. To maintain its patency, an active fibrinolytic system is essential. If fibrinolysis is impaired, vascular occlusion may contribute to tissue damage.

Fibrinolytic activity is regulated by plasminogen activators (PA), which form part of the group of serine proteases and are also involved in many protein-degrading processes, converting plasminogen into active plasmin. The tissue-type plasminogen activator (TPA), produced in the vascular endothelium, is a key enzyme in the fibrinolytic cascade. The urokinase-type plasminogen activator (UPA) plays a major part in extracellular matrix degradation, tumour invasion and inflammation, but also in tissue remodelling, angiogenesis and wound healing [18–24].

PA activity is controlled by plasminogen activator inhibitors, which are members of the serine protease inhibitors (serpin) family [25]. The PA inhibitor type-1 (PAI-1) is produced by endothelial cells and platelets, inhibits both TPA and UPA by forming a covalent inhibitor–enzyme complex [25,26].

Fibrinolytic activity was originally demonstrated in gastric and duodenal mucosa by a fibrin film method, used to localize the fibrinolytic activity in mucosal and submucosal blood vessels [27,28].

More recently, a semiquantitative method has been developed. With this method, a low fibrinolytic activity was found in gastroduodenal tissue surrounding the ulcers [29]. Finally, Wodzinski et al. [30] employed a sensitive quantitative spectrophotometric assay to measure TPA and UPA activity in gastric and duodenal mucosa biopsy homogenates, and they demonstrated impaired mucosal vascular fibrinolytic activity at the site of duodenal and gastric ulcers.

It had previously been shown by our group, as well as by others, that pepsinogens, cathepsins D (aspartic proteases) and also tryptase (a serine endoprotease) may play a part in the pathogenesis of peptic ulcer [31–33].

Indeed, we have been involved for some time in studying the pathogenesis of peptic ulcer disease [34–38] and the role of cysteine and serine proteases in gastric cancer and gastric precancerous conditions [39,40]. Since, to our knowledge, no clinical data are currently available on the possible relationship between cysteine proteases and peptic ulcer disease, and since cathepsins, UPA, TPA and PAI-1 have not been evaluated in the same ulcer patient, we decided to assess the antigen levels of CATB, CATL (cysteine proteases), UPA, TPA (serine proteases) and their inhibitor PAI-1 in duodenal ulcer disease (DU) and in control subjects.

PATIENTS AND METHODS

A total of 61 patients were included in the study. Twenty-six had active DU (15 males, 11 females; mean age 55 years, range 21–79); 26 had healed DU (19 males, 7 females; mean age 55 years, ranging 33–79); 12 of these (7 males, 5 females; mean age 64 years, range 33–79) were studied during different phases of their disease (in the active phase and also after ulcer scarring). Twenty-one control subjects (10 males, 11 females; mean age 41 years, range 25–66) with upper gastrointestinal complaints, with no history of ulcer and with either negative endoscopic and histological findings ($n = 7$) or only mild non-specific changes, such as superficial gastritis ($n = 14$), were also included in the study. Duodenal mucosa was always free from any significant change in this group of subjects.

During endoscopy, biopsy specimens were routinely taken from histological examination. In DU patients, for biochemical examination, one biopsy specimen was taken from the edge of the ulcer (or adjacent to the scar in patients with healed ulcer), and one biopsy at the antrum, about 5 cm from the pylorus. In control patients, one duodenal and one antral biopsy were also taken for biochemistry.

In preliminary studies, 5 control subjects' antral, angular, body, and fundic biopsies, and also specimens from the anterosuperior and posteroinferior halves of the duodenum, were taken to study the geographical distribution of protease and PAI-1 levels in gastric and duodenal mucosae.

The mean weight of one biopsy specimen was approximately 5 mg. Samples for biochemical determinations were snap-frozen at −70°C, while the material for histology was fixed in 5% buffered formaldehyde, and then observed blindly by the same pathologist for the presence of H. pylori infection by modified Giemsa, Warthin–Starry stain and by immunohistological confirmation with a peroxidase–antiperoxidase immunostaining (Dako-Milano, Italy).

All of the patients with active DU ($n = 26$) and 7 of the control subjects were H. pylori positive, while the remaining 14 control patients were H. pylori negative.

Informed consent was obtained from all patients taking part in the study.

Cysteine–serine protease and PAI-1 determination

The biopsy specimens were homogenized in melting ice in 1 ml (vol/vol) Tris Tween buffer (0.1 mol/L, 0.1% Tween 80, pH 7.5) per 25 mg wet tissue. After centrifugation for 10 min at 10 000g at 4°C, the supernatants were stored at −70°C before assay.

Protein concentrations of the supernatants were determined by the Bradford method [41] (Bio-Rad, Munich, Germany). Protease and PAI-1 antigen levels were measured using the ELISA method as follows.

Assay for cathepsin B and cathepsin L

Antigen concentrations of CATB and CATL were performed using a solid-phase ELISA based on the sandwich principle (BioAss, Diesen, Germany), as described before [39]. Briefly, 100 µl of tissue extract was added to a polyclonal, immunoselected anti-human-cathepsin antibody. A second anti-cathepsin antibody, labelled with horse-radish peroxidase (conjugate), was added.

Absolute quantities of CATB and CATL antigens on the samples were calculated from a 7-point standard curve of CATB and CATL (0–250 ng/ml). The lowest detectable concentration of CATB and CATL was estimated to be 10 ng/ml.

Assay for urokinase-type plasminogen activator (UPA)

Antigen quantification was measured using the TintElize UPA-ELISA (Biopool, Umea, Sweden) [39]. Briefly, a mouse monoclonal anti-urokinase-type plasminogen activator was used as a catching antibody. After incubation with the tissue homo-genates, a second goat anti-human UPA, conjugated with horseradish peroxidase, was used to form a 'sandwich' ELISA and ortho-phenylene-diamine was added as a substrate. The amount of UPA antigen in the samples was calculated from a 6-point standard curve of UPA (0–4 ng/ml). The detection limit was about 0.1 ng/ml for UPA.

Assay for tissue-type plasminogen activator (TPA)

TPA antigen was measured using the TintElize TPA-ELISA (Biopool, Umea, Sweden). Goat anti-TPA was used as a catching antibody, an anti-TPA horseradish peroxidase conjugate was used as the second antibody, and ortho-phenylene diamine dihydro-chloride was added as a substrate. Absolute quantities of TPA antigen in the samples were calculated from a 4-point standard curve (0–30 ng/ml). The detection limit was about 1.5 ng/ml for TPA.

Assay for plasminogen-activator inhibitor type-1 (PAI-1)

PAI-1 antigen was determined using Asserachrom PAI-1-ELISA (Diagnostica Stago, Asniéres-sur-Seine, France) [39], with mouse monoclonal anti-human PAI-1 as a captive antibody.

A second mouse monoclonal anti-PAI-1 is coupled with peroxidase and binds to another antigenic determinant at a distance from the first, forming the 'sandwich'. The bound enzyme peroxidase is then revealed, in the same way as for UPA, in the presence of hydrogen peroxide. Absolute quantities of PAI-1 antigen on the samples were calculated from a 5-point standard curve of PAI-1 (0–20 ng/ml). The detection limit is about 0.5 ng/ml for PAI-1. Antigen concentrations were expressed as ng of antigen/mg protein. Results are given as mean ± SD.

Statistics

Differences between groups were statistically tested using Student's *t*-test on paired and unpaired data, or the Mann–Whitney U test, where applicable and ANOVA one-way analysis of variance. Differences were considered significant when $2p < 0.05$.

RESULTS

Distribution of proteases in gastric and duodenal mucosa

There was no significant variation in the distribution of CATB, CATL, UPA, TPA and PAI-1 antigen levels in gastric antral, angular, body and fundic mucosa of the 5 control cases investigated. The antigen concentrations of cysteine–serine proteases and PAI-1 in mucosa from the anterosuperior wall of the duodenum were also similar to those in the mucosa from the opposite wall (Table 1). With respect to TPA levels in the 5 subjects who were studied in all the gastric and duodenal areas, a trend towards higher

TABLE 1
Distribution of cathepsin B, cathepsin L, urokinase-type plasminogen activator, plasminogen activator inhibitor type-1 and tissue-type plasminogen activator in control subjects, expressed in ng/mg protein (mean ± SD; $n = 5$)

	CATB	CATL	UPA	PAI-1	TPA
Antrum	137.9 ± 12.35	24.1 ± 4.61	0.53 ± 0.13	0.52 ± 0.04	7.5 ± 2.25
Angulus	140.3 ± 14.55	25.8 ± 7.93	0.58 ± 0.07	0.50 ± 0.06	7.6 ± 2.43
Body	138.1 ± 13.54	22.8 ± 6.68	0.56 ± 0.05	0.51 ± 0.03	7.1 ± 1.38
Fundus	135.2 ± 13.31	23.3 ± 7.44	0.60 ± 0.11	0.53 ± 0.07	7.7 ± 1.08
Duodenum					
Anterosuperior	144.7 ± 33.01	22.8 ± 1.82	0.61 ± 0.03	0.53 ± 0.08	9.0 ± 1.37
Posteroinferior	133.4 ± 26.12	23.3 ± 2.19	0.58 ± 0.06	0.54 ± 0.06	9.1 ± 3.00
ANOVA*	NS	NS	NS	NS	NS

CATB, cathepsin B; CATL, cathepsin L; UPA, urokinase-type plasminogen activator; PAI-1, plasminogen activator inhibitor type-1; TPA, tissue-type plasminogen activator

*ANOVA one-way analysis of variance

levels was observed in both the anterosuperior and the posteroinferior wall of the duodenum versus the levels detected in the antral, angular, body and fundic mucosa. This finding was confirmed by the fact that the antral mucosa showed significantly lower TPA levels than the duodenal mucosa when all the cases included in the control group were considered (7.63±2.24 vs. 9.89±3.66 ng/mg protein, $p = 0.01$). With respect to controls, no significant differences were found in protease and PAI-1 antigen levels between subgroups with a normal histology ($n = 7$) and those with mild superficial gastritis ($n = 14$; data not shown).

Duodenal ulcer

Cysteine proteases (CATB, CATL)

In patients with active DU, the antigen concentrations of CATB and CATL at the edge of the ulcers were significantly higher than in controls or in patients with healed DU in duodenal mucosa (Table 2). In patients with healed DU, CATB and CATL levels at the scar returned to normal (no differences being found between healed DU and controls; Table 2).

TABLE 2
Antigen concentrations of cathepsin B, cathepsin L, urokinase-type plasminogen activator, plasminogen activator inhibitor type-1 and tissue-type plasminogen activator from duodenal mucosa in patients with duodenal ulcer disease and in control subjects. Results expressed as ng/mg protein (mean±SD)

	CATB	CATL	UPA	PAI-1	TPA
Active DU edge (n = 26)	178.0±74.3	33.6±8.5	1.33±0.51	0.80±0.51	5.12±2.67
Healed DU scar (n = 26)	121.1±44.1	26.6±3.6	0.22±0.10	0.55±0.18	11.0±2.62
Control duodenum (n = 21)	109.5±31.8	24.7±3.6	0.58±0.36	0.49±0.17	9.89±3.66

Statistics (t-test): Active DU edge vs. control duodenum: CATB: $p < 0.01$; CATL: $p < 0.01$; UPA: $p < 0.01$; PAI-1, $p < 0.01$; TPA: $p < 0.01$. Active DU edge vs. healed DU scar: CATB: $p < 0.01$; CATL, $p < 0.01$; UPA: $p < 0.01$; PAI-1: $p = 0.02$; TPA: $p < 0.01$. Control duodenum vs. healed DU scar: UPA: $p < 0.01$.

CATB, cathepsin B; CATL, cathepsin L; UPA, urokinase-type plasminogen activator; PAI-1, plasminogen activator inhibitor type-1; TPA, tissue-type plasminogen activator; DU, duodenal ulcer

Serine proteases

At the edge of active DU, TPA antigen levels were significantly lower than in the biopsies from controls and patients with healed DU (Table 2). In patients with healed ulcer, duodenal TPA levels returned to normal and there was also a slight increase in the duodenum with respect to the control values but a significant difference was not reached. In contrast, the antigen levels of UPA at the edge of the ulcer of patients with active DU were significantly raised compared with controls and healed DU patients (Table 2). After healing, UPA levels showed a marked decrease in duodenal mucosa, becoming significantly lower than in controls.

Plasminogen activator inhibitor type-1

The antigen values of PAI-1 at the ulcer edge in patients with active DU were significantly higher than in controls and a significant difference was also found between ulcer edge and ulcer scar levels. After healing, PAI-1 levels returned to normal (Table 2).

When we considered only the 12 patients studied in both the active phase of their disease and after ulcer healing, the above-mentioned behaviour of the proteases and PAI-1 was strictly confirmed (data not shown).

Relationship between cysteine–serine proteases and PAI-1

Significant correlations were found in duodenal levels of CATB–CATL ($r = 0.45$, $p < 0.01$); UPA–PAI-1 ($r = 0.32$, $p < 0.01$); CATB–UPA ($r = 0.42$, $p < 0.01$); CATL–UPA ($r = 0.55$, $p < 0.01$) and CATL–PAI-1 ($r = 0.44$, $p < 0.01$). As expected, TPA antigen levels correlated inversely with PAI-1 ($r = -0.22$, $p = 0.02$) but also with UPA ($r = -0.64$, $p < 0.01$); with CATB ($r = -0.46$, $p < 0.01$), and finally with CATL ($r = -0.59$, $p < 0.01$).

DISCUSSION

To our knowledge, no previous studies have evaluated cysteine–serine proteases and PAI-1 in the same DU patients. In an attempt to assess any aggressive or protective roles of these proteases, the present study surveyed the relationship between antigen concentrations of CATB, CATL (cysteine proteases), UPA, TPA (serine proteases) and their inhibitor PAI-1 in DU.

In our study, ELISA methods rather than activity assays were used to measure proteases and PAI-1, due to the previous demonstration that UPA and TPA antigen and activity showed a significant correlation in both pathological and normal gastric and colonic mucosa [42,43] and to a specific previous experience by our group [39,40].

Intramucosal proteolysis may well be considered an aggressive factor with respect to the development of peptic ulcer. It has been suggested, for instance, that cysteine proteases (especially CATB) may contribute to the development of experimentally induced gastric mucosal injury [16,17] and that other proteases, such as pepsinogens, cathepsin D (aspartic proteases) and tryptase (a serine protease), may play a part in the pathogenesis of peptic ulcer [31,33].

We demonstrated that CATB and CATL are significantly higher in homogenates of biopsies taken from the ulcer's edge in patients with active DU than in those obtained from controls. We also found that, with healing, CATB and CATL levels return to within normal ranges, suggesting that these cysteine proteases are activated in the active phase of DU in the area directly involved in the ulcerous process.

The extracellular matrix may be damaged by cathepsins and this may contribute to an alteration of the mucosal barrier, thus favouring ulcer initiation and development.

The maintenance of an adequate blood flow in the gastric and duodenal mucosa is an essential protective factor. Indeed, an impaired fibrinolytic activity has been found in peptic ulcer disease, suggesting that vascular damage may play a part in ulcerogenesis [29,30]. TPA is a key enzyme in the fibrinolytic process and is essential for maintenance of the patency of blood vessels. We have found that, in duodenal mucosa of active DU, there is a significant reduction in TPA antigen concentration compared with controls. Our findings therefore confirm two previous studies reporting data obtained using endoscopic biopsy specimens, in both of which the fibrinolytic system was shown to play a part in DU. In the first, a low fibrinolytic activity was found in tissues obtained near ulcers [29]; in the latter, Wodzinski et al. [30] reported decreased TPA activity at the ulcer's edge by comparison with control mucosa.

It has been shown that the most vulnerable areas for peptic ulceration – the mucosa in the lesser curve of the stomach and the proximal duodenum – are supplied by end arteries [44,45], and microvascular disturbance and ischaemia have been thought to be closely related to ulceration [46–50].

The above, in association with our finding of reduced fibrinolysis at the ulcer's edge, provides a possible explanation for one of the mechanisms of ulcer development.

Reduced blood flow presumably leads to a tendency for thrombosis and, when fibrinolytic activity is impaired, mucosal ischaemia may result, especially in the areas supplied by end arteries. Acid and pepsin, or other proteases (such as CATB and CATL), can then further damage the ischaemic mucosa, leading to peptic ulcer, the size of which is limited by the vascular sufficiency of the surrounding mucosa [51]. Our finding that TPA antigen levels were significantly higher in duodenal mucosa than in gastric mucosa are consistent with reports from Sier et al. [43] and Wodzinski et al. [30] and may be linked to differences in mucosal blood supply.

While TPA is essentially linked to the fibrinolytic process, UPA is involved in a wider series of mechanisms, including tissue remodelling, angiogenesis and wound healing. We found that, in the duodenal mucosa of patients with active DU there was a significant increase in UPA antigen concentration compared with controls. Our results thus confirm the higher UPA activity demonstrated by Wodzinski et al. [30] and suggest that UPA may play a part in tissue remodelling and wound healing during the ulcer healing process. Tissue repair requires the development of new granulation tissue, which needs an efficient microcirculation to maintain blood flow and increased UPA levels – as suggested by our and other authors' results – for tissue remodelling. Similar results with respect to UPA were indeed reported in chronic leg ulcers by Stacey et al. [52] who detected raised UPA levels in venous and ischaemic ulcers, also concluded that UPA may play an important part in wound healing.

We found that PAI-1 antigen values were raised at the ulcer's edge of patients with active DU. The exact role of PAI-1 in this context is difficult to ascertain. In physiological conditions, PAI-1 inhibits the activity of TPA and may therefore play some part in impairing fibrinolysis [23,24,53] but the exact role of PAI-1 in pathological conditions is not well established. In tumour biology, it has been suggested that PAI-1 may serve to protect the transformed tissue from proteolytic degradation [54,55]. PAI-1, or UPA/PAI-1 ratio, might have a role in angiogenesis [56,57] and we know that an increased angiogenesis may lead to accelerated ulcer healing [58,59]. In the light of the above, PAI-1 may also be considered a protective factor in ulcerogenesis.

In terms of correlations, we found CATB, CATL, UPA and PAI-1 significantly related to each other. TPA was inversely and significantly correlated with all four of the other biological parameters, which is hardly surprising in view of their respective roles.

In conclusion, as Wodzinski et al. [30] have correctly suggested, DU investigation has been dominated by studies first of acid and peptic secretion and then of *H. pylori*, leaving very little room for studies investigating the intramuscular mechanisms of damage. Both Wodzinski et al. [30] and our own studies suggest that fibrinolytic and anti-fibrinolytic processes on the one hand, and intramucosal protease activity on the other, play an essential part in ulcer development and healing. The next essential step is to identify the factor(s) controlling these intramucosal attack and defence mechanisms.

REFERENCES

1. Rauws EAJ, Langenberg W, Houthoff HJ, Zanen HC, Tytgat GNJ. Campylobacter pyloridis-associated chronic active antral gastritis. A prospective study of its prevalence and the effects of antibacterial and antiulcer treatment. Gastroenterology. 1988;94:33–40.
2. Rauws EAJ, Tytgat GNJ. Cure of duodenal ulcer with eradication of Helicobacter pylori. Lancet. 1990;335:1233–5.
3. Axon AR. Duodenal ulcer: the villain unmasked? Br Med J. 1991;302:919–21.
4. Graham DY. Treatment of peptic ulcers caused by Helicobacter pylori. N Engl J Med. 1993;328:349–50.
5. Graham DY. Campylobacter pylori and peptic ulcer disease. Gastroenterology. 1989;96:615–25.
6. Slomiany BL, Piotroski J, Mojtahed DH, Slomiany A. Ebrotidine effect on the proteolytic and lipolytic activities of Helicobacter pylori. Gen Pharmacol. 1992;23:203–6.
7. Piotroski J, Czajkowski A, Yotsumoto F, Slomiany A, Slomiany BL. Sulglycotide effect of the proteolytic and lipolytic activities of Helicobacter pylori toward gastric mucus. Am J Gastroenterol. 1994;89:232–6.
8. Kominami E, Tsukahara T, Bando Y, Katunuma N. Distribution of cathepsin B and H in rat tissues and peripheral blood cells. J Biochem. 1985;98:87–93.
9. Bando Y, Kominami E, Katunuma N. Purification and tissue distribution of rat cathepsin L. J Biochem. 1986;100:35–42.
10. Howie AJ, Burnett D. The distribution of cathepsin B in human tissues. J Pathol. 1985;145:307–14.
11. Furuhashi M, Nakahara A, Fukutomi H, Kominami E, Grube D, Uchijama Y. Immunocytochemical localization of cathepsin B, H and L in the rat gastro-duodenal mucosa. Histochemistry. 1991;95:231–9.

12. Mason RW, Johnson DA, Barrett AJ, Chapman HA. Elastinolytic activity of human cathepsin L. J Biochem. 1986;233:925–7.
13. Okada Y, Yokota Y. Purification and properties of cathepsin B from sea urchin eggs. Comp Biochem Physiol. 1990;96:381–6.
14. Sloane BF. Cathepsin B and cystatins: evidence for a role in cancer progression. Semin Cancer Biol. 1990;1:137–52.
15. Jochum M, Machleidt W, Fritz H. Proteolysis-induced pathomechanisms in acute inflammation and related therapeutic approaches. Agents Actions (Suppl). 1993;42:51–69.
16. Nagy L, Johnson BR, Saha B et al. Correlation between gastroprotection and inhibition of cysteine proteases by new maleimide derivatives. Dig Dis Sci. 1990;35:1037a (Abstr).
17. Szabo S, Nagy L, Plebani M. Glutathione protein sulfhydryls and cysteine proteases in gastric mucosal injury and protection. Clin Chim Acta. 1992;206:95–105.
18. Dano K, Andreasen PA, Grondahl-Hansen J, Kristensen P, Nielsen LS, Skriver L. Plasminogen activators, tissue degradation and cancer. Adv Cancer Res. 1985;44:139–266.
19. Saksela O, Rifkin DB. Cell-associated plasminogen activation: regulation and physiological functions. Ann Rev Cell Biol. 1988;4:93–126.
20. Markus G. The relevance of plasminogen activators to neoplastic growth – a review of recent literature. Enzyme. 1988;40:158–72.
21. Nishino N, Aoki K, Tokura Y, Sakaguchi S, Takada Y, Takada A. The urokinase type of plasminogen activator in cancer of digestive tract. Thromb Res. 1988;50:527–35.
22. Scully MF. Plasminogen activator-dependent pericellular proteolysis. Br J Haematol. 1991;79:537–43.
23. Hart IR, Saini A. Biology of tumour metastasis. Lancet. 1992;339:1453–7.
24. Busso N, Nicodeme E, Chesne C, Guillouzo A, Belin D, Hyafil F. Urokinase and type 1 plasminogen activator inhibitor production by normal human hepatocytes: modulation by inflammatory agents. Hepatology. 1994;20:186–90.
25. Sprengers ED, Kluft C. Plasminogen activator inhibitors. Blood. 1987;69:381–7.
26. Hekman CM, Loskutoff DJ. Fibrinolytic pathways and the endothelium. Semin Thromb Hemost. 1987;13:514–27.
27. Cox HT, Poller L, Thomson JM. Gastric fibrinolysis. A possible aetiological link with peptic ulcer. Lancet. 1967;1:1300–2.
28. Eras P, Harpel P, Winawer SJ. Histological localization of plasminogen activator and proteolytic activity in human stomach and duodenum. Gut. 1970;11:851–4.
29. Helgstrand U. Fibrinolysis and peptic ulcer. Acta Chir Scand Suppl. 1988;547:39–41.
30. Wodzinski MA, Bardhan KD, Reilly JT, Cooper P, Preston FE. Reduced tissue type plasminogen activator activity in the gastroduodenal mucosa in peptic ulcer disease. Gut. 1993;34:1310–14.
31. Plebani M, Di Mario F, Battistel M et al. Measurement of tryptase in endoscopic biopsies: distribution and relationship with ulcer disease. Clin Chim Acta. 1992;206:107–14.
32. Plebani M, Basso D, Busatto G et al. Are tryptase and cathepsin D related to Helicobacter pylori infection and mucosal gastrin in peptic ulcer? Res Exp Med. 1994;194:1–8.
33. Samloff IM. Peptic ulcer: the many proteinases of aggression. Gastroenterology. 1989;96:586–95.
34. Di Mario F, Dotto P, Germanà B et al. Mucosal pepsin and group I pepsinogen concentration in peptic ulcer patients with a history of bleeding. Eur J Gastroenterol Hepatol. 1992;4:657–9.
35. Di Mario F, Plebani M, Gottardello L et al. Role of serum fasting gastrin in screening for hypergastrinemic syndromes in duodenal ulcer disease. Clin Biochem. 1992;25:121–4.
36. Di Mario F, Battaglia G, Grassi SA et al. Hemorrhagic duodenal ulcer disease: clinical and biochemical findings in a case–control pilot study. Curr Ther Res. 1993;54:494–9.
37. Vianello F, Germanà B, Plebani M et al. A preliminary report on Helicobacter pylori and antral gastrin concentration in patients with duodenal ulcer. Curr Ther Res. 1994;55:1–7.
38. Vianello F, Di Mario F, Plebani M et al. Pepsin concentration in gastroduodenal biopsy homogenates in chronic ulcer disease. Dig Dis Sci. 1994;39:301–8.
39. Plebani M, Herszényi L, Cardin R et al. Cysteine and serine proteases in gastric cancer. Cancer. 1995;76:367–75.
40. Farinati F, Herszényi L, Carraro P et al. Cysteine and serine proteases: behaviour in precancerous changes and prognostic value in gastric cancer. Meetings of the American Gastroenterological Association (AGA), AASLD at Digestive Disease Week, San Diego. Gastroenterology. 1995;108:465A (Abstr).
41. Bradford MA. Rapid and sensitive method for the quantitation of microgram quantities of protein utilizing the principle of protein-dye binding. Anal Biochem. 1976;72:248–54.
42. Sier CFM, Vloedgraven HJM, Ganesh S et al. Inactive urokinase and increased levels of its inhibitor type 1 in colorectal cancer liver metastasis. Gastroenterology. 1994;107:1449–56.

43. Sier CFM, Verspaget HW, Griffioen G, Ganesh S, Vloedgraven HJM, Lamers CBHW. Plasminogen activators in normal tissue and carcinomas of the human oesophagus and stomach. Gut. 1993;34:80–5.
44. Piasecki CK, Thrasivoulou C, Rahim A. Ulcers produced by ligation of individual gastric mucosal arteries in the guinea pig. Gastroenterology. 1989;97:1121–9.
45. Piasecki CK, Thrasivoulou C. Durations of complete focal mucosal ischaemia needed to produce gastric ulceration. Eur J Gastroenterol Hepatol. 1992;4:487–93.
46. Brooks FP. Pathophysiology of peptic ulcer disease. Dig Dis Sci. 1985;30:15S–29S.
47. Tarnawski A, Hollander D, Stachura J et al. Vascular and microvascular changes – key factors in the development of acetic acid-induced gastric ulcers in rats. J Clin Gastroenterol. 1990;12:148–57.
48. Nakamura M, Kitajima M, Tsuchiya M. Alteration of gastric microcirculation in ulcer healing and recurrence: significance of autonomic nervous regeneration and mesenchymal cell. Gastroenterol Jpn. 1993;28:139–44.
49. Kurose I, Suematsu M, Miura S et al. Involvement of superoxide anion and platelet-activating factor in increased tissue-type plasminogen activator during rat gastric microvascular damages. Thromb Res. 1991;62:241–8.
50. Sato N, Kawano S, Kamada T, Takeda M. Hemodynamics of the gastric mucosa and gastric ulceration in rats and in patients with gastric ulcer. Dig Dis Sci. 1986;31:35S–41S.
51. Wormsley KG. Aetiology of ulcers. Balliéres Clin Gastroenterol. 1988;2:555–71.
52. Stacey MC, Burnand KG, Alexandroni MM, Gaffney PJ, Bhogal BS. Tissue and urokinase plasminogen activators in the environs of venous and ischaemic leg ulcers. Br J Surg. 1993;80:596–9.
53. Eitzman DT, Fay WP, Lawrence DA et al. Peptide-mediated inactivation of recombinant and platelet plasminogen activator inhibitor-1 in vitro. J Clin Invest. 1995;95:2416–20.
54. Pyke C, Kristensen P, Ralfkiaer E, Eriksen J, Dano K. The plasminogen activation system in human colon cancer: messenger RNA for the inhibitor PAI-1 is located in endothelial cells in the tumor stroma. Cancer Res. 1991;51:4067–71.
55. Bouchet C, Spyratos F, Martin PM, Hacéne K, Gentile A, Oglobine J. Prognostic value of urokinase-type plasminogen activator (uPA) and plasminogen activator inhibitors PAI-1 and PAI-2 in breast carcinomas. Br J Cancer. 1994;69:398–405.
56. Vassali JD, Sappino AP, Belin D. The plasminogen activator/plasmin system. J Clin Invest. 1991;88:1067–72.
57. Montesano R, Pepper MS, Mohlesteinlein U, Risau W, Wagner EF, Orci L. Increased proteolytic activity is responsible for the abberrant morphogenetic behavior of endothelial cells expressing the middle T-oncogene. Cell. 1990;62:435–45.
58. Konturek SJ, Brzowski T, Majka T et al. Fibroblast growth factor in gastroprotection and ulcer healing: interaction with sucralfate. Gut. 1993;34:881–7.
59. Szabo S, Folkman J, Vattay P, Morales RE, Pinkus GS, Kato K. Accelerated healing of duodenal ulcers by oral administration of a mutein of basic fibroblast growth factor in rats. Gastroenterology. 1994;106:1106–11.

Section IV

CELL INJURY AND PROTECTION IN THE LIVER AND IN THE PANCREAS

G Mózsik et al. Cell Injury and Cytoprotection in the GI Tract. 273–278.

TREATMENT OF CHRONIC LIVER DISEASE. DO CYTOPROTECTIVE AGENTS INTERFERE WITH DRUG-METABOLIZING ACTIVITY?

A. BECCARELLO[1], L. BORTOLATO[1], C. PALEARI[2], C. TRICHES[1], M. AWASUM[1] AND F. LIRUSSI[1*]

[1]Institute of Internal Medicine, and [2]Clinical Chemistry, University of Padua, Italy
*Correspondence

ABSTRACT

There is evidence that interferon (IFN) depresses antipyrine and theophylline clearances, thus impairing the drug-metabolizing activity (DMA), whereas ursodeoxycholic acid (UDCA) treatment is associated with controversial findings regarding changes in quantitative liver function tests (LFTs). IFN (Intron A, 6 million units (MU) tiw), a membrane-stabilizing agent – UDCA (Deursil, 600 mg/day) and a new formulation of a free-radical scavenger – silibinin β cyclodextrin (IBI/S, 135 mg/day) were given to a total of 32 patients with chronic liver disease for 6 months. Liver function, as assessed by routine LFTs and the formation of monoethylglycinexylidide (MEGX) from lidocaine (1 mg/kg iv), was evaluated before and after treatment. For comparison, LFTs and MEGX were also estimated in 10 matched patients with chronic liver disease who received no therapy for 6 months. In the IFN-treated patients the 45-min MEGX values (normal value = 79.1 ± 3.3 ng/ml) were 58.2 ± 4.9 at time 0 and increased by 20% during treatment (69.8 ± 5.0); mean ALT levels decreased from 173 ± 20 U/L at time 0 to 98 ± 22 after treatment ($p < 0.02$); AST decreased by 27% whereas γ-GT levels did not vary significantly. MEGX values were virtually unchanged during UDCA and IBI/S administration (respectively, 45.5 ± 5.2 and 53.7 ± 7.6 at entry vs. 47.7 ± 6.3 and 57.4 ± 5.7 at month 6) whereas transaminase levels decreased by 16–30% after UDCA treatment and by 9–19% after IBI/S treatment. Moreover, UDCA and IBI/S caused a 36% and a 24% reduction of γ-GT levels, respectively. In the control group, MEGX values remained stable throughout the 6-month period and so did transaminase and γ-GT levels. Moreover, no correlation was found between the changes in LFTs and the 45-min MEGX values in any of the groups studied. Thus, in patients with chronic liver disease, a 6 months' treatment with different cytoprotective agents was associated with an improvement in the common markers of liver function but with no significant changes in MEGX formation. These results suggest a lack of interference of tested drugs with DMA and favour the association of various cytoprotective agents with improved treatment outcome.

Keywords: quantitative liver function tests, monoethylglycinexylidide (MEGX) formation, ursodeoxycholic acid, silibinin, interferon, hepatitis C virus

INTRODUCTION

There is no established effective treatment of chronic liver disease (CLD) to date. In fact, many factors may influence management and therapeutic options. These factors mainly concern the patient (age, general condition, stage of CLD, other concomitant diseases and treatments) and the aetiology of liver damage (viral, immune, toxic). Also, drug pharmacokinetics must be considered in patients with CLD because of possible side-effects and drug interactions.

This paper was presented at the Symposium on 'Cell injury and protection in the gastrointestinal tract: from basic science to clinical perspectives', October 8–11, 1995, Pécs, Hungary.

The liver plays a fundamental role in the metabolism of lipophilic substances and in particular in the metabolism of drugs. A number of different enzymes, including cytochromes P_{450}, oxidases, reductases, hydrolases and transferases, are involved in these reactions. Depending on genetic variations, there exist subpopulations of patients with either decreased, absent or increased activities of certain enzymes. Besides, environmental factors, including drugs, diet, alcohol and cigarette smoking, may induce or inhibit the drug-metabolizing activity (DMA) and cause intra-individual differences.

Current therapeutic options of CLD include a range of different cytoprotective agents. Ursodeoxycholic acid (UDCA) and its taurine conjugate TUDCA are used in the treatment of chronic cholestatic and non-cholestatic liver disorders [1–7]; anti-oxidant drugs (silymarin, glutathione) appear beneficial in CLD of toxic origin, including alcoholic liver disease [7–9] while methyl donors are especially indicated in cholestatic disorders [10]. In acute or chronic liver disease of viral aetiology (especially hepatitis B and C), antiviral drugs, such as interferon (IFN), are currently being explored [11–14]. In case of no response to IFN treatment, the possibility should be considered of combining IFN with other drugs, such as ribavirin [15,16], UDCA [17,18] or N-acetyl cysteine [19].

QUANTITATIVE LIVER FUNCTION TESTS

The so-called quantitative liver function tests (QLFTs) are used for the evaluation of CLD [20]. They provide information about the splanchnic flow (indocyanine green), the functioning liver mass (galactose elimination capacity) and the DMA as assessed by the administration of drugs metabolized by the cytochrome P_{450} enzyme system (antipyrine, aminopyrine, theophylline and lidocaine). In particular, the formation of monoethylglycinexylidide (MEGX) from lidocaine, which is mediated by a cytochrome P_{450} de-ethylation reaction [21] is a reliable index of DMA. Moreover, galactose elimination capacity and MEGX may have predictive value as regards the evolution of CLD [22] and the survival of patients after liver transplant [23], respectively. Thus, the monitoring of QLFTs may be used in the follow-up of the treatment of CLD as well as in the assessment of prognosis and/or the choice of optimal timing for liver transplantation.

There are conflicting results in the literature as regards the changes of QLFTs during UDCA treatment in chronic cholestatic and non-cholestatic disorders [1,2,7,24–26]. Moreover, little is known about the influence of silymarin or other antioxidant drugs on liver function.

A number of reports suggest that interferon (IFN) depresses DMA, at least after short-term administration of the drug [27–30]. Such an effect has been shown to occur after a single dose or following repeated doses of different types of IFN. The mechanism(s) by which IFN depresses hepatic DMA is still unclear, although it might be mediated by several cytokines [30]. Moreover, the depressant effect of IFN on DMA might be a property which is inseparable from its antiviral or antitumour activity.

ANTIVIRAL/CYTOPROTECTIVE AGENTS AND LIVER FUNCTION

We have investigated, in patients with CLD, the effect of 6 months' treatment with an antiviral drug – IFN, a membrane stabilizing agent – UDCA, and a highly absorbable formulation of a free-radical scavenger – silibinin β cyclodextrin (SBC) on liver function as assessed by routine LFTs and a QLFT, the formation of MEGX from lidocaine. For comparison, LFTs and MEGX were also evaluated in patients with CLD who received no therapy for 6 months. Inclusion criteria were: 1) aged between 18 and 70 years; 2) a biopsy-proven diagnosis of CLD; 3) a persistent increase of serum transaminase levels ($\geqslant 1.5$ times the upper limit of normal). All patients gave their informed consent to the study, which was approved by the Ethical Committee of our Teaching Hospital.

Forty-three patients with compensated CLD of different aetiology were enrolled in the study. Of these, 16 were positive for hepatitis C virus (HCV) antibodies (RIBA II test), ten had chronic active hepatitis (CAH) and six had liver cirrhosis. They received IFNα_{2b} given at a dose of 6 MU tiw for 6 months (Group I). Seven patients (5 anti-HCV-positive unsuitable for IFN therapy; CAH = 5; cirrhosis = 2) received 6 months' UDCA treatment (600 mg/day; Group II). Ten anti-HCV-negative patients (fatty liver = 8; cirrhosis = 2) received SBC at a dose of 135 mg/day for 6 months (Group III) and 10 matched patients (8 anti-HCV-positive; CAH = 7; cirrhosis = 3) received no therapy for 6 months (Group IV).

Routine LFTs and a biochemical profile were evaluated monthly by means of a multianalyser at the Central Laboratory of the University of Padua. The concentration of MEGX was measured at entry and at the end of the study in a blood sample obtained 45 min after 1 mg/kg body weight of lidocaine given iv as a bolus injection, according to the method described by Oellerich and Raude [21].

In the IFN-treated group, a complete (normalization of ALT) or partial response (ALT reduction $> 50\%$) was observed in 10 patients. ALT levels decreased significantly from 170 U/L± 25 SEM at entry to 43 ± 6 after 6 months of IFN treatment ($p < 0.01$) in the responders, whereas no significant changes were observed in the non-responders (Figure 1). Similarly, mean AST values normalized in responders and did not change in the non-responders (Figure 1). The mean γ-GT levels decreased by 31% in responders, whereas they increased by 57% in non-responders. As shown in Figure 1, the values of this enzyme at entry were much higher in non-responders than in responders.

As regards the evaluation of DMA, basal MEGX values were similar in the patients which showed a response to IFN therapy and in the non-responders. Unlike the previous reports in the literature, we did not find any changes in the DMA after IFN treatment either in the responders or in the non-responders (Figure 2). Moreover, we also evaluated the changes in MEGX values 6 months after IFN withdrawal and, again, the 45-min MEGX concentrations remained stable in comparison with the values observed at the end of IFN treatment or following IFN discontinuation for no response (pooled data, Figure 2).

In the UDCA-treated group, serum transaminase levels decreased by 16–30% and γ-GT by 35%. No significant changes in MEGX values were observed in these patients: from 45 ± 5 ng/ml at entry to 47 ± 4 ng/ml after UDCA treatment.

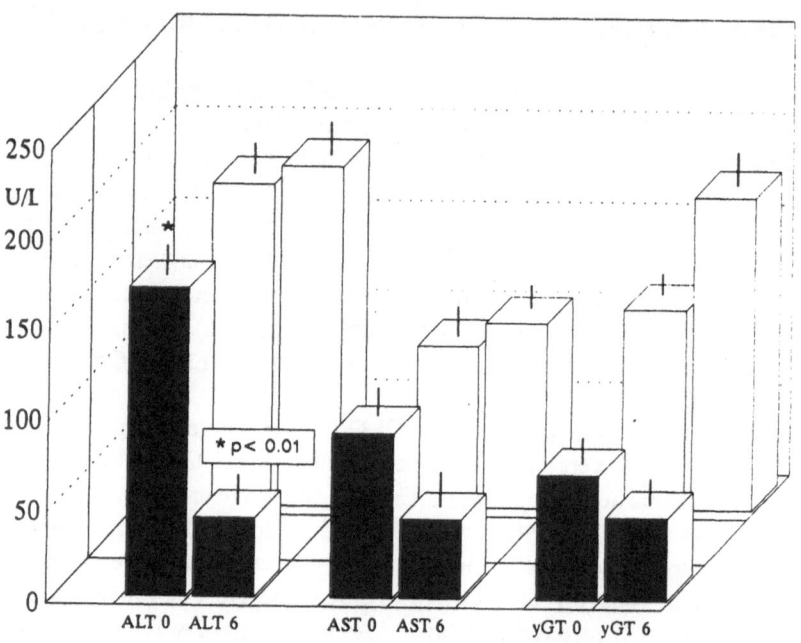

Figure 1. Changes in conventional liver function tests before and after 6 months of interferon treatment (6 MU three times a week). Mean ± SEM; ■ = responders; □ = non-responders

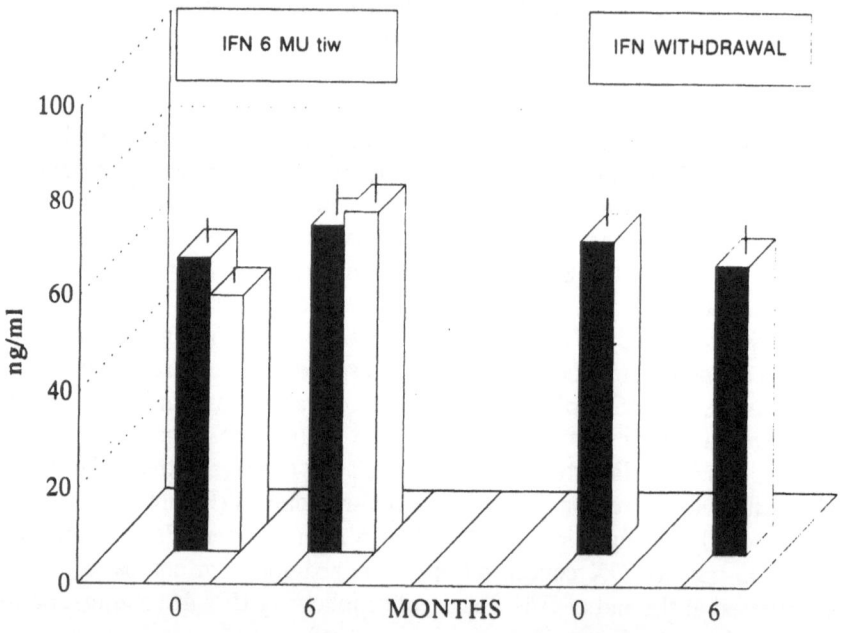

Figure 2. Changes in monoethylglycinexylidide values (45-min sample) during interferon treatment (6 MU three times a week) and after interferon withdrawal. Mean ± SEM; ■ = responders; □ = non-responders

Similar results were observed in the group of patients treated with SBC. In particular, transaminase levels decreased by 9–20% whereas γ-GT levels were reduced by 24%. Again, we found virtually no changes in MEGX values after SBC treatment (57 ± 5 ng/ml) compared with initial values (53 ± 7 ng/ml).

In the group of patients who received no treatment for 6 months, the serum transaminase and γ-GT values remained stable and so did MEGX values.

These results show that, in patients with chronic liver disease, 6 months' treatment with different cytoprotective agents is associated, in general, with an improvement in the conventional markers of liver function but with no significant changes in MEGX formation. Similarly, IFN treatment did not cause an impairment of liver function. Thus, although our findings confirm the beneficial effect of cytoprotective agents on liver dysfunction, our observations regarding the effect of IFN treatment on DMA do not support previous reports [27–30]. Possible explanations include differences in the dosage and the duration of therapy. The former was lower and the latter longer than in previous studies. Also, we evaluated MEGX formation 6 months after starting treatment. A depressant effect of the drug after short-term IFN treatment cannot be excluded and we are currently evaluating the short-term (1 month) effect of IFN treatment in patients with HCV-related CLD.

So far, our results suggest the lack of interference of tested drugs with the detoxification function of the liver and favour the association of various cytoprotective and/or antiviral agents with improved treatment outcome.

REFERENCES

1. Poupon R, Poupon RE, Calmous Y et al. Is ursodeoxycholic acid an effective treatment for primary biliary cirrhosis? Lancet. 1987;11:834–6.
2. Cotting J, Lentze MJ, Reichen J. Effects of ursodeoxycholic acid treatment on nutrition and liver function in patients with cystic fibrosis and longstanding cholestasis. Gut. 1990;31:918–21.
3. Podda M, Ghezzi C, Battezzati PM et al. Ursodeoxycholic acid, taurine or a combination of the two for chronic hepatitis. Gastroenterology. 1990;98:1044–50.
4. Plevris JN, Hayes PC, Bouchier IAD. Ursodeoxycholic acid in the treatment of alcoholic liver disease. Eur J Gastroenterol Hepatol. 1991;3:653–6.
5. Poupon RE, Poupon R, Balkau B and the UDCA–PBC Study Group. Ursodiol for the long-term treatment of primary biliary cirrhosis. N Engl J Med. 1994;330:1342–7.
6. Beccarello A, Lirussi F, Bortolato L et al. Effect of ursodeoxycholic acid (UDCA) and its taurine-conjugate (TUDCA) in HCV-related and unrelated cirrhosis. Gut. 1994;35(suppl 5):A153.
7. Lirussi F, Nassuato G, Orlando R et al. Treatment of active cirrhosis with ursodeoxycholic acid and a free radical scavenger: a two year prospective study. Med Sci Res. 1995;23:31–3.
8. Ferenci P, Dragosic B, Dittrich H et al. Randomized controlled trial of silymarin treatment in patients with cirrhosis of the liver. J Hepatol. 1989;9:105–13.
9. Meister A. New developments in glutathione metabolism and their potential application in therapy. Hepatology. 1984;4:739–42.
10. Frezza M, Surrenti C, Marzillo G et al. Oral S-adenosyl-L methionine in the symptomatic treatment of intrahepatic cholestasis: a double-blind, placebo controlled study. Gastroenterology. 1990;99:211–15.
11. Tinè F, Magrin S, Craxi A et al. Interferon for non-A non-B chronic hepatitis. A meta-analysis of randomised clinical trials. J Hepatol. 1991;13:192–9.
12. Chemello L, Alberti A, Rose K et al. Hepatitis C serotype and response to interferon therapy. N Engl J Med. 1994;330:143.
13. Lampertico P, Rumi MG, Romeo R et al. A multicentre randomized trial of recombinant interferon-alpha-2b in patients with acute transfusion-associated hepatitis C. Hepatology. 1994;19:19–22.

14. Booth JCL, Brown JL, Thomas HC. The management of chronic hepatitis C virus infection. Gut. 1995;37:449–54.
15. Di Bisceglie AM, Shindo M, Fong TL et al. A pilot study of ribavirin therapy for chronic hepatitis C. Hepatology. 1992;16:649–54.
16. Kakumu S, Yoshioka K, Wakita T et al. A pilot study of ribavirin and interferon beta for the treatment of chronic hepatitis C. Gastroenterology. 1993;105:507–12.
17. Angelico M, Gandin C, Pescarmona E et al. Recombinant interferon-α and ursodeoxycholic acid vs interferon-α alone in the treatment of chronic hepatitis C: a randomized clinical trial with long-term follow-up. Am J Gastroenterol. 1995;90:263–9.
18. Boucher E, Jouanolle H, Andre P et al. Interferon and ursodeoxycholic acid combined therapy in the treatment of chronic viral C hepatitis: results from a controlled randomized trial in 80 patients. Hepatology. 1995;21:322–7.
19. Beloqui O, Prieto J, Suarez M et al. N-Acetyl cysteine enhances the response to interferon-alfa in chronic hepatitis C: A pilot study. J Interferon Res. 1993;13:279–82.
20. Bircher J. Quantitative assessment of deranged hepatic function: A missed opportunity? Semin Liv Dis. 1983;3:275–84.
21. Oellerich M, Raude E. Monoethylglycinexylidide formation kinetics: a novel approach to assessment of liver function. J Clin Chem Clin Biochem. 1987;25:845–53.
22. Reichen J, Widmer T, Cotting J. Accurate prediction of death by serial determination of galactose elimination capacity in primary biliary cirrhosis: a comparison with the Mayo model. Hepatology. 1991;14:504–9.
23. Oellerich M, Burdelski M, Ringe B et al. Lignocaine metabolite formation as a measure of pre-transplant liver function. Lancet. 1989;i:640–2.
24. Leuschner U, Fischer H, Kurtz W et al. Ursodeoxycholic acid in primary biliary cirrhosis: results of a controlled double-blind trial. Gastroenterology. 1989;97:1268–74.
25. Lotterer E, Stiehl A, Raedsch R et al. Ursodeoxycholic acid in primary biliary cirrhosis: no evidence for toxicity in the stages I to III. J Hepatol. 1990;10:284–90.
26. Lirussi F, Okolicsanyi L. Cytoprotection with ursodeoxycholic acid: effect in chronic non-cholestatic and chronic cholestatic liver disease. Ital J Gastroenterol. 1992;24:31–5.
27. Williams SJ, Farrel GC. Inhibition of antipyrine metabolism by interferon. Br J Clin Pharmacol. 1986;22:610–12.
28. Williams SJ, Baird-Lambert JA, Farrel GC. Inhibition of theophylline metabolism by interferon. Lancet. 1987;ii:939–41.
29. Okuno H, Kitao Y, Takasu M et al. Depression of drug metabolizing activity in the human liver by interferon-α. Eur J Clin Pharmacol. 1990;39:365–7.
30. Okuno H, Takasu M, Kano H et al. Depression of drug-metabolizing activity in the human liver by interferon-β. Hepatology. 1993;17:65–9.

G Mózsik et al. Cell Injury and Cytoprotection in the GI Tract. 279–286.
© 1997 Kluwer Academic Publishers.

RECOMBINANT INTERFERON-α_{2b} TREATMENT FOR CHRONIC HEPATITIS C. A PROSPECTIVE MULTICENTRE STUDY IN HUNGARY

J. FEHÉR[1*], G. LENGYEL[1] (co-ordinators), L. DALMI[2], K. DÁVID[3], J. GERVAIN[4], Á GÓGL[4], J. LONOVICS[5], Zs. OZSVÁR[6], A. PÁR[7], F. SCHNEIDER[8] AND Zs. TULASSAY[1]

[1]2nd Department of Medicine, Semmelweis University, Budapest; [2]County Hospital, Department of Infectious Diseases, Debrecen; [3]BM Central Hospital, Department of Medicine, Budapest; [4]St. Georg Hospital, 1st Department of Medicine, Székesfehérvár; [5]Szent-Györgyi A. University, 1st Department of Medicine, Szeged; [6]City Hospital, Department of Infectious Diseases, Szeged; [7]Medical University, 1st Department of Medicine, Pécs; [8]Markusovszky L. Hospital, 1st Department of Medicine, Szombathely, Hungary
*Correspondence

ABSTRACT

Interferon-α_{2b} is widely used in the treatment of chronic hepatitis C. The aim of this multicentre study was to analyse the effect of prolonged recombinant interferon-α on liver functions and hepatitis C virus markers in serum. A further aim was to provide data on dosage and long-term administration of α-interferon. Eight liver units in universities and hospitals were involved in the open prospective study. Ninety-one patients were selected for the trial.

Therapy protocol: The patients with chronic C hepatitis were treated with α-interferon (Intron A) for one year and observed for another six months.

Efficacy of the therapy: There were 59 responders out of 91 patients (64.8%) with chronic C hepatitis. After one year of therapy, 37 out of 91 cases (40.6%) with chronic C hepatitis had completely responded: more patients under 40 years old had sustained a complete response than those over 40 years old. Side-effects, apart from a flu-like syndrome, were found only in a few cases.

Conclusion: The interferon-α therapy is a good modality for treatment of patients with hepatitis-C-virus-induced chronic hepatitis. It is more effective in younger patients than in older ones.

Keywords: chronic hepatitis, hepatitis C virus, interferon

About 20–35% of patients with chronic C hepatitis treated with interferon-α have long-term remission. Most authors have established that there is complete response with the normalization of alanine amino transferase (ALT) but have not given any attention to eradication of HCV-RNA from the serum. It seems more appropriate to consider both normalization of ALT in the serum and HCV-RNA eradication from the serum in order to evaluate the efficacy of interferon therapy [1–4]. When the complete remission lasts for six months post-treatment, it can be taken as a sustained complete response [5].

We studied the effect of interferon-α_{2b} over a 12-month period on serum ALT activities,

---

This paper was presented at the Symposium on 'Cell injury and protection in the gastrointestinal tract: from basic science to clinical perspectives', October 8–11, 1995, Pécs, Hungary.

on HCV eradication from the serum and on liver biopsy findings in patients with chronic C hepatitis. After the treatment period, follow-up continued for 6 months. We also studied the connection between age and complete response provided by interferon.

PATIENTS AND METHODS

Eight liver centres from universities and hospitals were involved in the open prospective multicentre study. Patient selection criteria were: ALT at least three times higher than the normal value in the last three months; positive serology for hepatitis C virus (anti-HCV antibody, HCV-RNA); chronic hepatitis in liver histology; age between 18 and 65 years; no contraindications (see exclusion criteria); and informed consent from the patient. Exclusion criteria include: any other kind of liver disease; severe metabolic alterations; severe cardiovascular disease; renal insufficiency; haematological disorders; pregnancy or lactation; HIV positive reaction; chronic alcoholism; mental disorders; and lack of compliance of patients.

Recruitment of patients involved at least six months observation period before starting therapy. Laboratory examinations included: routine haematological examinations; serum bilirubin; ALT; aspartate aminotransferase (AST); γ-glutamyl-transpeptidase; serum proteins; coagulation factors; as well as virus marker determinations in detail. Viral markers were: HBsAg, anti-HBs, HBeAg, anti-HBe, anti-HBc, anti-HCV, anti-EBV, anti-CMV and HIV reaction. In most cases, HCV-RNA in serum was tested.

In a case of suspicion of chronic C hepatitis, liver biopsy was carried out in all patients before starting the interferon therapy. After the interferon therapy and observation period, only some of the patients (25 cases) allowed us to make another liver biopsy. Morphological examinations were carried out by experts in pathology. Histological activity index (HAI) was determined by international criteria [6]. Score values were determined according to the severity of disease. Periportal and bridging necrosis was graded 0–10, intraglobular degeneration and focal necrosis 0–4, severity of portal inflammatory reaction 0–4, and fibrosis 0–4. The sum of the four values gives the so-called Knodell index, characterizing the liver histology of a patient.

Therapy of patients included in the study was the following: interferon-α_{2b} (Intron A, Schering–Plough Co.) was given at a dosage of 3 million units three times a week. The period of treatment was one year and the patients were followed up with clinical and laboratory examinations for another 6 months. If the patients were nonresponders after a three-month period, the dose of therapy was increased to 5 million units interferon three times a week.

Efficacy of treatment was analysed according to the literature [3,7,8,11]. Patients with normalization of ALT and lack of HCV-RNA were classed as having sustained complete remission at the end of the eighteen-month period. If either the value of ALT had increased or seroconversion was absent, this was called a partial response. Patients were non-responders if they had no normalization of ALT and no seroconversion.

All patients provided written informed consent before the trial. The protocol was approved by the ethics committee of all institutions involved in the study.

Statistical analysis was carried out by the χ^2-test and Student's t-test.

RESULTS

The multicentre study was carried out between 1992 and 1995. In total, 91 patients were selected for the trial. The mean age of patients was 45.9 years (range 18–65 years), among them 52 male and 39 female patients.

The possible modes of infection are shown in Figure 1. The transmission of infection was mostly by transfusion or surgical operation; rarely, sexual contact, risk of profession or acute hepatitis were the causative factors. In 33 cases out of 91, we were not able to identify the method of infection.

Duration of chronic hepatitis before the treatment is indicated in Table 1. Therapy was started within two years of the development of chronicity in about one third of patients. In one third of cases, the duration of the disease was longer than 5 years or unknown.

Thirty-seven cases (40.6%) with sustained complete remission and 22 cases (24.2%) with partial remission (among them 5 cases with complete remission and late relapse) demonstrate the efficacy of long-term interferon treatment. Eighteen patients were non-responders; the disease had progressed in three cases. Fourteen patients dropped out due to lack of compliance as well as haematological side-effects. Age and responder state is shown in Table 2; the rates of complete remission for patients under 40 and above 40 years old are shown in Table 3. It is clear from the tables that patients in the younger age group have a better response to interferon therapy. Serum ALT responses were significantly associated with clinical improvement and this value was one of the most important signs for predicting remission (Figure 2).

When we examined the age, sex and duration of disease according to responder state (Table 4) we concluded that the rate of remission is higher and the efficacy of therapy is better if the treatment is given after a shorter duration of disease.

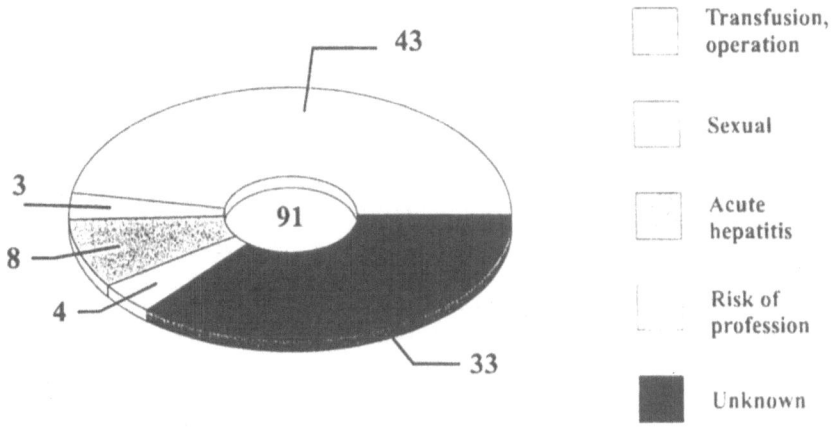

Figure 1. Possible modes of transmission of hepatitis C virus infection

TABLE 1
Duration of chronic hepatitis C before the interferon treatment

6 months–2 years	26
2–5 years	25
More than 5 years	26
Unknown	14
Total	91

TABLE 2
Responder status after interferon

	<40 years old	>40 years old	Total
Sustained complete remission	17	20	37
Partial response	12	10	22
Non-responder	6	9	15
Worsening	1	2	3
Dropped out	3	11	14
Total	39	52	91

TABLE 3
Rate of remission related to age (years)

	<40 years old	>40 years old	Total
Sustained complete remission			
Numbers	17/39	20/52	37/91
Percent	43.5%	38.4%	40.6%
Complete and partial remission together			
Numbers	29/39	30/52	59/91
Percent	74.3%	57.6%	64.8%

The difference between the number of patients <40 years old and >40 years old is statistically significant ($p < 0.05$) for total numbers of patients with sustained complete and partial remission. Statistical analysis was by χ^2-test

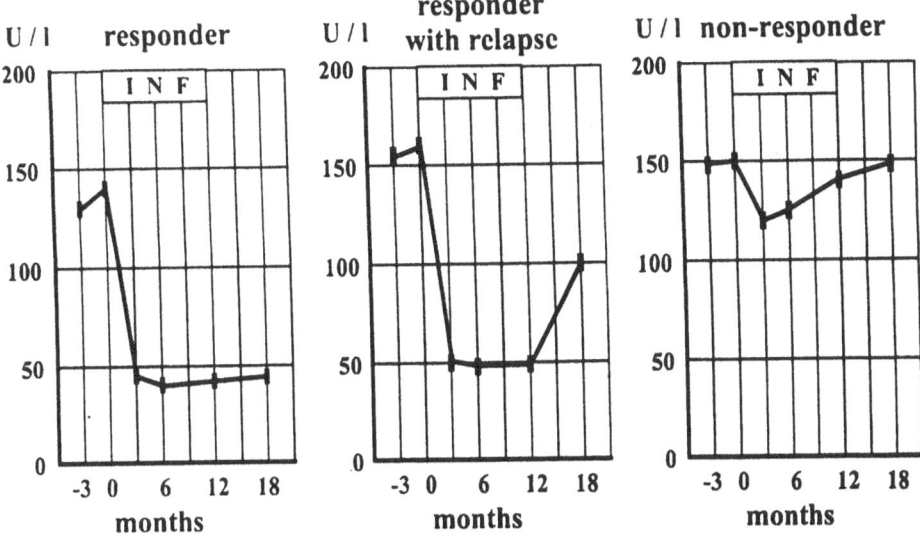

Figure 2. Typical ALT activity in chronic C hepatitis during interferon treatment. Each line shows a representative patient

At the end of the clinical trial, control liver biopsies were carried out in only 25 cases. In half of these cases, the liver tissue activity had decreased. The histological activity index (Knodell) was significantly smaller after the interferon therapy (Table 5).

The side-effects of interferon therapy are shown in Table 6. Flu-like syndrome, myalgia and joint complaints were found mostly. The table shows the different symptoms. In some cases, two or three different symptoms were found in the same patient. In total, 36 patients had at least one side-effect out of 91 cases.

DISCUSSION

In this multicentre study, we gave interferon-α_{2b} therapy to 91 patients with established chronic HCV infection, with HCV-RNA and anti-HCV detected in the serum. The majority of our patients responded with normalization of their serum ALT levels. This is a similar or better response rate than found in most previously published studies with shorter treatment courses. Furthermore, only a few responders (5 patients) relapsed during follow-up after treatment, corresponding to an overall sustained remission rate of 40.6%. This correlates well with the data of Hoofnagle et al. [7], as well as of Reichard et al. [8]. They have shown that long-term treatment with interferon produces better results than short-term therapy.

TABLE 4

Age, sex and responder status of patients with chronic C hepatitis after interferon treatment

	Total cases	Responders total	Response without relapse	Responsse with relapse	Non-responders
Number of cases	91	59	37	22	32
Relative rate (%)	100	64.8	40.6	24.1	35.1
Mean age (years)	45.9	43.1	42.5	43.7	50.4
Duration of disease					
<2 years	26	21 (80.7%)	12 (46.1%)	9	5
>2 years	65	38 (58.4%)	25 (38.4%)	12	27
Sex					
Male	52	35	21	14	17
Female	39	24	16	8	15

TABLE 5

Liver histology in patients with chronic hepatitis C

Activity decreased	11
No change	5
Progression	9

At the end of the clinical study control liver biopsy was carried out in only 25 cases

Histology activity index was scored in 15 cases. The difference between the Knodell index before (10.1) and after (7.0) treatment was statistically significant ($p < 0.05$) shown by the χ^2-test

Another important result of our clinical trial is the correlation between age and remission rate of patients, as well as the connection between the duration of disease and the responder status. Reichard et al. [5,8] widely studied the connection between the age and responder status of patients as well as the connection between the duration of the chronic C hepatitis before interferon treatment and the remission rate after therapy. In their study, they found no significant difference between the groups regarding age, but the proportion of responders was higher in patients with shorter duration of disease. Our results are in good accordance with these results regarding duration of chronic hepatitis. As the figures in Table 4 show, the remission rate is higher (80.7% for total remission and 46.1% for sustained complete remission) in patients with a shorter duration of disease (less than 2 years) than in patients with a longer duration of disease (more than 2 years; 58.4 and 38.4%, respectively). In the case of age, we obtained different results from those of Reichard et al. In our study, patients

TABLE 6
Side-effects of interferon treatment in chronic C hepatitis

*	Flu-like syndrome	16
*	Fatigue, weight loss	4
*	Alopecia (transitory)	4
*	Relapse of psoriasis	1
*	Leucocytopenia	7
*	Thrombocytopenia	1
*	Tbc activation	1
*	Worsening of diabetes mellitus	1
*	Myalgia, joint complaints	11
*	Transitory depression	1
*	Autoimmune thyroiditis	1

Number of patients with side-effects = 36. Some had more than one symptom

under 40 years showed a better rate of remission than those above 40. The differences for all cases with remission (complete and partial remission together) was statistically significant (Table 3). The mean age of non-responders was higher (Table 4). We have not seen any difference in response rate between the two sexes.

A significant proportion of patients do not respond to interferon using a standard regimen. Few alternatives exist for these patients. If the patient has not responded after the first 12 weeks of treatment, increasing the dose to 10 million units produces a response in about 20% of patients [2,7]. Other therapy modalities include ribavirin treatment [7,9] and ursodeoxycholic acid therapy [2]. Out of 91 of our patients, 15 did not respond and the clinical state of 3 patients worsened. The rate is similar to that in the literary data [7,9,11]. The causes of non-response and relapse are unclear. Neutralizing anti-interferon antibodies may be responsible in a few cases. However, it is likely that most cases result from the virus itself which is resistant to the effects of interferon [10].

The progression of chronic liver disease can be evaluated by pathological methods from liver biopsy material. In our study, we were able to take liver biopsy samples before and after treatment in only 25 cases, though we did take biopsies in all cases before starting the study. In eleven cases, we saw a decrease in tissue alterations. All of these belonged to the group with complete sustained remission. Histologically, the outcome was assessed in 15 cases by a scoring system comparing pretreatment histological findings with those at treatment cessation. Biochemical responders usually have a concomitant improvement in necroinflammatory parameters, including the fibrosis score, which is most pronounced in cases with sustained response. Histological activity scores in our patients were lower after interferon treatment than before the study. Examining the morphological alterations in individual cases together with the biochemical parameters and viral markers, we can also say that there is a correlation between the biochemical and the morphological changes.

On the basis of these results, we conclude that a prolonged interferon-α_{2b} treatment course may possibly reduce the tendency for relapse after treatment cessation. The rate of sustained complete remission is higher in patients under 40 years that in those above this age, and the effect of interferon treatment is relatively better if this therapy is used after a shorter duration of chronicity of hepatitis C.

ACKNOWLEDGEMENTS

We are very grateful to Schering–Plough Co. for providing the interferon-α_{2b} for these patients free of charge. The authors are grateful to the pathologists in the different institutions for helping in the establishment of the diagnosis.

REFERENCES

1. Di Bisceglie AM, Martin P, Kassiandies C et al. Recombinant interferon therapy for chronic hepatitis C. A randomized, double blind, placebo-controlled trial. N Engl J Med. 1989;321:1506–10.
2. Lengyel G, Fehér J. Interferon treatment in virus induced chronic active hepatitis (Hung.). Orv Hetil. 1995;136:1–7.
3. Poynard T, Bedossa P, Chevallier M and the Multicenter Study Group. A comparison of three interferon-α_{2b} regimens for the long-term treatment of chronic non-A non-B hepatitis. N Engl J Med. 1995;332:1457–62.
4. Thomas HC. Chronic Hepatitis C. F. Hoffmann–La Roche Ltd; 1994.
5. Reichard O, Glaumann H, Frydén A et al. Two-year biochemical, virological, and histological follow-up in patients with chronic hepatitis C responding in a sustained fashion to interferon-α_{2b} treatment. Hepatology. 1995;21:918–22.
6. Knodell RG, Ishak KG, Black WC et al. Formulation and application of a numerical scoring system for assessing histological activity in asymptomatic chronic active hepatitis. Hepatology. 1981;1:431–5.
7. Hoofnagle JH, De Bisceglie AM, Michiko Shindo. Antiviral therapy of hepatitis C – present and future. J Hepatol. 1993;17:130–6.
8. Reichard O, Foberg U, Frydén A et al. High sustained response rate and clearance of viremia in chronic hepatitis C after treatment with interferon-α_{2b} for 60 weeks. Hepatology. 1994;19:280–5.
9. Camps J, Garcia N, Riezn-Boj JI, Civeira MP, Prieto J. Ribavirin in the treatment of chronic hepatitisC unresponsive to a interferon. J Hepatol. 1992:19:408–12.
10. Davis GL, Balart LA, Schiff ER. Treatment of chronic hepatitis C with recombinant interferon alpha: A multicenter randomized, controlled trial. N Engl J Med. 1989;321:1501–6.
11. Zeuzem S, Roth WK, Herrmann G. Virushepatitis C. Z Gastroenterol. 1995;33:117–32.

G Mózsik et al. Cell Injury and Cytoprotection in the GI Tract. 287–303.
© 1997 Kluwer Academic Publishers.

IMMUNOLOGICAL FEATURES AND THE EFFECT OF INTERFERON TREATMENT IN CHRONIC HEPATITIS C

A. PÁR[1]*, M. PAÁL[3], Á. GÓGL[5], J. GERVAIN[5], J. SZEKERES-BARTHO[2], J. SIPOS[6], T. BERÓ[1], E. HÜTTER[7], Gy. BERENCSI[7], I. KÁDAS[4], G. HEGEDÜS[4], Gy. BRASCH[4], I. SZABOLCSI[5] AND Gy. MÓZSIK[1]

[1]First Department of Medicine and [2]Institute of Microbiology, University Medical School Pécs; [3]Blood Transfusion Centre and [4]Department of Pathology, Baranya County Hospital, Pécs; [5]St. George's Hospital, Székesfehérvár; [6]Department of Pathology, Zala County Hospital, Zalaegerszeg; [7]Johan Béla National Institute of Hygiene, Budapest, Hungary
*Correspondence

ABSTRACT

Clinical and immunological findings with 74 patients with chronic hepatitis C are reported. Transfusion or major surgery was noted in the case history of 69% of patients and the time elapsed from the transfusion to the diagnosis was 7.15 ± 8.1 years in the transfused subjects. The severity of the liver disease was recorded; chronic persistent hepatitis was present in 40%, active hepatitis in 45% and cirrhosis in 15% of the patients. Cholestasis was recorded in 32%, a significant elevation of serum immunoglobulin levels was noted in 83%, an antibody to liver specific protein (anti-LSP) occurred in 80%, cryoglobulinaemia in 44% and circulating immune complexes in 33% of the patients. Natural killer cell activity of peripheral blood mononuclear cells was significantly lower in the patients compared with the normal controls. HLA B8 and HLA DR3 antigens were found with an increased frequency (36.6% and 42.1%). Of the 74 patients, 31 were treated with recombinant interferon-α_2 injection sc at a dose of 3 million units (MU) three times a week (tiw) for six months. Interferon therapy normalized serum alanine aminotransferase in 45% of patients and a sustained remission was found in 26%. The treatment resulted in the clearance of HCV-RNA from the serum in 40% of patients and this correlated with complete remission. In the responders, a decrease in CD4+ cell count and a transient decrease in CD8+ cell count as well as a moderate rise in B cell count were seen during the treatment. Mitogen-induced lymphoproliferative response and natural killer cell activity increased. Predictors of response were as follows: female sex, shorter time elapsed since transfusion, absence of HLA A1, B8, DR3 and serum anti-HBc negativity.

Keywords: chronic hepatitis C, immune parameters, interferon treatment

INTRODUCTION

The discovery of hepatitis C virus (HCV), using molecular biological techniques was a milestone in modern virus hepatitis research [1]. Since then, it has been discovered that most of the diseases previously identified as non-A, non-B hepatitis and parenteral (post-transfusion) chronic hepatitis are of HCV origin and named as chronic hepatitis C [2]. In the past four years, we have observed large numbers of patients with chronic hepatitis C and, in many cases, we were able to perform continuous follow-up combined with detailed immunological examinations. Our first results have already been published [3–5].

This paper was presented at the Symposium on 'Cell injury and protection in the gastrointestinal tract: from basic science to clinical perspectives', October 8–11, 1995, Pécs, Hungary.

The present report summarizes clinical and immunological features of patients with chronic hepatitis C and also our experiences with the interferon treatment. We examined the immunological functions of patients with chronic hepatitis C and their changes during interferon (IFN) therapy, and whether there were any differences between the immunological parameters of good responders and of non-responders before and during therapy, that is predictors of response have been searched for.

PATIENTS

Between January 1990 and December 1993, 74 patients with chronic hepatitis C (40 males and 34 females) were observed. Their mean age was 48.4 years (range 16–74 years). Duration of the disease was between 6 and 240 months, with an average of 30.5 months. Transfusion or major surgery in the case history was noted in 49 cases (69%). Time elapsed from the transfusion to the diagnosis was a mean of 7.15 ± 8.15 years in the transfused patients. Criteria of diagnosis of chronic hepatitis C were serum GPT (ALT) elevation for at least 6 months at 1.5 times the normal upper limit. Histological findings of liver biopsy proved the liver disease. Second-generation anti-HCV ELISA verified HCV aetiology. The most important diseases, from the point of view of differential diagnosis, were the following: autoimmune (lupoid) hepatitis and primary biliary cirrhosis, HBV-, EBV-, CMV-origin hepatitis, Wilson's disease, α_1-antitrypsin deficiency and haemochromatosis.

Based on clinical, immunological and histological findings, chronic persistent hepatitis was diagnosed in 30 cases (biopsy: 26), chronic active hepatitis in 33 (biopsy: 28) and chronic hepatitis with cirrhosis in 11 (biopsy: 9) cases, respectively.

Among the above-mentioned patients, immunoserological studies were performed in 36 cases, complex humoral and cellular immune functions in 32 cases and HLA phenotyping in 30 cases, respectively.

Interferon-treated patients

Between January 1992 and June 1993, 31 patients (16 males and 15 females) were enrolled into an open interferon therapy programme (see later), and were followed-up clinically and immunologically. The patients' mean age was 45.7 years (range 17–64 years), and the average duration of disease was 23.4 months (range 6–120 months). Twenty-four patients had a history of blood transfusion. Histological findings revealed features of chronic persistent hepatitis in 12 cases, chronic active hepatitis in 13 cases and active hepatitis with cirrhosis in 6 cases.

Blood donors

A comparative immunological study was also performed in 16 asymptomatic anti-HCV-positive blood donors. All of them were asymptomatic and repeated conventional liver function tests (serum bilirubin, GOT, GPT, GGT) were found to be normal; thus no manifest liver disease was found.

METHODS

After taking the case history and physical examination, the following laboratory parameters were studied:

Biochemistry

Urine test, serum bilirubin, alanine aminotransferase (GPT/ALT), aspartate aminotransferase (GOT/AST), alkaline phosphatase (ALP), γ-glutamyl transpeptidase (GGT), pseudocholinesterase (PsCh), total protein, albumin, prothrombin complex, procollagen-III-peptide (P-III-P), α_1-antitrypsin, serum iron, iron-binding capacity, ferritin, coeruloplasmin, serum copper, urea, creatinine, cholesterol, plasma glucose.

Virology

Tests for hepatitis B surface antigen (HBsAg), antibody to hepatitis B core antigen (anti-HBc), HBeAg, anti-HBe, anti-Delta, anti-HIV, anti-HCV and anti-EBV were performed using ELISA test systems (Abbott, Ortho and Organon Technique) as recommended by the manufacturers. Detection of HCV-RNA was performed by polymerase chain reaction (PCR) from frozen sera samples.

The detailed methods of purifying of primers and RNA have been described and published by Telegdy et al. [6].

We used the enzyme system created by the Perkin Elmer Cetus (Gene Amp RNA PCR kit) and followed the manufacturer's instructions. The PCR products were identified by HpaII restrictive enzyme digestion (Hütter et al., unpublished results).

Serum samples from the same patient – obtained several times – were examined and deviations were evaluated in the same studies of line intensity. Based on semiquantitative comparative studies, the decrease in intensity – made visible with photography – allowed us to predict a 100-fold decrease in virus titre.

Immunology

a) Humoral parameters: serum immunoglobulins (IgA, IgG, IgM) and complement factors (C3, C4); β_2-microglobulin; autoantibodies: antinuclear (ANA), antimitochondrial (AMA), smooth muscle (SMA), liver cell membrane (LMA), anti-LSP, liver–kidney microsomal (LKM), parietal cell (PCA), anti-DNA, thyroid gland microsoma and thyroglobulin, pancreas islet cell, and anti-SSA antibodies (detected by indirect immunofluorescence and ELISA techniques), rheumatoid factor, lymphocytotoxic antibodies, circulating immune complexes (PEG-precipitation) and serum cryoglobulin level were determined.

b) Cellular immunity: blood picture, absolute granulocyte and lymphocyte count, E-rosette-forming T-cell count, CD4+, CD8+, CD16+ cell and B-cell count, mitogen-induced (phytohaemagglutinin = PHA) lymphoproliferative response (lymphoblast transformation), and natural killer (NK) cell activity (single cell method on K562 target cell).

c) HLA, A, B, C, DR and DQ determinations were carried out by the serological method using standardized microlymphocytotoxicity tests according to the National Institute of Health (NIH).

Histology

Liver biopsy specimens from the patients treated with IFN were studied, based on standard criteria and scored for histological activity, according to Knodell's numerical scoring system [7] evaluating the degree of portal inflammation, periportal activity, and necrosis, lobular necrosis and fibrosis, scored from 0 to 22.

Interferon treatment

Thirty-one patients with chronic hepatitis C were entered in the study. The trial was approved by the National Institute of Pharmacy and by the Ethics Committees of the Hospitals. According to the original protocol, patients were given 3 million units (MU) of recombinant α-interferon three times a week. (Twenty-nine patients received IFN-α-2b Intron-A (Schering-Plough/USA), 2 patients IFN-2a Roferon-A (Roche) injection sc.) In the first week, IFN was given in the institute; after that, the patients were taught how to self-administer the interferon at home. In the first month of treatment, the patients were checked weekly, twice during the second month, and, from the third month, once a month. The duration of the treatment was scheduled for 6 months.

Inclusion criteria

– Age: 18–65 years
– Serum GPT level three times higher than the upper limit of normal for at least six months
– Chronic hepatitis proven histologically
– Anti-HCV-positivity and presence of HCV-RNA by PCR
– Informed consent of the patient

Exclusion criteria

- Pregnancy, lactation
- Antiviral or immunosuppressive therapy within the last 6 months
- Severe haematological alterations (Hgb <11 g/dl, WBC $<3000/mm^3$, platelets $<70\,000/mm^3$
- Cardiovascular disease, untreated hypertension ($>170/100$ mmHg)
- Decompensated liver cirrhosis (serum bilirubin >2.5 mg/dl, albumin <30 g/L, prothrombin activity $<60\%$)
- Renal failure
- Neuropsychiatric alterations, alcohol and drug abuses
- HIV-positivity
- Autoimmune hepatitis, primary biliary cirrhosis
- Haemochromatosis, Wilson's disease, α_1-antitrypsin deficiency

Statistical analysis

Two-sample (unpaired) Student's *t*-test was performed to evaluate the statistical significance of differences between the data series of groups. The Pearson χ^2 contingency analysis was used to test the significance of the relationships between our categorical variables.

RESULTS

Clinical findings in chronic hepatitis C

Among the 74 HCV-positive patients with liver disease, 10 patients (13.5%) had a history of post-transfusion acute hepatitis with icterus, manifested 5–8 weeks after transfusion. Serious fatigue was the main complaint of 18 patients (24%). Alcohol abuse (more than 60 g daily) occurred in 6 cases (8%). In 8 patients (10.8%), HBsAg-positivity was verified at the same time. In 23 patients (31.1%), anti-HBc- and/or anti-HBs-positivity suggested a previous HBV hepatitis in the history. Hepatomegaly was found in 55 cases (74.3%), splenomegaly in 10 (13.5%) and cholestasis in 24 cases (32.4%).

Ascites occurred in 4 cases (5%), oesophageal varicosity in 4 cases (5%) and diabetes in 12 cases (16.2%).

Hepatocellular carcinoma was diagnosed in two cases; furthermore, in one case, a patient who had had chronic hepatitis for 18 years, hepatocellular carcinoma developed during the study period.

During the four-year follow-up of 74 patients, four died (5%): two patients due to hepatocellular carcinoma, one due to stroke and one due to liver failure after oesophageal varix rupture.

At the time of diagnosis, the pathological serum bilirubin level was noted in 21 cases (28.4%), GOT was twice the normal upper limit (NUL) in 38 cases (51.3%), GPT was >2× NUL in 55 cases (74.3%), GGT was >2× NUL in 36 cases (48.6%) and increased ALP occurred in 17 cases (22.9%).

Abnormally low (<70%) prothrombin activity was seen in 9 patients (12.1%) and a high level (>20 g/L) of serum γ-globulin in 62 (83.7%).

Leukopenia was found in 10 cases (13.5%); lymphopenia (<1500) in 16 cases (21.6%); granulocytopenia (<2000) in 8 cases (10.8%); and thrombocytopenia in 16 cases (21.6%).

During follow-up, progression of chronic hepatitis C to cirrhosis or clinical signs of decompensation of the cirrhosis were not observed.

Procollagen-III-peptide examinations

The serum P-III-P level is an accepted marker for collagen metabolism and for monitoring fibrogenesis in liver disease [8]. P-III-P levels from sera of 44 patients with chronic hepatitis C (12 persistent hepatitis, 24 active hepatitis and 8 cirrhosis) were determined with radio-immunoassay (RIA-guost, Behring, Marburg, Germany). (The normal serum level of P-III-P is 0.3–0.8 U/ml.) Among 12 patients with persistent hepatitis, pathological P-III-P levels (>0.8 U/ml) were found in 8 cases, with a mean of 1.13 ± 0.38 U/ml. An increased serum P-III-P level was found in 23 cases of 24 patients with active hepatitis (mean: 1.35 ± 0.51 U/ml) and in all 8 patients with cirrhosis (mean: 1.47 ± 0.46 U/ml).

During the course, P-III-P levels were determined repeatedly in 39 patients. Out of the 15 patients not treated with IFN, the serum P-III-P level decreased in 3 cases, did not change in 7, and increased in 5 cases. Of 24 IFN-treated patients, the serum P-III-P level decreased in 10 cases, did not change in 8 and increased in 6 cases.

Immunological examinations

Humoral immunity

Mean values of serum immunoglobulin and complement factors are summarized in Table 1.

IgG, IgA and IgM were significantly increased in patients with chronic hepatitis C. Examined individually, an abnormally high (>16.0 g/L) serum IgG level was found in 23/36 cases (63.8%); a significantly increased IgA level (>3.0 g/L) in 14/36 (38.8%); and a high IgM level (>2.0 g/L) in 18/36 (50%). An increased level of any of the immunoglobulin classes was found in 30 cases (83%).

Serum immunoglobulin and complement levels in asymptomatic HCV-positive blood donors scarcely deviated from the normal level, though increases occurred in 4/16 cases for IgG, in 1/16 case for IgA and in 2/16 cases for IgM.

TABLE 1
Serum immunoglobulins and complement factors

	Healthy controls (n = 50)	Anti-HCV-positive donors (n = 13)	Chronic hepatitis C patients (n = 36)
IgG (g/L)	12.25 ± 2.00	15.65 ± 3.65	18.40 ± 4.42*
IgA (g/L)	2.13 ± 0.65	2.05 ± 0.59	3.09 ± 1.60*
IgM (g/L)	1.37 ± 0.42	1.80 ± 0.82	2.77 ± 1.71*
C3 (mg/dl)	86.80 ± 13.0	80.76 ± 22.92	84.90 ± 19.7
C4 (mg/dl)	27.90 ± 11.0	29.82 ± 10.77	32.60 ± 15.3

*$p < 0.05$ compared with the controls

Autoantibodies: ANA was observed in 4/36 cases (11%), SMA in 8/36 (22%), anti-SSA in 6/25 (24%), anti-DNA in 13/30 (43.3%), anti-LPS in 29/36 (80.5%), rheumatoid factor in 15/36 (41.6%), parietal cell antibody in 8/36 (22%), cryoglobulin in 16/36 (44.4%), and circulating immune complex in 12/36 (33.3%), but no AMA, thyroid gland microsomal antibodies, thyroglobulin antibodies and lymphocytotoxic antibodies were found in chronic hepatitis C patients.

Of 16 anti-HCV-positive blood donors, circulating immune complexes were found in 5 subjects, cryoglobulin-positivity also in 5 cases, and rheumatoid factor in 2 cases but no other autoantibodies.

Cellular immune parameters

Lymphocyte subsets: No significant difference was noted in cell counts of patients with chronic hepatitis C compared with the control group (Table 2), though a moderate decrease in mean values of CD16+ (NK cell) count and B cell count was seen.

Considering individual values, absolute lymphocyte count was lower than the lower limit of normal ($< 1500/\mu l$) in 8 cases, T-cell count was lower in 3 cases and higher in one case than the normal level (750–2000/μl). CD4+ cell count (normal: 500–1000/μl) was low in six cases, CD8+ cell count (normal: 150–750/μl) in one case and CD16+ (NK) cell count (normal: 200–300/μl) in 10 cases. B cell count did not reach the lower limit of normal (100/μl) in 9 cases.

In asymptomatic anti-HCV-positive blood donors, either the lymphocyte count or the T-cell count and the mean values of T-subsets significantly increased, and the CD4/CD8 ratio decreased ($p < 0.05$). Alterations in B cell and NK cell counts were not significant.

Lymphoproliferative response: Mean values of PHA-stimulation index in patients with chronic hepatitis C showed a minimal (statistically non-significant) decrease compared with the control. Lymphoblast transformation in anti-HCV-positive blood donors did not differ significantly from the control.

TABLE 2

Cellular immunity parameters in chronic hepatitis C

a) *Lymphocyte subsets*

	Healthy controls (n = 40)	Anti-HCV- positive donors (n = 16)	Chronic hepatitis C patients (n = 32)
Total lymphocyte/μl	1860 ± 345	2912 ± 1155*	1856 ± 556
Total T cell	1125 ± 325	1905 ± 753*	1314 ± 421
CD4+ cell	757 ± 350	1195 ± 532*	711 ± 268
CD8+ cell	447 ± 314	954 ± 276*	432 ± 181
CD4/CD8 ratio	1.9 ± 0.70	1.1 ± 0.2*	1.7 ± 0.6
B cell	192 ± 92	275 ± 174	183 ± 144
NK cell	360 ± 217	317 ± 163	276 ± 157

*$p < 0.05$ compared with the controls

b) *Lymphocyte function*

	Healthy controls (n = 40)	Anti-HCV- positive donors (n = 12)	Chronic hepatitis C patients (n = 32)
PHA			
10 μg SI	122 ± 52	111 ± 68	103 ± 53
50 μg/SI	114 ± 55	121 ± 85	107 ± 48
NK activity (%)	3.44 ± 1.10	ND	2.06 ± 1.67*

*$p < 0.05$

NK-cell activity: Mean NK-cell activity of the subjects studied was significantly decreased compared with control ($p < 0.05$); NK activity did not reach the lower level of normal in 6/16 (37.5%) cases.

HLA determinations: Results of HLA typings are summarized in Table 3. HLA B8, HLA DR3 and HLA DQw2 antigens occurred with significantly increased frequency in patients with chronic hepatitis C.

TABLE 3
Results of HLA studies

	Healthy controls	Chronic hepatitis C
HLA A1, B8	36/340 (10.59%)	7/30 (23.3%)
HLA B8	52/340 (15.29%)	11/30 (36.6%)*
HLA DR3	16/77 (20.59%)	8/19 (42.1%)*
HLA DR4	14/77 (18.18%)	4/19 (21.05%)
HLA DR5	30/77 (38.96%)	4/19 (21.05%)
HLA DQw2	14/77 (18.1%)	8/19 (42.1%)*

*$p < 0.05$

In anti-HCV-positive blood donors, we determined only HLA Class I antigens; results did not differ from control. (Here, we present only the frequency of HLA A1 and HLA B8.)

Results of interferon therapy

Clinical–biochemical changes related to IFN treatment are summarized in Table 4. Of 14 patients who achieve complete remission, in 11 cases, normalization of serum GPT occurred in the first three months of the treatment. Relapse occurred in 6 patients relatively early, within 3 months after the end of six months' therapy. A sustained remission (in 8 patients) means that the GPT level remained normal six months after the withdrawal of IFN.

In the case of partial remission, the GPT level decreased more than 50% relative to the initial values, but did not normalise.

Examining the relationships between biochemical and virological changes, we established the following: of 14 patients achieving complete remission, in 11 cases, serum HCV-RNA (PCR) became negative; in 2 cases, the HCV-RNA level decreased; and in one case, it did not change. Of 17 partial or non-responders, in one anti-HCV-positive patient, the HCV-RNA test was negative which is why HCV-RNA changes were examined in 16 patients: one patient became HCV-RNA negative permanently; one temporarily negative but later positive again; in 5 cases, serum HCV-RNA level decreased; and, in 9 cases, did not change.

Histological observations

Six months after the end of IFN treatment (up to now 12 cases), a second liver biopsy was carried out: in 7 patients with complete remission and in 5 non-responders.

TABLE 4

The effect of interferon treatment on clinical–biochemical and virological parameters

	Number of patients/total
Complete remission (normalization of ALT/GPT)	14/31 (45%)
Partial remission	4/31 (13%)
No response or drop-out	13/31 (42%)
Sustained complete remission	8/31 (26%)
Serum	
HCV-RNA (PCR) became negative	12/30 (40%)
HCV-RNA level decreased	8/30 (27%)
HCV-RNA level did not change	10/30 (33%)

Of the good responders, in 6 cases, the Knodell index decreased, indicating histological improvement; in one case, it did not change. (Mean value before treatment 7.9; after treatment 4.7.)

Of the 5 non-responders, in 3 cases, the Knodell index did not change, and, in 2 cases, it increased, one of them with signs of progression to cirrhosis (mean value before treatment 8.1; afterwards 9.0).

P-III-P changes indicating fibrogenesis

During IFN treatment, we examined changes in the serum P-III-P level of 24 patients. An abnormally high initial level was observed in 20 patients.

After IFN treatment, the P-III-P level normalized in one case, significantly (>0.3 U/ml) decreased in 9 cases, increased in 6 cases and did not change in 8 cases. A significant decrease was observed in 6/12 good responders and in 4/12 non-responders.

Changes in immunological parameters during IFN treatment

Humoral immunity studies: An abnormally increased serum IgG level was normalized in 6/15, IgA level in 1/7 and IgM level in 3/10 cases.

With regard to autoantibodies, no ANA could be seen before the treatment in any case. During IFN therapy, temporary ANA positivity occurred in one patient. SMA was positive in 6/28 cases before and in 1/28 after the treatment. Frequency of LKM positivity (5/28) did not change. Anti-DNA of low titre occurred in 13/28 cases before and in 12/28 after the therapy. Thyroid microsomal antibodies and antibodies against thyroglobulin were not found either before or after the therapy.

Cryoglobulin was found in 7/19 cases before the IFN therapy, among them 3 patients in whom it disappeared after the treatment. Circulating immune complexes were found in 5/19 cases before the therapy; in two cases the test became negative. Rheumatoid factor was bound in 12 patients before the therapy; in 3 cases the test became negative.

Lymphocyte subsets and cellular immunity: The peripheral blood lymphocyte count in 5/25 cases permanently decreased; furthermore, in 7 patients it decreased temporarily. T cell count decreased permanently in 2 cases, temporarily in 5 cases; CD4+ cell count decreased permanently in 6/12 cases, temporarily in a further 3 cases; and a CD8+ cell count decrease was found permanently in 2 and temporarily in 3 cases.

The PHA-induced lymphoproliferative response increased in 6/12 cases, and NK-cell activity in 9/12 cases after IFN therapy.

In good responders, relative to the others, either the CD4+ or CD8+ cell levels were lower after the first month of therapy, and the CD4+ cell level was also lower in the sixth month of the therapy. B-cell count was significantly higher in good responders than in others by the end of third month (Figures 1, 2 and 3).

β_2-Microglobulin (B-2-m): B-2-m is a subunit of the HLA I membrane protein and found in the serum during normal circumstances in low concentrations (ng/L), but its serum level increases in renal disease and malignancies as well as in autoimmune diseases. B-2-m level may indicate lymphocyte activation, and, in liver diseases, the mesenchymal reaction. In our earlier studies in chronic active hepatitis, we established that there is a significant B-2-m increase in parallel with the level of circulating immune complexes [9].

To our knowledge, we were the first to examine B-2-m level to monitor the immunological effects of IFN therapy. Before treatment in 14/20 (70%) cases abnormally high serum B-2-m levels were noted. After IFN therapy, the abnormal B-2-m values normalized in 6 cases; in a further 2 cases, it did not normalize but a decrease was found, while in 5 cases the serum B-2-m level increased.

The decrease in B-2-m level was significant in both responders and non-responders but there was no difference between the two subgroups of patients. (Significant B-2-m level decrease occurred with similar frequency, but B-2-m level increase occurred more frequently among non-responders.)

'Predictors' of response to IFN

Comparison of the most important feature of patients with complete remission with the remainder are summarized in Table 5. Female sex, shorter time elapsed since blood transfusion, absence of HLA A1, B8 and DR3 haplotypes and anti-HBc negativity are predictors of good response.

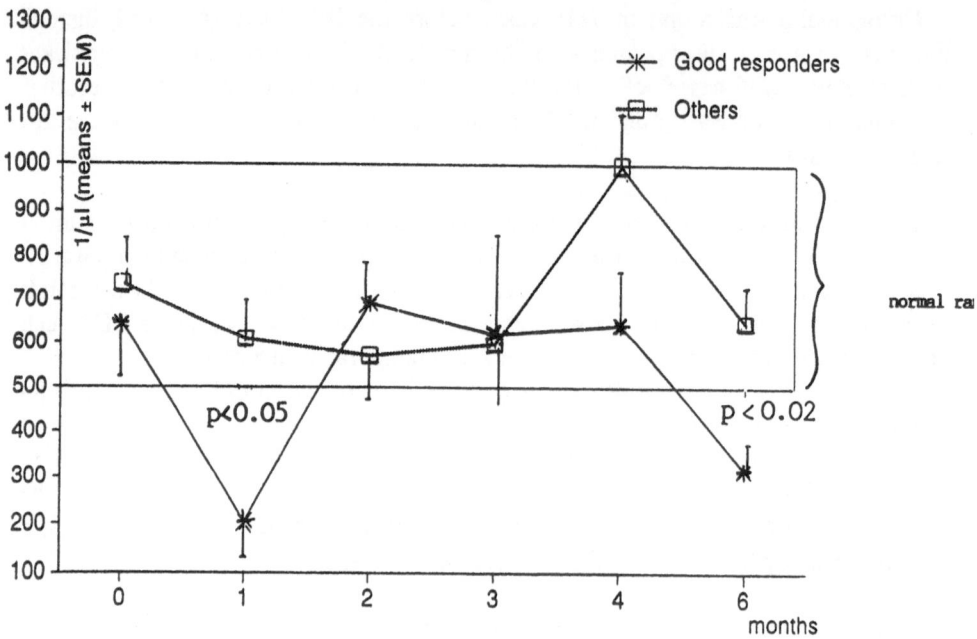

Figure 1. Changes in CD4+ cell number in chronic HCV hepatitis during interferon-α treatment

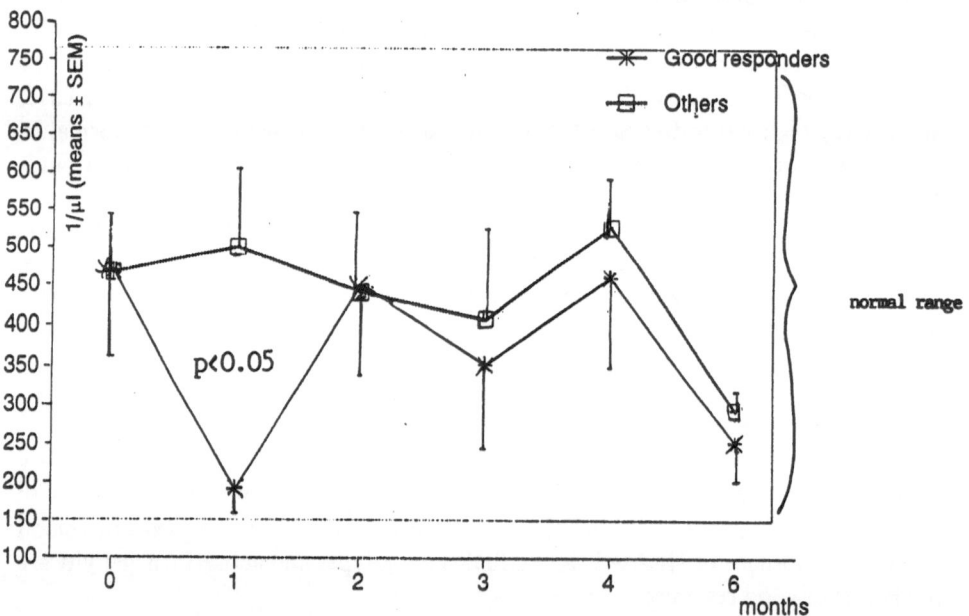

Figure 2. Changes in CD8+ cell number in chronic HCV hepatitis during interferon-α treatment

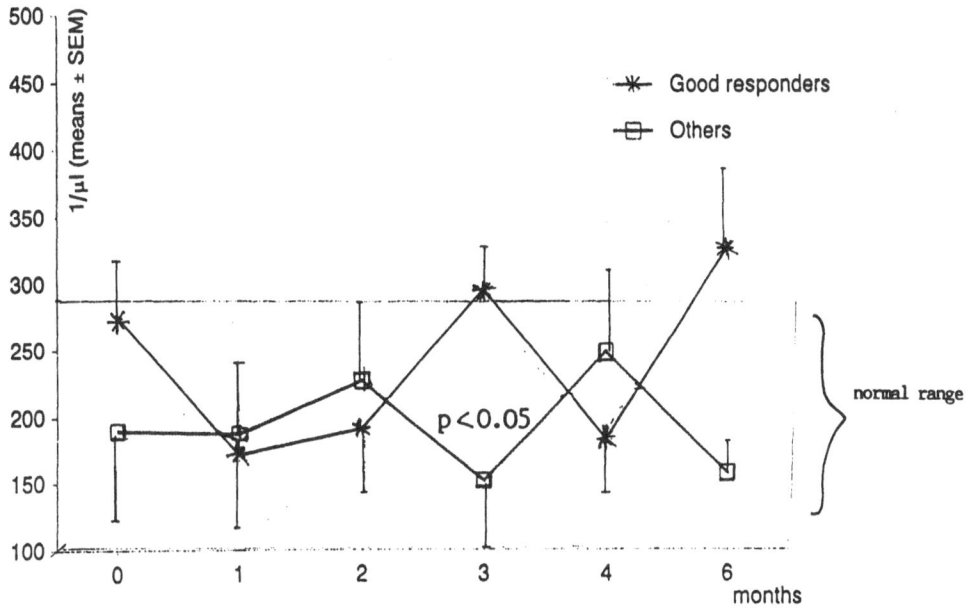

Figure 3. Changes in B cell number in chronic HCV hepatitis during interferon-α treatment

Side-effects of IFN treatment

In the first month of treatment, IFN had to be suspended in 3 patients due to repeated severe leukopenia (<3.000). (It is to be noted that in these cases pretreatment leukocyte counts were also decreased, about 4000).

Since leukopenia remained below 3.000 for more than 2 weeks after withdrawal, no more IFN was administered to these patients.

In 2 patients, therapy was withdrawn after 3 months: in one case due to the reactivation of pulmonary tuberculosis; in the other case due to failure of compliance. (In these two cases, therapy did not result in remission; thus they were placed in the group of non-responders.)

Further side-effects: reactivation of psoriasis, depression and hypertension occurred in one case, and anorexia, loss of weight, dermatological symptoms and alopecia occurred in two cases (of each), respectively. Fever ('flu-like syndrome') occurred only in about a third of cases and mostly only in the first weeks of therapy. Paracetamol given before IFN injection prevented the complaints.

DISCUSSION

Recent studies on the pathogenesis of chronic hepatitis C, besides showing the direct cytopathogenic effect of HCV, show that the role of immune mechanisms seems to be

TABLE 5
Results concerning the predictors for response

Sex:		
Good response: 4 males, 10 females	$\chi^2 = 5.427$	
Bad response: 12 males, 5 females	$p < 0.05$	
Time from transfusion:		
Good response: 2.3 ± 2.3 years		
Bad response: 12.9 ± 14.0 years	$p < 0.05$	
HLA A1, B8, DR3 haplotype:		
Good response: 1/7 cases	$\chi^2 = 4.219$	
Bad response: 7/11 cases	$p < 0.05$	
Anti-HBc positivity:		
Good response: 2/14 cases	$\chi^2 = 4.514$	
Bad response: 13/17 cases	$p < 0.05$	

more important [10–15]. In autoimmune hepatitis, the presence of anti-HCV antibodies and in chronic hepatitis C the presence of liver–kidney microsomal antibody (LKM₁) [16] was detected [17]. Immunological alterations observed in HCV infection and accompanying diseases such as cryoglobulinaemia [18], periarteritis nodosa [17], membranoproliferative glomerulonephritis [19] and Sjögren's syndrome [20] were also reported. We were the first to describe the high prevalence of the antibody against liver specific protein (anti-LSP) together with circulating immune complexes and hyper-γ-globulinaemia in patients with chronic hepatitis C [3]. The present results confirm our previous findings, even though now we often found such autoantibodies as anti-DNA, anti-SSA, and antibodies against parietal cells, which are known as serological markers of 'real' autoimmune diseases. Thus, it was not surprising that in the HLA typing a high frequency of HLA A1, B8, DR3 antigen was observed which may predispose to autoimmune reactions (and to decreased suppressor function) in our patients with chronic hepatitis C. Previously, this was reported in individual patients with autoimmune hepatitis [21] and in anti-HCV negative nonA, nonB hepatitis [22]. Based on our serological findings, it is unlikely that our HCV cases have a 'sui generis' autoimmune disease, but there may be an association of 'real' autoimmune disease and chronic hepatitis C from a genetic predisposition to autoimmunity and this may play a role in the process of developing a self-sustained chronic hepatitis after HCV infection. It is known that cross-reactions occur between HCV-proteins and autoantigens of the host organism [13,15] and these may also be of importance.

Another interesting observation may support the concept of genetic predisposition to hepatitis C autoimmune disease. Kawamoto et al. reported high frequency of HLA-DR4 phenotype in patients with chronic hepatitis C [12]. The frequent presence of the same MHC II antigen is known in a proportion of patients with autoimmune hepatitis, and most of all in Japanese populations [23]. This finding also confirms our supposition that genetic factors predisposing to autoimmune hepatitis can play a key role in the pathogenesis of chronic hepatitis C.

In contrary studies in Italy it has been suggested that the presence of HLA DR5 phenotype may have a 'protective effect' against developing liver disease after HCV infection. Peano et al. found liver disease after HCV infection with lower frequency in HLA DR5-positive subjects than in HLA DR5-negative ones, in whom the risk of developing liver disease was greater. In asymptomatic anti-HCV-positive subjects, HLA DR5 occurred in 52.8%, while in chronic hepatitis C it was 13.7%, and in the control population was 32.9% [24]. Our results are in accordance with the above mentioned studies, namely while in the control population a 38.9% HLA DR5 frequency was found, in chronic hepatitis C, a decreased frequency (21.5%) was noted.

In asymptomatic anti-HCV-positive subjects, we had no opportunity to determine HLA DR. It is interesting that a similar 'protective effect' of HLA DR5 related to primary biliary cirrhosis has been observed. Thus, in primary biliary cirrhosis, HLA-DR5-positivity occurred with lower frequency than in the healthy population [25]. Among our asymptomatic anti-HCV-positive blood donors, the HLA A1, B8 prevalence was equal to that of the normal controls. In this group, except for rheumatoid factor, no autoantibodies were found although circulating immune complexes and cryoglobulinaemia occurred. At the same time, in the peripheral blood of anti-HCV-positive donors, either lymphocyte or T and B cell counts increased while the CD4/CD8 ratio decreased relative to the healthy control values.

The therapeutic effect of IFN observed in this study corresponds to other published data. The majority of good responders became HCV-RNA-negative too after 9–12 months, i.e. complete remission correlated well with clearance of HCV-RNA.

Considering the nature of 'predictive factors', among our good responders, there were more females, the time elapsed since the transfusion was shorter, fewer subjects had haplotype HLA A1, B8, DR3 and the number of anti-HBc-positive patients (i.e. suffering from both HBV and HCV infection) was smaller.

There was no significant difference in histological findings between good responders and non-responders. However, more patients showing signs of cirrhosis were from the latter group. According to the literature the most important predictors for IFN response are as follows: female sex, shorter duration of disease, younger, absence of cirrhosis, and certain HCV genotypes (other than HCV1) [26–29]. The anti-HCV-positive subjects in Hungary are infected mainly with HCV genotype 1 (personal communication of Dr M. Héjjas).

IFN treatment resulted in a long-lasting remission in only about a quarter of patients with chronic hepatitis C. This fact suggests the use of combinations of treatments and search for non-toxic possibly orally administered, drugs as alternatives to IFN.

First of all, the question of changing the dosage arose. IFN treatment which begins with 3×6 ME weekly for 3 months, then continues with a lower dose for at least six months longer [5,27] seems to be of more efficacy.

The meta analysis of Ferenci also favours higher IFN doses and longer duration of treatment [30].

Studies in Japan have suggested that long-lasting IFN therapy increases not the number of patients responding primarily to IFN therapy but also the ratio of patients remaining in sustained remission [3]. Our studies agree with this view. Telegdy et al. [6] gave an account of favourable results with a Hungarian-manufactured natural human leucocyte IFN (Egiferon, EGIS) and think that, from using an optimal individual treatment protocol, more successful therapies can be expected.

Based on a multicentre study coordinated by Fehér and Lengyel in Hungary, the efficacy of recombinant IFN in chronic hepatitis C was also found where the ratio of good responders was 43% [32].

As an alternative to IFN, firstly a synthetic nucleoside analogue, ribavirin (Virasole) has been used as this antiviral drug is able to stop the synthesis of viral RNA. In chronic hepatitis C, ribavirin can induce remission but its effect, similarly to IFN, is often temporary: after withdrawal a relapse follows [33]. Recently it was also suggested that IFN combined with ribavirin may be of more efficacy than IFN alone in chronic hepatitis C.

A controlled study was reported on the combination of ursodeoxycholic acid with IFN. This kind of treatment increased the remission rate to 69% from 55%, and decreased the occurrence of relapses from 70% to 40% [34]. In our results published by Vincze et al. a remission-inducing effect of ursodeoxycholic acid in chronic hepatitis C with severe cholestasis was found [35]. Ursodeoxycholic acid is a non-toxic, secondary bile acid with known ability to influence cell membrane fluidity and modify MHC expression, thus having an immunomodulating capacity. Further controlled clinical studies are required with ursodeoxycholic acid combined with IFN in chronic hepatitis C.

REFERENCES

1. Choo Q-L, Kuo G, Weiner A et al. Isolation of a cDNA clone derived from a blood-borne non-A, non-B viral hepatitis genome. Science. 1989;244:359–62.
2. Alter HJ, Purcell RH, Shih W et al. Detection of antibody to hepatitis C virus in prospectively followed transfusion recipients with acute and chronic non-A, non-B hepatitis. N Engl J Med. 1989;321:1494–500.
3. Pár A, Sipos J, Paál M et al. Antibody to hepatitis C virus (HCV) in high risk groups and various liver diseases and humoral immunity in non-A, non-B (NANB) hepatitis. Z Gastroenterol. 1991;29(Suppl):80–3.
4. Pár A, Beró T, Brasch Gy et al.. Isoprinosine treatment with chronic hepatitis C. (In Hungarian). Orv Hetil. 1993;134:1015–19.
5. Pár A. Management of patients with chronic hepatitis C. (In Hungarian). Transfuzió. 1993;26:75–85.
6. Telegdy L, Dávid K, Falus A et al. Effect of human leukocyte interferon in chronic hepatitis C. (In Hungarian). Infektol Klin Mikrobiol. 1994;1:46–51.
7. Knodell RG, Ishak KG, Black WC et al. Formulation and application of a numerical scoring system for assessing histological activity in asymptomatic chronic active hepatitis. Hepatology. 1981;1:431–5.
8. Weigand K, Zangg PY, Frei A et al. Long term follow up of serum N-terminal propeptide of collagen type III levels in patients with chronic liver disease. Hepatology. 1984;4:835–8.
9. Pár A, Falus A, Jávor T. Serum beta-2-microglobulin and anti-B2m antibodies in chronic liver disease. In: Okolicsányi L, Csomós G, Crepaldi G, eds. Assessment and Management of Hepatobiliary Diseases. Berlin-Heidelberg: Springer Verlag; 1987:349–54.
10. Botarelli P, Brunetto MR, Minutello MA et al. T-lymphocyte response to hepatitis C virus in different courses of infection. Gastroenterology. 1993;104:580–7.

11. Camps J, Cordoba J, Esteban JI. Pathophysiology of chronic hepatitis C. In: Miguet JP, Dhumeaux D, eds. Progress in Hepatology. Paris: John Libbey Eurotex; 1993:63–8.
12. Kawamoto H, Sakaguchi K, Takaki A et al. Autoimmune responses as assessed by hypergammaglobulinaemia and the presence of autoantibodies in patients with chronic hepatitis C. Acta Med Okayama. 1993;47:305–10.
13. Manns MP. Autoimmunity and hepatitis C virus. In: Miguet JP, Dhumeaux D, eds. Progress in Hepatology. Paris: John Libbey Eurotex; 1993:79–87.
14. Michel G, Ritter A, Gerken G et al. Anti-GOR and hepatitis C virus in autoimmune liver disease. Lancet. 1992;339:267–9.
15. Mishiro S, Hoshi Y, Takeda K et al. Non-A,non-B hepatitis specific antibodies directed at host derived epitope: implication for an autoimmune process. Lancet. 1990;336:1400–3.
16. Vento S, Di Perri G, Luzzati R et al. Type 2 autoimmune hepatitis and hepatitis C virus infection. Lancet. 1990;335:921.
17. Cacoub P, Lunel-Fabiani F, Huong-Du LT. Polyarteritis nodosa and hepatitis C virus infection. Ann Intern Med. 1992;116:605–6.
18. Agnello V, Chung RT, Kaplan LM. A role for hepatitis C virus infection in type II cryoglobulinemia. N Engl J Med. 1992;327:1490–5.
19. Rollino C, Roccatelo D, Giachino O et al. Hepatitis C virus infection and membranous glomerulonephritis. Nephron. 1991;59:319–20.
20. Haddad J, Deny P, Munz-Gotheil C et al. Lymphocytic sialadenitis of Sjögren's syndrome associated with hepatitis C virus liver disease. Lancet. 1992;339:321–3.
21. Nouri-Aria KT, Donaldson PT, Hegarty JS et al. HLA A1/B8/DR3 and suppressor cell function in first degree relatives of patients with autoimmune chronic active hepatitis. J Hepatol. 1985;1:235–41.
22. Lenzi M, Mantovani W, Cataleta M et al. HLA typing in autoimmune hepatitis (AI-CAH) type 2. J Hepatol. 1992;16:59.
23. Seki T, Kiyosawa K, Inoko H et al. Association of autoimmune hepatitis with HLA Bw54 and DR4 in Japanese patients. Hepatology. 1990;12:1300–4.
24. Peano GM, Fenoglio LM, Ponzetto A et al. Does HLA DR5 protect patients infected by hepatitis C virus from evolution towards chronic liver disease. Second United European Gastroenterology Week, Barcelona, 19–24 July, 1993.
25. Gores GJ, Moore SB, Fischer LD et al. Primary biliary cirrhosis association with class II major histocompatibility complex antigen. Hepatology. 1987;7:889.
26. Kanai K, Kako M, Okamoto H. Hepatitis C virus genotypes in chronic hepatitis C and response to interferon. Lancet. 1992;339:1543.
27. Métreau JM, and the French Group for the Study of NANB/C hepatitis treatment. Results of a long-term interferon treatment in non-A,non-B/C chronic active hepatitis. Gut. 1993;34(Suppl.2):S112–13.
28. Trepo C, Habersetzer F, Bailly F et al. Factors of response to antiviral treatment in chronic hepatitis C. In: Miguet JP, Dhumeaux D, eds. Progress in Hepatology. Paris: John Libbey Eurotex; 1993:69–77.
29. Yoshioka K, Kakumu S, Wakita T et al. Detection of hepatitis C virus by polymerase chain reaction and response to interferon-alpha therapy. Relationship to genotype of hepatitis C virus. Hepatology. 1992;16:293–9.
30. Ferenci P. Treatment of chronic viral hepatitis with interferon-alpha. (In Hungarian). Orv Hetil. 1992;133(Supp.1):66–71.
31. Nakano Y, Kiyosawa K, Sodeyama T et al. Anti-c100 antibodies to hepatitis C virus in patients with chronic hepatitis C virus infection treated with interferon. Scand J Gastroenterol. 1993;28:335–42.
32. Fehér J, Lengyel G (coordinators). Recombinant interferon-alpha treatment of chronic viral hepatitis C. (In Hungarian). Orv Hetil. 1996;137:1179–85.
33. Reicherd O, Anderson J, Schvarz R et al. Ribavirin treatment for chronic hepatitis C. Lancet. 1991;337:1058–61.
34. Angelico M, Gandin C, Goffredo F et al. Interferon-alpha and urso-deoxycholic acid vs interferon-alpha alone in the treatment of chronic hepatitis C: a randomized, controlled clinical trial. Hepatology. 1992;16:513.
35. Vinczé A, Patty I, Jávor T, Pár A. Clinical evidence of hepatoprotection induced by ursodeoxycholic acid. Acta Phys Hung. 1992;80:369–74.

G Mózsik et al. Cell Injury and Cytoprotection in the GI Tract. 305–311.
© 1997 Kluwer Academic Publishers.

LONG-TERM INTERFERON-α2b THERAPY IN CHRONIC HEPATITIS B. A PROSPECTIVE MULTICENTRE STUDY IN HUNGARY

G. LENGYEL[1*], J. FEHÉR[1] (co-ordinators), L. DALMI[2], K. DÁVID[3], J. GERVAIN[4], Á GÓGL[4], J. LONOVICS[5], Zs. OZSVÁR[6], A. PÁR[7], F. SCHNEIDER[8] AND Zs. TULASSAY[1]

[1]2nd Department of Medicine, Semmelweis University, Budapest; [2]County Hospital, Debrecen; [3]BM Central Hospital, Budapest; [4]St. György Hospital, Székesfehérvár; [5]1st Department of Medicine, Szent-Györgyi A. University, Szeged; [6]City Hospital, Szeged; [7]1st Department of Medicine, Medical University Pécs; [8]Markusovszky L. Hospital, Szombathely, Hungary
*Correspondence

ABSTRACT

Several controlled trials have shown that administration of interferon-α for some months with a dosage about 3 million units three times weekly induces normalization of alanine aminotransferase (ALT) activity and seroconversion of patients in about 40% of cases with B-virus-induced hepatitis at the end of treatment. The aim of this prospective open multicentre study is to give further data about the dosage and the long-term administration of α-interferon. Eight liver units in universities and hospitals have been involved in this trial. Twenty-one patients with chronic B hepatitis were selected for study.

Therapy protocol: The patients with chronic B hepatitis were treated with interferon-α2b (Intron A) for one year. If the patients had no response after three months, the dose was increased. After one year of therapy, the patients were observed for another six months.

Efficacy of the therapy: Sustained complete remission occurred in ten cases (47.6%); partial remission in five; four patients had no response; in one case, the disease had progressed; and one patient dropped out. Side-effects, apart from a flu-like syndrome, occurred in only a very few cases.

Conclusion: Long-term therapy with interferon-α2b for one year produced sustained complete remission in about half of the patients. In non-responders after three months' therapy, increasing the dose of interferon had a beneficial effect. On the basis of these data, long-term therapy and higher dosage in non-responders can be recommended.

Keywords: chronic hepatitis B, interferon-α, complete remission

Chronic hepatitis induced by hepatitis B virus (HBV) leads very frequently to liver cirrhosis, and this virus is also an important pathogenic factor in the development of primary liver cancer. The mechanism behind the development of chronicity is not yet fully understood but factors involved include infection at an early age, the state of the immune system and virus heterogeneity. The most important factor in the pathogenesis of chronicity is the insufficiency of endogen interferon (IFN) response. The HBV selectively inhibits the IFN production in the mononuclear cells [1–5].

This paper was presented at the Symposium on 'Cell injury and protection in the gastrointestinal tract: from basic science to clinical perspectives', October 8–11, 1995, Pécs, Hungary.

The aim of interferon treatment in chronic hepatitis B is to inhibit the replication of hepatitis B virus (HBV), that is the clearance of HBV-DNA, HBeAg from the serum as well as to produce seroconversion. The sign of this seroconversion is proved by the manifestation of anti-HBe antibody in the serum [6–8].

The first study of IFN-α in chronic hepatitis B was reported in 1975 [9]. After several years' experience, the effectiveness of IFN (natural and recombinant) has been firmly established at smaller and higher doses given thrice weekly, usually within a short (3–6 months) period. In these circumstances, complete remission may be achieved in 30–40% of cases. After cutting down the treatment, the activity of alanine aminotransferase (ALT) increased, showing the inflammatory process [10–12].

The purpose of this prospective multicentre study is to answer the question of whether long-term (one year) treatment with IFN is able to increase the rate of remission and whether an increased therapeutic dose of IFN can influence the response reaction of patients. Eight of the most important liver units in Hungary have taken part in the clinical study.

PATIENTS AND METHODS

Eight university or regional liver centres were involved in this open multicentre prospective study. Selection criteria for patients were: ALT at least three times higher than the normal value in the last six months, positive serology for HBV (HBsAg, HBeAg, HBV-DNA), chronic hepatitis with liver histology, age between 18 and 65 years, absence of contraindications and informed consent from the patients. Exclusion criteria were: involvement of any other kind of liver disease, severe metabolic alterations, severe cardiovascular disease, renal insufficiency, haematological disorders, pregnancy or lactation, chronic alcoholism, mental disorders, and absence of compliance.

Recruitment of patients was carried out after an observation period of at least six months. Laboratory examinations included: routine haematological examinations, serum bilirubin, ALT, aspartate aminotransferase (AST), γ-glutamyl-transpeptidase, serum protein, coagulation factor and virus marker determinations. These markers were: HBsAg, anti-HBs, HBeAg, anti-HBe, anti-HBc, anti-HCV, anti-CMV, anti-EBV and HIV reaction. In a few cases, the level of serum HBV-DNA was determined. The diagnosis of chronic hepatitis B was confirmed by histological examination of liver biopsy material before starting the treatment. We wanted to repeat the histological examination at the end of the treatment and observation period, but some of the patients did not agree to a control liver biopsy. In the histological examination, we studied the inflammatory reaction in the portal region, piecemeal necrosis, development of fibrosis, incomplete or complete septal alterations as well as nodular lesions.

The treatment protocol for patients involved in the study was: 3 million units of interferon-α$_{2b}$ (Intron A, Schering–Plough Co.) three times a week for one year; the observation period lasted for 6 months after therapy had finished. In non-responder cases, the dosage of IFN was increased to 5 million units after three months.

The effectiveness of the therapy was evaluated according to the literature [6,15]. Complete remission means normalization of ALT and seroconversion of patients treated. In partial response, either normalization of ALT or seroconversion was absent. Patients were non-responders if neither seroconversion nor normalization of ALT followed the IFN treatment.

The interferon-α_{2b} preparation (Intron A) for treatment of patients was provided by Schering–Plough Co. Ethical approval for the study was given by the appropriate university or hospital ethical committee as well as by the National Institute of Pharmacy (0162/41/92). Statistical analysis was carried out by the χ^2-test.

RESULTS

The multicentre study was carried out between 1992 and 1995. Twenty-one patients were selected for the trial. The mean age of patients was 45.1 years (range 18–65 years); 14 men and 7 women.

Transmission of HBV infection is demonstrated in Figure 1. In more than half of the patients, the mode of infection was verified, but the type of infection was unknown in the remainder. The infection was acquired by transfusion with or without operation in 4 cases; by sexual contact in 3 cases; in two patients, the chronic hepatitis developed after acute hepatitis within 6 months; and, in 3 cases, the risk of profession of the patients (medical workers) was presumed to be responsible for the infection.

The duration of the disease before treatment is shown in Table 1. This period was between six months and two years for the majority of patients. In six cases, the duration of the disease is unknown.

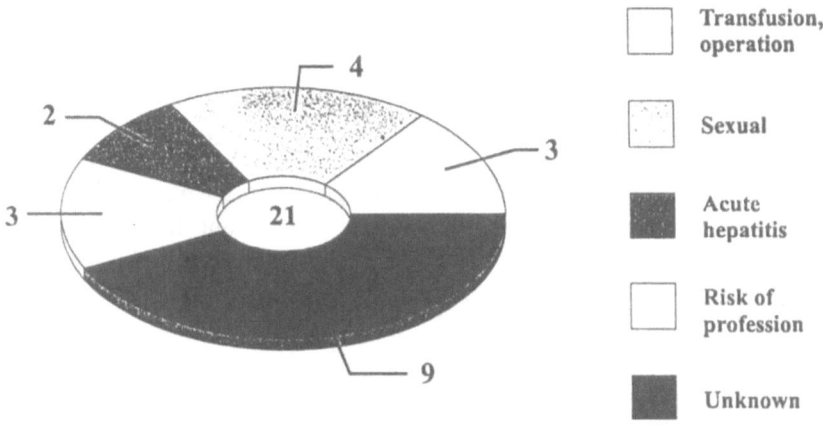

Figure 1. Possible modes of transmission of hepatitis B virus infection

TABLE 1
Duration of chronic hepatitis B before the interferon treatment

6 months–2 years	9
2–5 years	4
More than 5 years	2
Unknown	6
Total	21

TABLE 2
Responder status after interferon

	Number of cases	< 40 years old	> 40 years old
Sustained complete remission	10	3	7
Partial response	5	3	2
Non-responder	4	4	–
Worsening	1	–	1
Drop out	1	–	1
Total	21	10	11

The difference between the numbers under 40 years and over 40 years is not statistically significant. Statistical analysis was by χ^2 test

IFN treatment was effective in 15 cases out of 21: 10 cases (47.6%), sustained complete remission, and in 5 cases, partial remission was observed. Concerning the age of patients we found no differences in the response reactions of patients under 40 and above 40 years old (Table 2).

Typical changes in ALT activities are shown in Figure 2. Each line shows the response of a representative patient. After administration of IFN, normalization of ALT was found and sustained within the normal range over the observation period. In partial remission, the activity of ALT increased after ending the therapy. In non-responders, the activity of ALT remained high, even with the higher dosage of IFN.

Sustained complete remission was found in 10 cases at the end of one year of IFN therapy and 6 months' observation period.

In these cases, the markers for HBV did not show virus replication; the patients became HBeAg negative, and, in some cases, anti-HBe and anti-HBs antibodies could be demonstrated, and the activities of serum ALT remained in the normal range over the 6-month observation period. In the partial responders (5 patients), the values of ALT repeatedly increased after cutting down the IFN treatment.

Before the clinical trial, liver biopsy was carried out in all 21 cases. Morphological examination proved the diagnosis of chronic hepatitis. At the end of the study, only

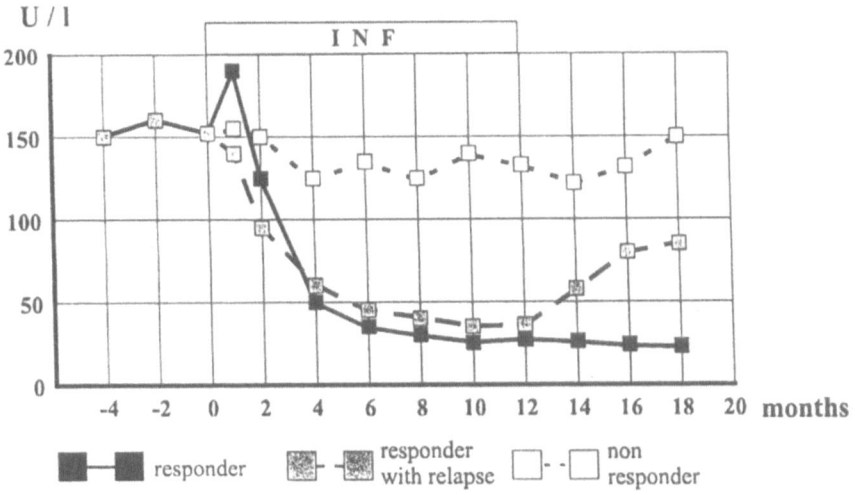

Figure 2. Typical ALT activities in chronic B hepatitis during interferon treatment. Each line is that of a representative patient

seven patients agreed to a control liver biopsy. On the basis of periportal lymphocytic infiltration, piecemeal necrosis, partial or total bridge building and of necrotic alterations in the liver cells, we found a significant decrease in the tissue reaction in three patients; in another three cases, the morphological signs had not changed; and, in one patient, primary hepatocellular carcinoma had developed. The tissue alteration characterized by the Knodell index was measured in only a few cases; thus the results have little value. All the three cases with a decreased reaction on morphological examination belonged to the group of patients with sustained complete response.

Side-effects during IFN treatment were found to be rare. A transitory flu-like syndrome occurred in 5 cases, and in another three cases, loss of appetite, joint complaints and myalgia could be observed. These problems were mild and treatment was continued. One patient dropped out from treatment due to lack of compliance.

DISCUSSION

The characteristics of interferons, being endogenous or exogenous therapeutic preparations are to have antiviral, immunosuppressive and antiproliferative effects in the organism. The antiviral effect may be induced by IFNs binding to a specific membrane receptor. IFNs stimulate the synthesis of several proteins, among them oligoadenylate synthase. This enzyme activates the ribonuclease which degrades the virus RNS inhibiting virus replication. The immunosuppressant effects of IFNs are explained by various theories. The most important effect is that IFN potently activates both natural and macrophages which can destroy virally infected cells. IFNs also exert antiproliferative activity by inducing cell differentiation, thus affecting oncogenic expression and the interaction of growth factors.

The therapeutic use of IFN was limited to clinical practice in several malignant and virus diseases. Here, we report results only in chronic hepatitis B. One of the first studies was carried out by Hoofnagle and co-workers [13,14]. They used the IFN-α treatment in 45 patients with HBV-induced chronic hepatitis for 16 weeks in a dosage of 5–10 million units three times a week. Virus replication decreased in a third of patients together with normalization of serum ALT and a beneficial effect on the liver inflammatory process. Following these observations, several authors reported successful treatment with IFN (endogen or recombinant) in chronic B hepatitis. Today it is generally accepted that, in this disease, the higher dosage of IFN given for at least 6 months is associated with more successful clinical results [15–18].

In this multicentre study, we have especially examined whether the long-term (one year) IFN treatment is able to increase the rate of sustained complete remission compared with short-term experience. It is clear that, in our patients, the long-term treatment was more effective, in that better results were achieved. Sustained remission occurred in nearly half the cases (10 out of 21), and a partial response was observed in a quarter of patients. This rate is significantly better than the results with short-term treatment [2,13,20].

We especially looked for a connection between ages of patients, duration of disease and response to IFN treatment. It is known from the literature that in younger patients and/or in chronic disease of shorter duration, IFN treatment is more effective. We did not reach this conclusion from these results, but, from another clinical trial with chronic hepatitis C [19] we have observed that IFN treatment of patients with shorter duration of disease and under 40 years old produced a greater rate of sustained remission than that in patients above 40 years [19].

On the basis of this multicentre clinical trial in Hungary, we can conclude that long-term treatment with interferon-α_{2b} in non-responder cases with higher dosage, is able to produce a higher rate of sustained complete remission in chronic B hepatitis. According to the data in the literature and our results in chronic hepatitis C, we can recommend use of this treatment, if it is possible for increasing the rate of remission in disease of shorter duration. In non-responder cases, other therapeutic modalities (thymostimulin, ursodeoxycholic acid, ribavirin) can be recommended.

ACKNOWLEDGEMENTS

The interferon-α_{2b} preparation for treatment of patients was given free of charge to participating liver centres by Schering–Plough Co. The authors are grateful to the pathologists of the various institutions for helping in the establishment of the diagnosis.

REFERENCES

1. Bonino F. The Role of Interferon in Chronic Viral Hepatitis. F. Hoffmann–La Roche Ltd; 1992.
2. Lengyel G, Fehér J. Interferon kezelés vírus okozta krónikus aktív hepatitisben. Orv Hetil. 1995;136:3–7.
3. Morgersen SC, Virilizer JL. Interferons. In: Gressor I, ed. Interferon. London: Academic Press; 1987:55.
4. Pár A. Krónikus vírushepatitisek: pathogenesis, prevencio, prognózis. Orv Hetil. 1992;133(Suppl. 1):137–40.
5. Samuel CE. The interferons. In: Pfeffer LM, ed. Mechanism of Interferon Action. Florida: CMC Press; 1987:111.
6. Chen G, Karayiannis P, McGarvay MJ et al. Subclasses of anti-HBe in chronic HBV infection: changes during treatment with interferon and predictors of response. Gut. 1989;30(Part 8):1123–8.
7. Samuel CE. Molecular mechanism of interferon action: ribosome associated protein P1 and protein synthesis initiation factor e1F-2. Texas Rep Biol Med. 1982;41:463–70.
8. Sréter L, Fehér J. Az interferon klinikai alkalmazása. Orv Hetil. 1991;132:507–12.
9. Isaacs A, Lindermann L. Virus interference. 1. The interferons. Proc R Soc London (Biology). 1975;147:258–67.
10. Fattovich G, Farci P, Rugge M et al. A randomized controlled trial of lymphoblastoid interferon-α in patients with chronic hepatitis B lacking HBeAg. Hepatology. 1992;15:584–9.
11. Revel M, Chabath J. Interferon activated genes. Trends Biochem Science. 1986;11:166–70.
12. Saksela E. In: Gressor I, ed. Interferon 3. London: Academic Press; 1981:45.
13. Hoofnagle JH, Peters M, Mullen KD et al. Randomized, controlled trial of recombinant human α-interferon in patients with chronic hepatitis B. Gastroenterology. 1988;95:1218–325.
14. Hoofnagle JH, Mullen KD, Jones DB et al. Treatment of chronic non-A non-B hepatitis with recombinant human α-interferon: a preliminary report. N Engl J Med. 1986;315:1575–8.
15. Barbera C, Bortolotti F, Crivellaro C et al. Recombinant interferon-α2b hastens the rate of HBe-Ag clearance in children with chronic hepatitis B. Hepatology. 1994;20:287–90.
16. Ibrányi E, Nagy E, Szalay F et al. Krónikus aktiv B hepatitis interferon (Egiferon) kezelése. Orv Hetil. 1993;134:2645–7.
17. Poynard T, Bedossa P, Chevallier M et al. A comparison of three interferon-α2b regimens for the long-term treatment of chronic non-A non-B hepatitis. N Engl J Med. 1995;322:1457–62.
18. Reichard O, Glaumann H, Hrydén A et al. Two-year biochemical, virological and histological follow-up in patients with chronic hepatitis C responding in a sustained fashion to interferon-α2b treatment. Hepatology. 1995;21:918–22.
19. Fehér J, Lengyel G, Dalmi L et al. Interferon-α2b kezelé chronicus C hepatitisben. Orv Hetil. 1996;137:1179–85.
20. Jacyna MR, Thomas HC. Antiviral therapy: hepatitis B. Br J Med Bull. 1990;446:368–82.

G Mózsik et al. Cell Injury and Cytoprotection in the GI Tract. 313–322.
© 1997 Kluwer Academic Publishers.

NEW EMPHASIS IN THE TREATMENT OF PANCREATIC INSUFFICIENCY

A. PAP

2nd Department of Medicine, St. Imre Hospital, H-1115 Budapest, Hungary

ABSTRACT

Pancreatic secretion has a considerable reserve capacity due to adaption to the diet by non-parallel synthesis, transport and secretion of pancreatic enzymes. Regeneration of acinar cells also supports the economic function of pancreas. However, exocrine insufficiency due to chronic pancreatitis, cystic fibrosis or pancreatic cancer is difficult to manage because of susceptibility of lipase to acid and/or proteolytic inactivation. The role of trypsin and chymotrypsin in lipase inactivation became evident only recently, changing our concept about dietetic treatment and enzyme substitution therapy significantly. These considerations, together with the new enteric-coated microspheric pancreatin preparations, can correct nowadays steatorrhoea and maldigestion in pancreatic insufficiency.

Keywords: adaptation, non-parallel secretion, regeneration, lipase survival, dietetic considerations

BACKGROUND

The incidence of chronic pancreatitis [1,2] as well as pancreatic cancer [3,4] responsible for most pancreatic insufficiency cases is constantly increasing. The contribution of cystic fibrosis to the frequency of pancreatic insufficiency has also become more important over the last decade [5] as survival with this inherited multiorgan disease has increased due to effective care of pulmonary complications, and the slower-developing pancreatic lesions more frequently evolve to endocrine and exocrine insufficiency. Among chronic pancreatitis patients, the predominant alcoholic forms result in earlier calcification with higher incidence of exocrine and endocrine pancreatic insufficiency [6]. Overt steatorrhoea occurs in approximately 30% of patients with chronic calcific pancreatitis; manifest diabetes can rise to 70% in this special group.

The pancreas has a considerable reserve functional capacity. Steatorrhoea and azotorrhoea do not occur until there is at least 90% reduction in secretion of pancreatic lipase and trypsin [7]. Amylase secretion and carbohydrate malabsorption have been rarely correlated but results of the starch tolerance test [8] and the newer H_2 breath test [9] give indirect measures of carbohydrate malabsorption in pancreatic insufficiency. In chronic pancreatitis, lipase secretion decreases more rapidly than the secretion of proteolytic enzymes [10], influencing sensitivity of diagnostic methods of pancreatic function as well as appearance of steatorrhoea and azotorrhoea. Changes of amylase secretion are somewhat less sensitive and specific for pancreatic damage [1]. The

This paper was presented at the Symposium on 'Cell injury and protection in the gastrointestinal tract: from basic science to clinical perspectives', October 8–11, 1995, Pécs, Hungary.

surprisingly large reserve capacity of the exocrine pancreas has been demonstrated in patients with pancreatic cancer too, the proximal 40% of the pancreas being able to give maximal secretory response to cholecystokinin (CCK) [12].

Accumulating evidence supports a role for non-parallel enzyme synthesis, transport and secretion in the maintenance of the economic function of the pancreas [13–15].

Non-parallel secretion of enzymes is based on functional and structural differences of acinar cells [14,15].

A whole orchestra of hormones and neurotransmitters is released postprandially from the intestine. Thus proteins and amino acids release CCK [16], GIP [17] and cholinergic stimuli [18], lipids stimulate CCK, secretin, neurotestin [19], GIP [20] and cholinergic mechanisms [18], while carbohydrates liberate insulin, GIP [21] and some CCK [16]. The combination of this intestinal hormone release in response to different meals together with different pool and stimulus-specific regulation of enzyme secretion modified by digestive end-products [14,15] and changing metabolism of acinar cells [22] results in an economic adaptation to the actual diet in normal and pathological conditions.

Besides non-parallel pancreatic enzyme secretion, unco-ordinated enzyme synthesis and intracellular transport have also been clearly demonstrated during recent years. Early changes of enzyme synthesis in response to CCK are regulated at translational levels; after 6-h continuous stimulation transcription of mRNAs of proteases increases and expression of amylase mRNAs decreases [23]. Similar changes can be observed during long-term adaption to the diet in the functional mRNA level [24]. Short-term translational adaptation of enzyme synthesis to different meals can be further modified by non-parallel intracellular enzyme transports. In rats, amylase transport is the slowest, and that of proteases is the fastest during the CCK-stimulated [25] and basal phase [26].

Non-parallel changes in enzyme synthesis, transport and secretion in response to a specific stimulus act together in the same direction, resulting in more effective and economic adaption to the diet. Thus CCK stimulates prevalent protease synthesis, transport and secretion at the same time, while also releasing pancreatic polypeptide [27] which inhibits overall pancreatic secretion, having a role in preventing exhaustion of the gland and further modifying enzyme content of the acinar cells.

Reserve capacity of the pancreas is greatly enhanced by the capability of acinar cells to regenerate. Depending on the extension of pancreatic resection, 20–70% regeneration of the remnant was demonstrated in different animals [28] and also in humans with chronic pancreatitis [29]. An even more pronounced increase in pancreatic secretion was demonstrated after release of ductular obstruction in animal experiments [30] and in patients with papillary stenosis [31]. A duodenopancreatic feedback mechanism and CCK release [28,32] seem to be involved in pancreatic regeneration. CCK treatment successfully accelerated regeneration in animal models [33–35] and also in patients with chronic pancreatitis [36,37]. Hyperplasia of the acinar cells together with protease prevalent enzyme synthesis, transport and secretion can ameliorate mainly protein digestion during the treatment and also the overall enzyme secretion for some time thereafter [36–38].

The regeneration of endocrine pancreas is slow [39] and functionally contradictory.

In chronic pancreatitis, ductular hyperplasia is frequently accomplished by ductoendo-crine proliferation. The newly formed insulae contain more A and less B cells in diabetic patients than in non-diabetic patients and in controls [40]. Release of glucagon seems to be somewhat delayed from the old and/or newly formed A cells but the decrease in insulin secretion is even more important and not compensated for by regeneration of B cells. The tendency to severe hypoglycaemia in alcoholic pancreatitis may reflect impared glucagon release and/or inappropriate insulin secretion beside alcoholic liver damage [41]. The somatostatin-producing D cells have a further modulating effect on glucagon secretion and less on insulin release [42].

PITFALLS OF SUBSTITUTION THERAPY IN STEATORRHOEA

Manifestation of pancreatic insufficiency depends on pancreatic function as well as on gastrointestinal motility, gastric, biliary and intestinal secretions, absorption, hormone releases and postoperative situations. The secondary factors may need special correc-tions to achieve significant amelioration of resistant steatorrhoea. Thus, pylorus-preserving pancreatoduodenectomy mainly with duodenojejunostomy restoring nor-mal gastrointestinal passage and preserving reservoir function of the stomach can contribute to successful treatment of pancreatic insufficiency [43] which is rarely achieved after Whipple's operation. Even better results can be expected after duodenum-preserving techniques [44]. Antibiotic treatment of afferent loop syndrome after Billroth II resection [45] or in bacterial overgrowth [46] may also be necessary in specific cases.

Supplying enough lipase to the duodenum to achieve more than 5–10% of normal enzyme concentrations is associated with abolition of steatorrhoea in most cases [47]. However, recovery experiments in patients who have ingested different preparations have demonstrated uneven lipase, somewhat more trypsin and amylase activities in the duodenum [48,49]. There are two factors involved in rapid disappearance of enzyme activities during passage through the intestinal tract: gastric acid secretion and proteolytic inactivation.

Gastric function and duodenal pH

Gastric emptying is essentially normal in patients with severe pancreatic insufficiency [50], although even rapid gastric emptying of a liquid meal has been reported previously [51]. Decreased gastric secretion, and postprandial volume might result in erroneous calculations of emptied volume. In alcoholic chronic pancreatitis, reduced parietal cell mass due to alcoholic gastritis and smoking may explain decreased gastric secretion with antral cell hyperplasia and high gastrin levels [50]. The decreased postprandial gastric secretion occurs only during the first hour after ingestion of a meal; later it parallels that of controls. When the food has been emptied, gastric secretion is not further buffered by the meal, and the intragastric then intraduodenal pH falls to 4 or less as delivered acid cannot be equilibrated by decreased bicarbonate secretion of the diseased pancreas [52]. The low duodenal pH may decrease micellar concentrations of bile acids and lipids by precipitating bile acids, although post-prandial secretion of bile is normal in patients with pancreatic insufficiency. Raising intraduodenal pH by giving H_2 blockers prevents precipitation of bile acids and improves lipid digestion [53].

The major problem with unbuffered postprandial gastric secretion in pancreatic insufficiency is that the decreased duodenal enzyme activity delivered by the diseased acinar cells can be further diminished by acid inactivation. Amylase and lipase are more sensitive to low pH. Between pH 5 and pH 4, first amylase then lipase are inactivated irreversibly while trypsin activity remains intact [54]. At lower pH, proteases may also be inactivated. Indeed, in chronic pancreatitis patients, 35% of ingested trypsin of Viokase reached the duodenum compared with only 17% of lipase [55]. Amylase was not measured in this study but it has proved to be more resistant than lipase in other studies [48,49]. Thus, acid inactivation of lipase can only partially explain the uneven results of substitution therapy in steatorrhoea when azotorrhoea and carbohydrate malabsorption cause no problems in the same patients. H_2 blockers, or antacid therapy, were proposed and used as adjuvant treatment but published results are contradictory [56] and total abolition of steatorrhoea was only rarely achieved with the different schedules although gastric and duodenal pH was maintained above pH 5 for a long time [47,55]. The results of replacement therapy [57] and duodenal recovery of enzymes [49] were not influenced by hyperacidity or anacidity of patients and bypassing the stomach by duodenal application of Viokase did not abolish steator-rhoea better than oral administration [58]. Enteric-coated tablets protecting the preparation from acid secretion of the stomach proved useless; only the newer enteric-coated microspheres resulted in dose-dependent amelioration of steatorrhoea [59,60] and normalization of duodenal amylase and trypsin activity with less but significant increase in lipid activity [48,49]. Although amylase is even more sensitive to acid than lipase, normalization of amylase activity was easily achieved with these preparations and replacement therapy of carbohydrate maldigestion was not difficult with older preparations either. Lastly, acid-stable fungal lipase proved to be no more effective than the enteric-coated microspheres for amelioration of steatorrhoea [61].

Proteolytic inactivation of lipase

A role of pepsin, as well as of acid, in the inactivation of pancreatic enzymes was presumed earlier [47,52] but its clinical significance has not been separately proven. In-vitro experiments have demonstrated that rapid inactivation of lipase by different pancreatin preparations is in inverse relationship with trypsin activation, and inhibit-ing trypsin activity with soybean trypsin inhibitor has significantly prolonged survival of lipase during incubation in buffer solution and in secretin–pancreozymin- or Lundh test-meal-stimulated duodenal juice [62]. The lipase activity of secretin–pancreozymin-stimulated duodenal juice itself decreased faster than that stimulated by a Lundh meal, and a protein-containing meal prevented inactivation of lipase of the duodenal juice and most of the pancreatin preparations examined. Indeed, several milligrams of soybean trypsin inhibitor significantly enhanced the effectiveness of crushed Panpur tablets, which were without effect in enteric-coated tablet form on steatorrhoea of the same patients. Amylase proved to be stable; some autoinactivation of trypsin was demonstrated at a later phase. It was proposed that proteolytic inactivation of lipase has to be prevented by increasing the lipase–trypsin ratio to physiological levels and by amelioration of mixing the pancreatin with protein-containing meals [60,62].

In-vivo studies in human using non-absorbable markers have demonstrated that 74% of amylase, 22% of trypsin and only 1% of lipase from activities delivered to the duodenum survived transit to the ileum [63]. Enzymatic activity and immunoreactivity of trypsin and lipase disappeared at different rates: specific immunoreactivity of lipase did not change during intestinal transit while that of trypsin decreased faster than trypsin activity; thus, intestinal absorption of intact enzymes cannot explain the loss of activities, but splitting into fragments with separated enzyme activity and immuno-reactivity has to be inferred. Indeed, in-vitro experiments with cholecystokinin-stimulated human duodenal juice and specific inhibitors of trypsin and chymotrypsin have demonstrated that chymotrypsin is responsible for lipase inactivation while the partial inhibitory effect of trypsin requires chymotrypsin [64]. The porcine lipase of pancreatin preparations is resistant to trypsin and other proteases but chymotrypsin splits it at the Phe 335/Ala 336 bond into two fragments; the first maintains its ability to adsorb to interfaces, the other seems to be responsible for lipolytic activity [65].

However activation of chymotrypsinogen needs trypsin. Moreover, trypsin has an important role in lipase survival when pancreatin preparations are dissolved [66] and also postprandially as colipase required for lipase activity in the presence of bile acids [67] can be activated than destroyed by trypsin [68]. During intestinal transit, about 55% of lipase, more than 40% of colipase was destroyed although casein, triolein and starch solution was perfused into the duodenum [69]. In-vitro triolein and bile acids had some protective effect on lipolytic activity [70]. The proteolytic inactivation of lipase and colipase can be prevented by proteins giving alternative substrates for proteases [60,62,70]. Large concentrations of hydrophobic proteins, however, competi-tively inhibit lipase activity by displacing it from the interface of emulsified triglycer-ides [71]. Bile salts can clear the interface from proteins including lipase but colipase binds to the lipase substrate even in the presence of bile and anchors lipase to its substrate. Thus, the protecting effect of triglyceride also needs colipase to form a substrate–colipase–lipase complex for fat digestion mainly in the presence of bile.

Proteolytic digestion of lipase may be of physiological significance in humans as loss of lipase activity during aboral small intestinal transit might reduce fat digestion [64] so that more fat enters the distal small intestine, delaying gastric and gallbladder emptying, intestinal transit and modifying pancreatic secretion by a feedback mechan-ism involving PYY, neurotensin and GIP [72,73]. The same process is even more important in maldigestion and malabsorption states due to pancreatic insufficiency [63,64] when proteolytic inactivation of lipase can further contribute to diminishing lipase activity below the critical value for manifest steatorrhoea. Carbohydrate maldigestion could aggravate syndromes but the ileal break of gastrointestinal motility with increased amylase secretion [74,75] supports adaptation to the maldigestion of carbohydrates with decreased calorie intake.

In patients with alcoholic chronic pancreatitis, the ratio of protease to lipase activity is high in the duodenal juice because of trypsin and chymotrypsin prevalent pancreatic secretion [10]. Proteolytic inactivation of lipase in these patients must be more important than in normals. Treating them with pancreatic supplements containing a high proportion of proteases may contribute to an even faster inactivation of lipase [60,62,64] and to the often-noted difficulty in correcting steatorrhoea [55–62,76]. In addition, the orthodox clinical dogma about a high-carbohydrate, low-protein and low-fat diet advised for chronic pancreatitis patients may further aggravate lipase survival. Although relapsing pancreatitis with pain may indicate restrictions in fat intake [77], medium-chain triglycerides, which are particularly suitable substrates for lingual lipase [68] and can absorb even without digestion less stimulating pancreatic secretion, could successfully substitute long-chain triglycerides in dietetic treatment of chronic pancreatitis. Other phospholipid- and cholesterol-containing meals (brain, egg yolk, liver) using carboxylester lipase and phospholipase A_2 for digestion may also contribute to survival of pancreatic lipase by ameliorating formation of the micellar phase [68].

Ingestion of pancreatic supplements with increased proteolytic activity was recently proposed to diminish pain of chronic pancreatitis by suppressing pancreatic secretion via the aforementioned duodenopancreatic feedback mechanism [56].

This treatment which proved to be effective only in patients with mild to modertate pancreatic insufficiency [78,79] might produce steatorrhoea in severe insufficiency by diminishing survival of lipase [64] as well as blocking the trophic effect of CCK release [32] and/or cholinergic mechanism [80] involved in the duodenopancreatic feedback regulation. Individual administration of high lipase- or high protease-containing pancreatin preparations [64] adapted to the degree of pancreatic insufficiency and to the different meals in a galenic form which allows fast mixing and segregation of proteases and lipase to their substrate could possibly ameliorate substitution therapy in pancreatic insufficiency.

MODERN TREATMENT OF PANCREATIC INSUFFICIENCY

Reserve capacity of the exocrine pancreas can be effectively increased by adaptation to the diet via non-parallel enzyme synthesis, transport and secretion of enzymes. To increase the proportion of lipase in the pancreatic juice which is needed for decreasing steatorrhoea – the most important failure in pancreatic maldigestion – an optimal level of unsaturated long-chain fatty acid supply should be given which maximally stimulates lipase synthesis and secretion due to release of a mixture of CCK, secretin, GIP and cholinergic stimuli. Protein digestion products release the same factors except secretin, potentiating lipase production with a parallel increase in protease secretion which has to be equilibrated by protein meals as substrates for proteases preventing proteolytic inactivation of lipase. Optimal protein and fat supply releasing CCK also contribute to maintaining trophism of the pancreas, regenerating acinar cells until a certain limit caused mainly by ductular structure and fibrosis. In relapsing pancreatitis, although the intake of long-chain triglycerides, the most powerful stimuli of pancreatic secretion, may be restricted, and substituted by medium-chain fats, in order to rest the pancreas, more effort should be made to eliminate the causes of relapses, such as alcohol consumption, stones, strictures and pseudocysts, whenever possible. In cases of painless chronic pancreatitis, no rationale for a carbohydrate-prevalent diet can be supported nowadays. The high buffer capacity of proteins with some fat consumed at least five times daily as snacks may avoid the need for further antacid therapy, diminishing secretin release and provoking concentrated pancreatic juice and protein plugs. Beside the short acid spikes of duodenal pH, fatty acids potentiated by proteins are even more important for maintaining secretin release and an optimal water and bicarbonate secretion; thus the same meal mixture, stimulating the highest lipase secretion, also contributes to its longer survival.

Optimal supply of patients with insulin is as important for proportionate enzyme synthesis and secretion of acinar cells as for prevention of diabetic disturbances and complications. Spiking of blood sugar levels or reactive hypoglycaemia must be avoided by equilibrated carbohydrate intake and individualized, thorough insulin treatment if required (human insulin given four times daily).

Replacement therapy of exocrine insufficiency can be managed well in most patients with modern enteric-coated microspheres with diameters of less than 1–2 mm, emptying from the stomach well mixed with meal. The lipase–protease ratio of preparation, however, has to respect physiological levels of postprandial pancreatic secretion and units of lipase delivered to the duodenum ought to achieve at least 10% of normal activity. In unsuccessful cases, duodenal delivery of pancreatic enzymes and gastric acid in response to a test meal and after pancreatin supplementation needs to be examined and replacement therapy modified according to the results, by elevating dose and/or ratio of lipase administered or by antacid therapy. In patients with intestinal bacterial overgrowth, afferent loop syndrome, short bowel or other postoperative situations, supplementary treatment could be necessary.

REFERENCES

1. Worning H. Incidence and prevalence of chronic pancreatitis. In: Beger HG, Büchler M, Ditschuneit H, Malfertheiner P, eds. Chronic Pancreatisis. Berlin: Springer–Verlag; 1990:8–14.
2. Riela A, Zinsmeister AR, Melton LJ, DiMagno EP. Trends in the incidence and clinical characteristics of chronic pancreatitis. Pancreas. 1990;5:727.
3. Boyle P, Hsieh C-C, Maisonneuve P et al. Epidemiology of pancreas cancer (1988). Int J Pharmacol. 1989;5:327–46.
4. Riela A, Melton LJ, Twomey CK, Zinsmeister AR, DiMagno EP. Has the natural history of pancreatic cancer (CP) changed during the past 46 years? Pancreas. 1989;5:639.
5. Lebenthal E, Lerner A, Heitlinger L. The pancreas in cystic fibrosis: In: Go VLW, Gardner JD, Brooks FP, Lebenthal E, DiMagno EP, Scheele GA, eds. The Exocrine Pancreas. Biology, Pathobiology, and Diseases. New York: Raven Press; 1986:783–817.
6. DiMagno EP, Glain JE. Chronic pancreatitis. In: Go VLW, Gardner JD, Brooks FP, Lebenthal E, DiMagno EP, Scheele GA, eds. The Exocrine Pancreas. Biology, Pathobiology, and Diseases. New York: Raven Press; 1986:541–75.
7. DiMagno EP, Go VLW, Summerskill WHJ. Relations between pancreatic enzyme outputs and malabsorption in severe pancreatic disease. N Engl J Med. 1973;288:813–15.
8. Pap Á, Berger Z, Varró V. Tubeless pancreatic function tests used in combination for screening of pancreatic disease. Acta Med Hung. 1986;43:39–43.

9. Mackie RD, Levine AS, Levitt MD. Malabsorption of starch in pancreatic insufficiency. Gastroenterology. 1981;80:1220.

10. DiMagno EP, Malagelada JR, Go VLW. Relationship between alcoholism and pancreatic insufficiency. NY Acad Sci. 1975;252:200–7.

11. Goldberg DM, Wormsley KG. The interrelationships of pancreatic enzymes in human duodenal aspirate. Gut. 1970;11:859–66.

12. DiMagno EP, Malagelada JR, Go VLW. The relationships between pancreatic ductal obstruction and pancreatic secretion in man. Mayo Clin Proc. 1979;54:157–62.

13. Rothmann SS. "Non-parallel transport" of enzyme protein by the pancreas. Nature (London). 1967;213:460–2.

14. Adelson JW, Miller PE. Heterogeneity of the exocrine pancreas. Am J Physiol. 1989;256:G817–25.

15. Liebow C. Non-parallel pancreatic secretion: its meaning and implications. Pancreas. 1988;3:343–51.

16. Liddle R, Goldfine I, Rosen M, Taplitz R, Williams J. Cholecystokinin bioactivity in human plasma: molecular forms, responses to feeding and relationship to gall bladder contraction. J Clin Invest. 1985;75:1144–52.

17. Thomas F, Sinar D, Mazzaferi E et al. Selective release of gastric inhibitory polypeptide by intraduodenal amino acid perfusion in man. Gastroenterology. 1978;74:1261–5.

18. Singer MV, Solomon TE, Grossman MI. Effect of atropine on secretion from the intact and transplanted pancreas in the dog. Am J Physiol. 1980;238:G18–22.

19. Lluis F, Gomez G, Hashimoto T, Fujimura M, Greeley GH Jr, Thompson JC. Pancreatic juice enhances fat stimulated release of enteric hormones in dogs. Pancreas. 1988;4:23–30.

20. Rogers W, O'Dorisio T, Johnson S, Cataland S, Stradley R, Sherding R. Postpandrial release of gastric inhibitory polypeptide (GIP) and pancreatic polypeptide in dogs with pancreatic acinar atrophy. Correlation of blunted GIP response by addition of pancreatic enzymes to a meal. Dig Dis Sci. 1983;28:345–9.

21. Pederson R, Schubert H, Brown J. Gastric inhibitory polypeptide – its physiological release and insulinotropic action in the dog. Diabetes. 1975;24:1050–6.

22. Nagy I, Pap Á, Takács T. Evidence for a metabolic regulation of pancreatic lipase synthesis during starvation in the rat. Digestion. 1989;43:165–6.

23. Steele G. Regulation of gene expression in the exocrine pancreas. In: Go VLW, Gardner JD, Brooks FP, Lebenthal E, DiMagno EP, Scheele GA, eds. The Exocrine Pancreas. Biology, Pathobiology, and Diseases. New York: Raven Press; 1986:55–67.

24. Schick J, Verspohl R, Kern H, Scheele G. Two distinct adaptive responses to the synthesis of exocrine pancreatic enzymes to inverse changes in protein and carbohydrate in the diet. Am J Physiol. 1984;246:G611–16.

25. Iovanna J, Giorgi D, Dagorn JC. Newly synthesized amylase, lipase and serine proteases are transported at different rates in rat pancreas. Digestion. 1986;34:178–84.

26. Keim V, Rohr G, Stöckert HG. Asynchronous secretion of newly synthesized pancreatic proteins in the rat. Digestion. 1986;33:211–18.

27. Beglinger C, Taylor I, Grossman MI, Solomon T. Pancreatic polypeptide release: role of stimulants of exocrine pancreatic secretion in dogs. Gastroenterology. 1984;87:530–6.

28. Pap Á, Boros L, Hajinal F. Essential role of cholecystokinin in pancreatic regeneration after 60% distal resection in rats. Pancreas. 1991;6:412–18.

29. Pap Á, Flautner L, Karácsonyi S, Szécsény A, Varró V. Recovery of pancreatic function after distal resection for chronic pancreatitis: Regeneration or merely functional amelioration? Mt Sinai J Med. 1987;54:409–12.

30. Tiscorina OM, Dreiling DA. Does the pancreatic gland regenerate? Gastroenterology. 1966;5:1267–71.

31. Pap Á, Tihanyi T, Flautner L, Széchény A, Varró V. Recovery of pancreatic function after surgical choledocho-wirsungoplasty or double endoscopic papillotomy. Int J Pancreatol. 1988;3(Suppl 2, S270):70.

32. Fölsch UR, Cantor P, Wilms HM, Schafmayer A, Becker HD, Creutzfeldt W. Role of cholecystokinin in the negative feedback control of pancreatic enzyme secretion in conscious rats. Gastroenterology. 1987;92:449–58.

33. Majumdar AP, Vesenka GD, Dubick MA. Acceleration of pancreatic regeneration by cholecystokinin in rats. Pancreas. 1987;2:199–204.

34. Steinberg WM, Burns MK, Henry JP, Nochomovitz LE, Anderson KK. Cerulein induces hyperplasia of the pancreas in a rat model of chronic pancreatic insufficiency. Pancreas. 1987;2:176–80.

35. Pap Á. Pancreatic adaptation, growth, and regeneration in experimental chronic pancreatitis. In: Beger HG, Büchler M, Ditschuneit H, Malfertheiner P, eds. Chronic Pancreatitis. Berlin: Springer–Verlag; 1990:122–33.

36. Pap Á, Berger Z, Varró V. Trophic effect of cholecystokinin octapeptide in man. A new way in the treatment of chronic pancreatitis? Digestion. 1981;21:163–8.

37. Pap Á, Berger Z, Varró V. Complementary effect of cholecystokinin octapeptide and soyflour treatment in chronic pancreatitis. Mt Sinai J Med. 1984;51:254–7.

38. Oates PS, Morgan RGH. Pancreatic growth after partial resection of normal and enlarged pancreas in rats fed soyaflour. Am J Physiol. 1988;255:G670–5.

39. Martin JM, Lacy PE. The prediabetic period in partially pancreatectomized rats. Diabetes. 1963;12:238–42.

40. Lászik Z, Pap Á, Farkas Gy, Ormos J. Endocrine pancreas in chronic pancreatitis. A qualitative and quantitative study. Arch Pathol Lab Med. 1989;113:47–51.

41. Glasbrenner B, Malfertheiner P, Ditschuneit H. Diabetes mellitus in chronic pancreatitis. In: Beger HG, Büchler M, Ditschuneit H, Malfertheiner P, eds. Chronic Pancreatitis. Berlin: Springer–Verlag; 1990:358–67.

42. Owyang C. Endocrine changes in pancreatic insufficiency. In: Go VLW, Gardner JD, Brooks FP, Lebenthal E, DiMagno EP, Scheele G, eds. The Exocrine Pancreas. Biology, Pathobiology, and Diseases. New York: Raven Press; 1986:577–85.

43. Pap Á, Flautner L, Szécsény A, Varró V. Pancreato-duodenectomy preserving a functioning pylorus, the stomach and a pancreatic remnant: a complex functional evaluation. Mt Sinai J Med. 1987;54:409–12.

44. Beger HG, Büchler M, Ditschuneit H, Malfertheiner P. Chronic Pancreatitis. Berlin: Springer–Verlag; 1990.

45. Meyer JH. Peptic ulcer: complications and surgical treatment. In: Wyngaarden JB, Smith LH Jr, eds. Philadelphia: WB Saunders; 1982:650–4.

46. Balgha V, Pap Á. Bacterial overgrowth of small intestine demonstrated by H2 test in patients with pancreatitis. Z Gastroenterol. 1991;29:179–80.

47. Regan PT, Malagelada JR, DiMagno EP, Glanzman SL, Go VLW. Comparative effects of antacids, cimetidine, and enteric coating on the therapeutic response to oral enzymes in severe pancreatic insufficiency. N Engl J Med. 1977;297:854–8.

48. Ihse I, Lilja P, Lundquist I. Intestinal concentrations of pancreatic enzymes following pancreatic replacement therapy. Scand J Gastroenterol. 1980;15:137–44.

49. Worning H. The effect of enzyme substitution in patients with pancreatic insufficiency. Scand J Gastroenterol. 1980;15:529–33.

50. Regan PT, Malagelada JR, DiMagno EP, Go VLW. Postprandial gastric function in pancreatic insufficiency. Gut. 1979;20:249–54.

51. Long WB, Weiss JB. Rapid gastric emptying of fatty meals in pancreatic insufficiency. Gastroenterology. 1974;67:920–5.

52. DiMagno EP, Malagelada JR, Go VLW, Moertel CG. Fate of orally ingested enzymes in pancreatic insufficiency: comparison of two dosage schedules. N Engl J Med. 1977;296:1318–22.

53. Regan PT, Malagelada JR, DiMagno EP, Go VLW. Reduced intraluminal bile acid concentrations and fat maldigestion in pancreatic insufficiency: correction by treatment. Gastroenterology. 1979;77:285–9.

54. Legg EF, Spencer AM. Studies on the stability of pancreatic enzymes in duodenal fluid to storage temperature and pH. Clin Chim Acta. 1975;65:175–9.

55. DiMagno EP. Medical treatment of pancreatic insufficiency. Mayo Clin Proc. 1979;54:435–42.

56. Robert IM. Enzyme therapy for malabsorption in exocrine pancreatic insufficiency. Pancreas. 1989;4:496–503.

57. Pap Á, Varró V. Acid versus proteolytic inactivation of lipase. Comparison of the results of pancreatic replacement therapy with Panpur and Creon. Dig Dis Sci. 1987;32:1182.

58. Zerega J, Lerner S, Meyer JH. Direct duodenal delivery of large doses of pancreatin fails to normalize fat absorption in pancreatic insufficiency. Gastroenterology. 1987;92:1709.

59. Dobrilla G. Management of chronic pancreatitis. Focus on enzyme replacement therapy. Int J Pancreatol. 1989;5:17–29.

60. Pap Á, Varró V. Replacement therapy in pancreatic insufficiency with a new pancreatin preparation respecting the physiological ratio of lipase/trypsin activity. Hepato-gastroenterology. 1988;35:83–6.

61. Schneider MU, Knoll-Ruzicka ML, Domschke S, Heptner G, Domschke W. Pancreatic enzyme replacement therapy: comparative effects of conventional and enteric-coated microspheric pancreatin and acid stable fungal enzyme preparations on steatorrhea in chronic pancreatitis. Hepato-gastroenterology. 1985;32:97–102.

62. Pap Á, Varró V. Proteolytic inactivation of lipase as a possible cause of the uneven results obtained with enzyme substitution in pancreatic insufficiency. Hepato-gastroenterology. 1984;31:47–50.

63. Layer P, Go VLW, DiMagno EP. Fate of pancreatic enzymes during small intestinal aboral transit in humans. Am J Physiol. 1986;251:G475–80.

64. Thiruvengadam R, DiMagno EP. Inactivation of human lipase by proteases. Am J Physiol. 1988;255:G476–81.

65. Bousset-Risso M, Bonicel J, Rovery M. Limited proteolysis of porcine pancreatic lipase. Lability of the Phe 335–Ala 336 bond towards chymotrypsin. FEBS Lett. 1985;182:323–6.

66. Pap Á, Nagy I. Trypsin inhibitors and bile acids promote lipase release from pancreatin preparations. Gastroenterology. 1990;98:9.

67. Borgström B, Erlanson C. Pancreatic lipase and colipase. Interactions and effects of bile salts and other detergents. Eur J Biochem. 1973;37:60–8.

68. Borgström B. Luminal digestion of fats. In: Go VLW, Gardner JD, Brooks FP, Lebenthal E, DiMagno EP, Scheele GA, eds. The Exocrine Pancreas. Biology, Pathobiology, and Diseases. New York: Raven Press; 1986:361–73.

69. Kelly DG, Sternby B, DiMagno EP. Fate of pancreatic lipase and colipase during aboral small intestinal transit in humans. Pancreas. 1989;4:623.

70. Kelly DG, Bentley KJ, Sandberg RJ, Zinsmeister AR, DiMagno EP. Do nutrients and bile in human duodenal juice affect the survival of lipase activity? Possible clinical implications. Gastroenterology. 1988;94:222.

71. Borgström B, Erlanson C. Interactions of serum albumin and other proteins with porcine pancreatic lipase. Gastroenterology. 1978;75:382–6.

72. Jain NK, Boivin M, Zinsmeister AR, Brown ML, Malagelada JR, DiMagno EP. Effect of ileal perfusion of carbohydrates and amylase inhibitor of gastrointestinal hormones and emptying. Gastroenterology. 1989;96:377–87.

73. Soper NJ, Chapman NJ, Kelly KA, Brown ML, Phillips SF, Go VLW. The "ileal brake" after ileal pouch–anal anastomosis. Gastroenterology. 1990;98:111–6.

74. Tohno H, Nelson DK, Sarr MG, DiMagno EP. Does peptide YY (PYY) mediate postprandial feedback regulation on amylase secretion induced by carbohydrate (CHO) perfusion into the ileum? Gastroenterology. 1988;96:513.

75. Tohno H, Chung JB, Sandberg RJ, Bentley KJ, Sarr MG, DiMagno EP. Does fat in the ileum exert feedback regulation of canine pancreatic enzyme secretion postprandially? Pancreas. 1989;4:645.

76. Layer P, Holtmann G. Pancreatic enzymes in chronic pancreatitis. Int J Pancreatol. 1994;15:1–11.

77. Adler G, Arnold R, Kern HP. Supramaximal hormonal or neural stimulation – does it occur in humans? In: Gyr KE, Singer NV, Sarles H, eds. Pancreatitis Concepts and Classification. Amsterdam: Elsevier; 1984:153–7.

78. Isakson G, Ihse I. Pain reduction by an oral pancreatic enzyme preparation in chronic pancreatitis. Dig Dis Sci. 1983;28:97–102.

79. Slaff J, Jacobson D, Tillman CR, Curlington C, Toskes P. Protease-specific suppression of pancreatic exocrine secretion. Gastroenterology. 1984;87:44–52.

80. Adler G, Reinshagen M, Koop I et al. Differential effects of atropine and cholecystokinin receptor antagonist on pancreatic secretion. Gastroenterology. 1989;96:1158–64.

G Mózsik et al. Cell Injury and Cytoprotection in the GI Tract. 323–333.

METABOLIC RESPONSES TO OPEN AND LAPAROSCOPIC CHOLECYSTECTOMY

I. GÁL[1*], E. RŐTH[2] AND J. LANTOS[2]

[1]Department of Surgery, Bugát Pál Hospital, POB 177, Dózsa Gy.u. 22, H-3201 Gyöngyös; [2]Department of Experimental Surgery, University Medical School of Pécs, Kodály Z.u. 20, H-7624 Pécs, Hungary
*Correspondence

ABSTRACT

This study was designed to differentiate the free-radical-mediated reactions, the changes of endogenous antioxidant defence mechanism and activation of leucocytes following open (OC: $n = 21$) and laparoscopic cholecystectomy (LC: $n = 21$) in an unselected group of patients. The indication for surgery was chronic cholecystitis in all cases. Peripheral venous blood samples were taken 3 h before the operation and every day for 4 days following the operation. The measured biochemical parameters are the following: malondialdehyde (MDA) as a marker of the free-radical-induced lipid peroxidation, reduced and oxidized glutathione (GSG–GSSG), as endogenous scavengers as well as markers of oxidative stress and myeloperoxidase activity (MPO) of leucocytes. Our results showed that MDA continuously increased during the whole observation period in the OC group (393.08 ± 19.8 to 462.28 ± 22 nmol/ml), while the elevation in the LC group was apparent only on the first two days. There was a marked fall in the value of reduced glutathione measured in plasma fraction during the first 3 postoperative days in the OC group (0.89 ± 0.05 to 0.76 ± 0.03 nmol/ml); in contrast, the laparoscopic intervention caused only a temporary depletion of GSH. The same tendency was detected while measuring GSH–GSSG in the whole-blood samples. MPO activity of leucocytes significantly differed in the two groups. Increased MPO activity showed stimulation of leucocytes in the OC group from 1.25 ± 0.18 OD/ml, reaching a peak of 1.98 ± 0.2 OD/ml on the 4th day, while enzyme activity remained basically unchanged in the LC group. Our results suggested that the better clinical outcome following LC versus OC can be partially explained by diminished free-radical reactions.

Keywords: laparoscopic surgery, free radicals, scavengers, leucocytes

INTRODUCTION

The magnitude of the metabolic response to injury has been shown to be proportional to the degree of surgical trauma [1–5]. For this reason many investigators have henceforth tried to find ways of reducing the metabolic response to surgery [6–9].

Laparoscopic cholecystectomy is a minimal invasive procedure and has become the operation of choice in cases of uncomplicated gall stones [10]. Such a laparoscopic technique results in faster patient recovery and earlier discharge from hospital [11,12]. Whereas significant hormonal, metabolic and inflammatory responses following open cholecystectomy are well documented [13,14], the responses to laparoscopic cholecystectomy have only been investigated in a few studies [15–18].

This paper was presented at the Symposium on 'Cell injury and protection in the gastrointestinal tract: from basic science to clinical perspectives', October 8–11, 1995, Pécs, Hungary.

It is already established that the laparoscopic approach improves perioperative respiratory function [19] and diminishes the acute-phase response to surgery [15]. However, investigation of other pathological factors may be useful for better understanding of these processes. The aim of this study was to compare the free-radical-mediated mechanism and activation of leucocytes after open and laparoscopic cholecystectomy in an unselected group of patients.

PATIENTS AND METHODS

Patients

Forty-two otherwise healthy patients scheduled for elective cholecystectomy participated in the study. Of these, 21 underwent open cholecystectomy (OC) and 21 laparoscopic cholecystectomy (LC). The study was not randomized and patient selection was determined by the availability of laparoscopic equipment. Criteria for exclusion from the study included acute cholecystitis, any concurrent illness or the need to perform common bile duct exploration or an additional procedure during the operation. The study was approved by the ethics committee and informed consent was obtained from each patient.

Anaesthesia and operative technique

Anaesthetic techniques were similar in the two groups. Patients fasted for 8 h and were given premedication (diazepam and atropinum sulphuricum) 1 h prior to surgery. General anaesthesia was induced with midazolam and fentanyl and maintained with a mixture of 70% nitrous oxide in oxygen, supplemented with thiopental-Na. Fluid replacement during and for the first 24 h after operation was similar in both groups. Normal saline solution was given during surgery and later free fluids and normal diet was allowed. After the operation, patients received pain killers if necessary. Ceftriaxon (2 g) was administered as antibiotic prophylaxis 2 h before surgery.

Open cholecystectomy was performed via a standard subcostal incision and, in these cases, intraoperative cholangiography was performed routinely. Laparoscopic cholecystectomy was performed by a four-cannula technique using electrocautery. Intraoperative cholangiography was carried out on a selective basis in six such patients. All patients made an uneventful postoperative recovery.

Experimental protocol

Peripheral venous blood samples were taken 3 h before the operation from an indwelling venous cannula and every day for 4 days following the operation, at the same time. One part of the collected blood samples was analysed freshly and the other part was immediately centrifuged at +4°C. The plasma and sera were then separated and stored at –20°C for subsequent estimation of the investigated parameters.

Biochemical assays

Malondialdehyde (MDA) concentration was determined by the spectrophotometric method at 532 nm according to Placer et al. [20] in the whole blood, while, for measurement of plasma MDA content, we used the Ohkawa et al. [21] method at 535 nm. The amounts of reduced glutathione (GSH) and oxidized glutathione (GSSG) in the plasma as well as in whole blood was determined as described by Tietze [22] and slightly modified according to Guarnieri et al. [23] using an enzymatic method for spectrophotometric evaluation at 412 nm. The amount of serum myeloperoxidase was determined in sera [24] with colorimetric reaction at 560 nm.

Statistical analysis

To evaluate the results, mean and standard errors (SE) were calculated. The statistical significance of changes was determined by the Student's paired t-test and the preoperative values served as control.

RESULTS

The two groups were similar in number and in patient age, weight and sex. On average, the duration of anaesthesia and surgery was 15 min longer with open cholecystectomy, which was not statistically significant. There was only one significant difference between the two groups, namely the duration of postoperative stay in the hospital (Table 1).

TABLE 1
Patients characteristics and details of hospital stay

	Laparoscopic cholecystectomy (LC)	Open cholecystectomy (OC)
Number of patients	21	21
Sex (M/F)	5/16	3/18
Age (years)*	52.6	54.5
Weight (kg)*	69.6	76.8
Duration of surgery (min)*	66.8	81.2
Duration of postoperative hospital stay (days)*	3.2**	8.1

*Values are means, **$p < 0.01$

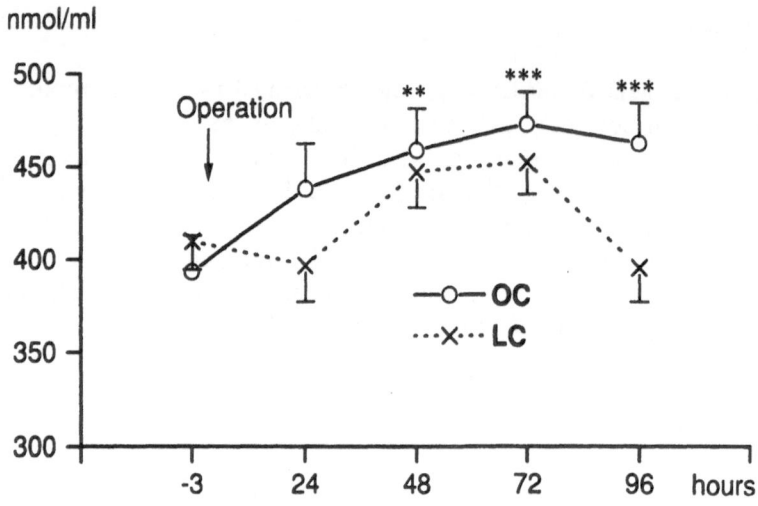

Figure 1. Mean±SE values of malondialdehyde (MDA) concentration in whole blood after open (OC) and laparoscopic (LC) cholecystectomy. Significant value presented as **$p<0.02$, ***$p<0.01$

According to our results, the level of MDA in the whole blood in the OC group continuously increased during the observation period from 393.08 ± 19.8 to 462.28 ± 22 nmol/ml by the fourth postoperative day. This elevation was significant ($p<0.01$) compared with only a small rise seen in the LC group. From an initial value of 409.69 ± 15.1 to 447.06 ± 18.9 and 452.39 ± 16.9 nmol/ml by the second and third days, respectively, decreasing to around the starting value (395.19 ± 18.9 nmol/ml) by the fourth day (Figure 1).

The MDA plasma level in the OC group increased only on the first postoperative day (0.92 ± 0.1 to 1.1 ± 0.15 nmol/ml), while the level of MDA in plasma decreased significantly during the same period in the LC group (1.03 ± 0.11 to 0.87 ± 0.11 nmol/ml; Figure 2).

There was a marked fall ($p<0.01$) in values of reduced glutathione in the OC group measured in the plasma fraction during the first three postoperative days (0.89 ± 0.05 to 0.7 ± 0.04, 0.73 ± 0.05 and 0.76 ± 0.36 nmol/ml, respectively). In contrast, the laparoscopic intervention caused only a temporary depletion of GSH (0.90 ± 0.04 to 0.77 ± 0.04, 0.83 ± 0.08 and 0.92 ± 0.06 nmol/ml; Figure 3). The level of GSH in whole blood decreased significantly ($p<0.05$) on the third postoperative day in the OC group (1357.0 ± 107.1 to 1190.3 ± 87.6 nmol/ml), while it remained practically unchanged in the laparoscopic group (Figure 4).

The values of GSSG in the plasma fraction were elevated significantly ($p<0.001$) in both groups during the first three postoperative days and reached the starting values by the end of the observation period (Figure 5). The value of oxidized glutathione in whole blood changed significantly ($p<0.05$) only in the OC group on the third postoperative day (Figure 6).

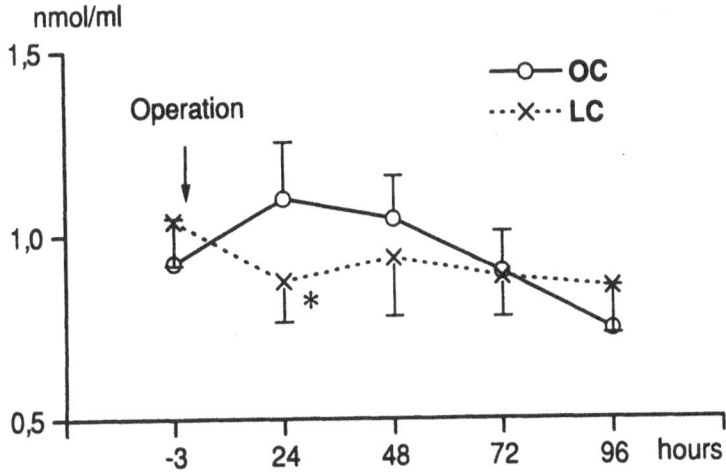

Figure 2. Mean ± SE values of malondialdehyde (MDA) concentration in plasma after open (OC) and laparoscopic (LC) cholecystectomy. Significant value presented as *$p < 0.05$

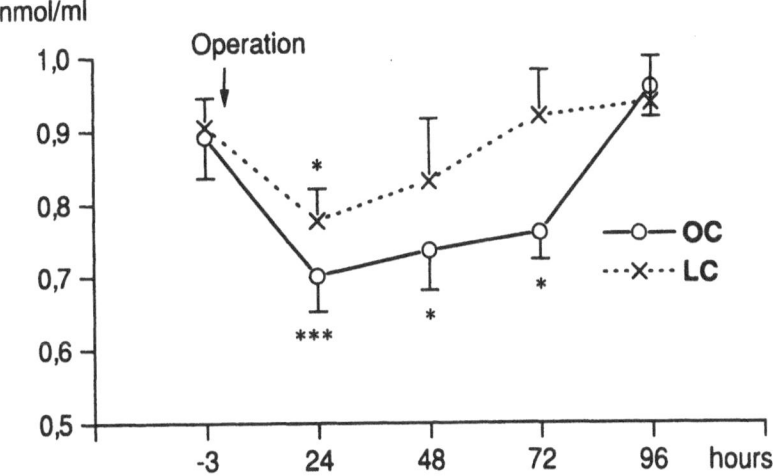

Figure 3. Mean ± SE values of reduced glutathione (GSH) concentration in plasma after open (OC) and laparoscopic (LC) cholecystectomy. Significant value presented as *$p < 0.05$, ***$p < 0.01$

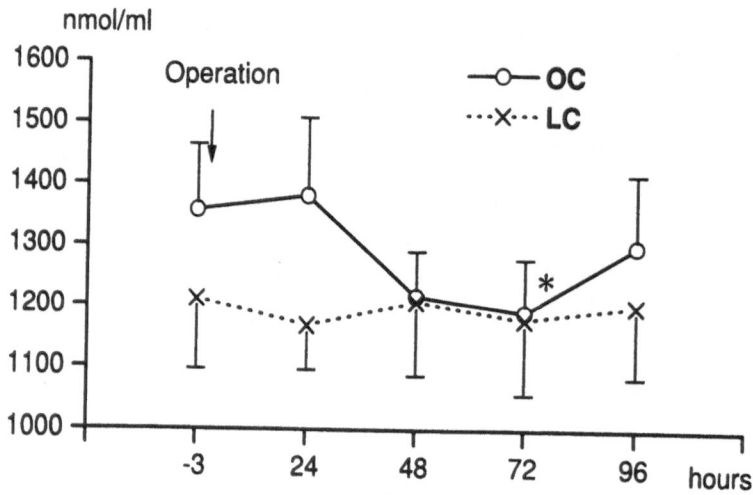

Figure 4. Mean ± SE values of reduced glutathione (GSH) concentration in whole blood after open (OC) and laparoscopic (LC) cholecystectomy. Significant value presented as *$p < 0.05$

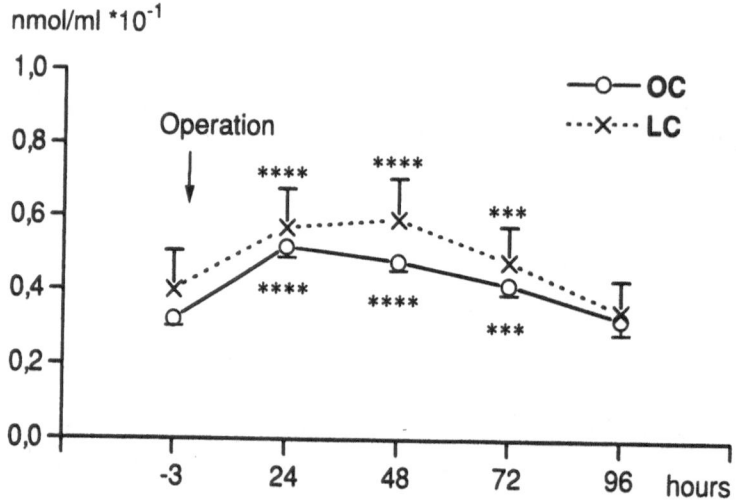

Figure 5. Mean ± SE values of oxidized glutathione (GSSG) concentration in plasma after open (OC) and laparoscopic (LC) cholecystectomy. Significant value presented as ***$p < 0.01$, ****$p < 0.001$

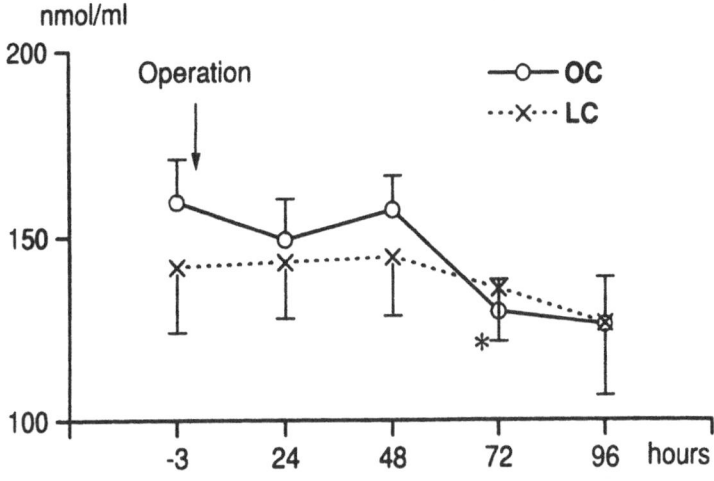

Figure 6. Mean ± SE values of oxidized glutathione (GSSG) concentration in whole blood after open (OC) and laparoscopic (LC) cholecystectomy. Significant value presented as *p < 0.05

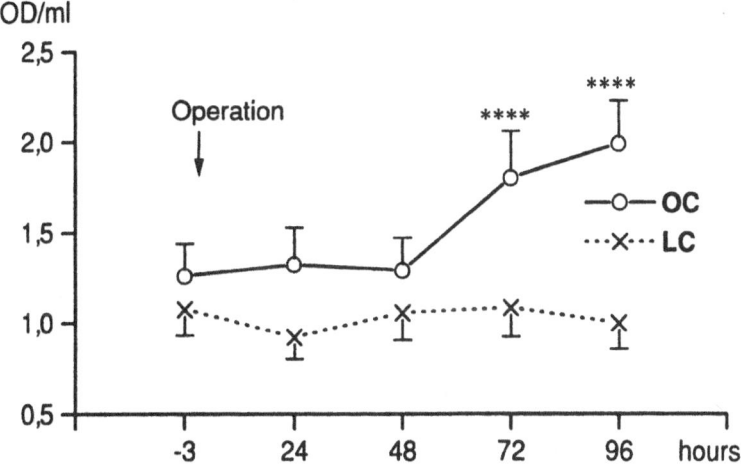

Figure 7. Mean ± SE values of myeloperoxidase activity in sera after open (OC) and laparoscopic (LC) cholecystectomy. Significant value presented as ****p < 0.001

MPO activity of leucocytes significantly ($p < 0.001$) differed in the two groups. Increased MPO activity showed stimulation of leucocytes in the OC group from 1.25 ± 0.18 OD/ml, reaching a peak of 1.98 ± 0.2 OD/ml on the fourth day (Figure 7), while MPO activity remained basically unchanged in the LC group.

DISCUSSION

This study has demonstrated characteristic metabolic responses to both laparoscopic and open cholecystectomy on the basis of the measured parameters with significant differences between the two types of procedure. It has been recently acknowledged that a laparoscopic intervention results in less postoperative pain [10,12,25], a smaller decline in pulmonary function after operation, better postoperative oxygen saturation [18,19] and a speedier return to normal activity [11,26] than open cholecystectomy. Three recent papers compared selected aspects of the metabolic response to laparoscopic and standard open cholecystectomy, using historical [27] and non-randomized [18,19] controls. Joris et al. [27] found that the metabolic and acute-phase response (glucose, leucocytosis, C-reactive protein) were less after laparoscopy compared with laparotomy, although plasma cortisol and catecholamine concentrations were not significantly different between the two groups. A similar cortisol response was demonstrated in the study of Rademaker et al. [19] following open and laparoscopic cholecystectomy. The catecholamine changes have not shown as consistent a pattern as that found by Mealy et al. [18]. These observations suggest that the neuroendocrine stimulation induced by the two surgical procedures may be similar. The interleukin-6 concentration using an immunoradiometric assay [1] was also lower in the laparoscopy group although measurements were made at only three time points and the data on the control group was historical.

Some aspects of the free-radical-mediated reactions after laparoscopic procedures have not yet been reported.

Reactive radicals can abstract H atoms from allelic sites in lipid membranes, and in the presence of oxygen, this leads to chain reactions propagating to involve lipid peroxy radicals and hydroperoxides. This process leads to lipid breakdown and the production of highly reactive aldehydes [28]. The MDA level measured in whole blood and/or in the plasma fraction is an indirect marker of such a process. The level of this marker differed significantly between the two groups in our series. According to these results, it seems that the surgical trauma of laparoscopic procedures induced only an attenuated response in lipid peroxidation compared with open surgery.

Reduced glutathione is a tripetide ubiquitous in mammalian systems, and has many functions within the cell, including its contribution to regulation of DNA and protein synthesis and its role as an essential cofactor for many enzymes [29], as for GSH-transferases and the GSH-peroxidase/GSSG-reductase system. The GSH-peroxidase/GSSG-reductase system is critical as a cellular defence mechanism against oxidizing molecules, such as hydroperoxides. During oxidative stress, GSH is oxidized to GSSG [28]. The surgical trauma induced stress affects this process.

In our series, a marked decrease in GSH values in the plasma fraction was observed accompanied by a reciprocal rise in GSSG following open cholecystectomy, while the laparoscopic intervention caused only a temporary fall in reduced glutathione. Our data reflects the changes in GSH values which can be taken as a good indication of the oxidative stress which in itself is a good demonstrator of patients postoperative recovery.

As it is already established, the amount of reduced glutathione in erythrocytes is an important factor in endogenous antioxidant defence mechanisms. Our observation was that the amount of reduced glutathione in whole blood diminished significantly following OC, allowing us to assume that the endogene antioxidant protection would have been seriously compromised, whilst following LC, no such decrease was recorded.

Major surgery appears to suppress leucocyte function but this recovers by the sixth or seventh day after uncomplicated procedures [4,30,31]. For this reason, any change of neutrophil function was investigated over the first four days after surgery in the two patient groups described.

MPO activity of leucocytes differed significantly in the two groups. There was continuous increase in the OC group, while enzyme activity closely maintained its original level in laparoscopically operated patients. These data suggest that neutrophil function was preserved in the patients undergoing minimally invasive surgery. Carey et al. [17] published that more factors might have a role in determining the differences between neutrophil function after open and laparoscopic or laparoscopically assisted surgery. One such factor might be the size of the abdominal incision, another the period of time during which the peritoneum was opened.

The differences in neutrophil function between patients in the two groups were observed in the absence of postoperative complications and it cannot be speculated, how it would change in postoperative septic complications. Yet it seems to be that laparoscopic cholecystectomy is less disruptive to neutrophil function than conventional open procedures.

Even though patient groups were not randomized in this study, it is clear that the physiological responses to laparoscopic and open cholecystectomy differ significantly. This observation is supported by others [12,15,17–19,27]. Metabolic assessment of laparoscopic surgery increases our knowledge about the physiological responses to surgery. Greater understanding of the components of these responses and their initiating stimuli requires subsequent randomized trials.

ACKNOWLEDGEMENTS

The assistance of Mrs Szalai, Miss Horváth, Mrs Csík, Mrs Tóth, Mrs Gelencsér and Mrs Abrudbányay during the course of this study is appreciated. We thank Mrs Csizmadia and Miss Ballagó for typing this manuscript.

REFERENCES

1. Cruickshank AM, Fraser WD, Burns HJG, Van Damme J, Shenkin A. Response of serum interleukin-6 in patients undergoing elective surgery of varying severity. Clin Sci. 1990;79:161–5.
2. Baigrie RJ, Lamont PM, Kwiatkowski D, Dallman MJ, Morris PJ. Systemic cytokine response after major surgery. Br J Surg. 1992;79:757–60.
3. Chernow B, Alexander R, Smallridge RC et al. Hormonal responses to graded surgical stress. Arch Intern Med. 1987;147:1273–8.
4. Wakefield CH, Carey PD, Foulds S, Monson JRT, Guillou PJ. Changes in major histocompatibility complex class II expression in monocytes and T cells of patients developing infection after surgery. Br J Surg. 1993;80:205–9.
5. Faist E, Storck M, Hültner L et al. Functional analysis of monocyte activity through synthesis patterns of proinflammatory cytokines and neopterin in patients in surgical intensive care. Surgery. 1992;112:562–72.
6. Schulze S, Roikjaer O, Hasselstrom L, Jensen NH, Kehlet H. Epidural bupivacaine and morphine plus systemic indomethacin eliminate pain but not systemic response and convalescence after cholecystectomy. Surgery. 1988;103:321–7.
7. Rutberg H, Hakanson E, Anderberg B, Jorfeldt L, Martensson J, Schildt B. Effects of the extradural administration of morphine or bupivacaine on the endocrine response to upper abdominal surgery. Br J Anaesth. 1984;56:233–7.
8. Scott NB, Mogensen T, Bigler D, Kemlet H. Comparison of the effects of continuous intrapleural vs epidural administration of 0.5% bupivacaine on pain metabolic response and pulmonary function following cholecystectomy. Acta Anaesthesiol Scand. 1989;33:535–9.
9. Klingstedt C, Giesecke K, Hamberger B, Jarnberg PO. High and low-dose fentanyl anaesthesia: circulatory and plasma catecholamine responses during cholecystectomy. Br J Anaesth. 1987;61:184–8.
10. Paterson-Brown S, Garden OJ, Carter OC. Laparoscopic cholecystectomy. Br J Surg. 1991;78:131–2.
11. Vitale GC, Collet D, Larson GM, Cheadle WG, Miller FB, Perissat J. Interruption of professional and home activity after laparoscopic cholecystectomy among French and American patients. Am J Surg. 1991;161:396–8.
12. Myers WC. The Southern Surgeons Club. A prospective analysis of 1518 laparoscopic cholecystectomies. N Engl J Med. 1991;324:1073–8.
13. Giesecke K, Hamberger B, Jarnberg PO, Klingstedt C, Persson B. High and low dose fentanyl anaesthesia: hormonal and metabolic responses during cholecystectomy. Br J Anaesth. 1988;61:575–82.
14. Colley CM, Fleck A, Goode AW, Muller BR, Myers MA. Early time course of the acute phase response. J Clin Pathol. 1983;36:203–7.
15. Jakeways MSR, Mitchell V, Hashim IA et al. Metabolic and inflammatory responses after open or laparoscopic cholecystectomy. Br J Surg. 1994;81:127–31.
16. McMahon AJ, O'Dwyer PJ, Cruikshank AM et al. Comparison of metabolic responses to laparoscopic and minilaparotomy cholecystectomy. Br J Surg. 1993;80:1255–8.
17. Carey PD, Wakefield CH, Thayeb A, Monson JRT, Darzi A, Guillou PJ. Effects of minimally invasive surgery on hypochlorous acid production by neutrophils. Br J Surg. 1994;81:557–60.
18. Mealy K, Gallagher H, Barry M, Lennon F, Traynor O, Hyland J. Physiological and metabolic responses to open and laparoscopic cholecystectomy. Br J Surg. 1992;79:1061–4.
19. Rademaker BM, Ringers J, Odoom JA, TDe Wit L, Kalkman CJ, Oosting J. Pulmonary function and stress response after laparoscopic cholecystectomy: Comparison with subcostal incision and influence of thoracic epidural analgesia. Anesth Analg. 1992;75:381–5.
20. Placer ZA, Cusahan LL, Johnson BC. Estimation of product of lipid peroxidation (malondialdehyde) in biochemical systems. Anal Biochem. 1966;16:359–64.
21. Ohkawa H, Ohishi N, Yagi K. Assay for lipid peroxides in animal tissues by thiobarbituric acid reaction. Anal Biochem. 1979;95:351–8.
22. Tietze F. Enzymatic method for quantitative determination of nanogram amounts of total and oxidized glutathione: applications to mammalian blood and other tissues. Anal Biochem. 1969;27:502–22.
23. Guarnieri C, Flamigni F, Caldarera R. Glutathione peroxidase activity and release of glutathione from oxygen deficient perfused rat heart. Biochem Biophys Res Commun. 1979;89:678–84.
24. Schultz J, Kaminker K. Myeloperoxidase of the leucocyte of normal human blood. Meth Enzymol. 1986;132:265–7.
25. McMahon AJ, Baxter JN, Anderson JR et al. Assessment of pain after laparoscopic and minicholecystectomy: a randomised controlled trial. Br J Surg. 1992;79:1224 (Abstract).

26. McMahon AJ, Ross S, Russel IT et al. Return to normal activity after laparoscopic and minicholecys-tectomy: a randomised trial. Gastroenterology. 1993;104:A370.
27. Joris J, Cigarini I, Legrand M et al. Metabolic and respiratory changes after cholecystectomy performed via laparotomy or laparoscopy. Br J Anaesth. 1992;69:341–5.
28. Ross D. Glutathione, free radicals and chemotherapeutic agents. Pharmac Ther. 1988;37:231–49.
29. Kosower NS, Kosower FM. The glutathione status of cells. Int Rev Cytol. 1978;54:109–60.
30. Lennard TWJ, Shenton BK, Borzotta A et al. The influence of surgical operations on components of the human immune system. Br J Surg. 1985;72:771–6.
31. Wakefield CH, Carey PD, Foulds S, Monson JRT, Guillou PJ. Polymorphonuclear leucocyte activation: an early marker of the post surgical sepsis response. Arch Surg. 1993;128:390–5.

G Mózsik et al. Cell Injury and Cytoprotection in the GI Tract. 335–339.
© 1997 Kluwer Academic Publishers.

OCTREOTIDE IN THE PREVENTION OF INCREASED SERUM AMYLASE AFTER ENDOSCOPIC CHOLANGIOPANCREATOGRAPHY. A PROSPECTIVE, RANDOMIZED AND MULTICENTRE STUDY IN HUNGARY

Z. DÖBRÖNTE[1]*, L. JUHÁSZ[2] AND Z. TULASSAY[3]

[1]Markusovszky Teaching Hospital, Szombathely; [2]Teaching Hospital, Miskolc;
[3]Semmelweis University Medical School, Gastroenterological and Endocrinological
Research Unit, Budapest, Hungary
*Correspondence

ABSTRACT

There are controversial data about the efficacy of the long-acting somatostatin analogue octreotide in the prevention of pancreatic enzyme changes following endoscopic retrograde cholangiopancreatography (ERCP).

Aim: The aim of this multicentre trial was to study the effect of octreotide (Sandostatin) on increased serum pancreatic amylase in a large number of patients.

Method: The study was carried out in a prospective random manner in 2102 patients in 11 endoscopic centres. Patients in the study received 0.1 mg octreotide acetate and those in the control group received isotonic sodium chloride subcutaneously before and 45 min after the ECRP. Serum amylase was determined before the endoscopic procedure and 6 and 24 h later.

Results: Of the total number of patients involved, data of 1199 patients (599 in the study group, and 600 in the control group) could be evaluated. Octreotide decreased the frequency of hyperamylasaemia after endoscopic sphincterotomy (EST) and in patients with chronic obstructive pancreatitis ($p < 0.01$). In all other cases, no significant difference was observed between the two groups. There were no differences in the clinical symptoms following ERCP between the two groups.

Conclusion: The prophylactic use of long-acting somatostatin may diminish the increase in serum amylase after ERCP in patients with chronic obstructive pancreatitis and in those patients who subsequently undergo EST.

Keywords: octreotide, hyperamylasaemia, ERCP, endoscopic sphincterotomy

BACKGROUND AND AIM OF THE STUDY

Acute pancreatitis with a frequency of about 2% is the most common complication of endoscopic cholangiopancreatography while an asymptomatic increase in pancreatic enzyme activity may occur in 40–70% of patients. Somatostatin and its long-acting analogue, octreotide acetate, are potent inhibitors of pancreatic secretion. Nevertheless, data of their efficacy in the prevention of pancreatic enzyme changes following

---

This paper was presented at the Symposium on 'Cell injury and protection in the gastrointestinal tract: from basic science to clinical perspectives', October 8–11, 1995, Pécs, Hungary.

ERCP are controversial [1–10]. However, the results are based on a relatively small number of patients. The aims of our multicentre trial, therefore, were: to study the effect of octreotide on the rise of pancreatic amylase in the serum after ERCP based on a large number of patients, and to search for subgroups of patients who may be candidates for preventive treatment with octreotide during ERCP.

PATIENTS AND METHODS

The study was conducted in a prospective random manner in 11 centres. A total of 2102 patients undergoing ERCP were allocated to two groups. Patients in the study group received 0.1 mg octreotide acetate, Sandostatin, while those in the control group received isotonic sodium chloride sc before the ERCP and 45 min later. Serum samples for amylase activity were collected from each patient before the ERCP and 6 and 24 h after.

A total of 508 cases were excluded for lack of data and also 395 cases because of initial elevation of serum amylase level. Data from 1199 patients could thus be statistically evaluated. The two groups were well matched regarding the patients' characteristics, the mean amount of contrast material given (Table 1), and the endoscopic diagnoses. Cases of endoscopic sphincterotomy (EST), chronic obstructive pancreatitis, those with normal pancreatic ducts and cases with only bile duct opacification were evaluated separately.

Percentage changes in amylase activities were analysed instead of absolute values because of the different normal ranges in the individual centres. Student's t-test, Mann–Whitney U-test and χ^2 test were used for statistical analyses respectively.

TABLE 1

Comparison of patients characteristics and the mean amount of contrast material in the study and control groups

	Study group	Control group
Number of patients	599	600
Male/female (n)	215/384	222/378
Mean age (y)	61.2	61.5
Mean amount of contrast material (ml)	16.0	15.5

TABLE 2
The effect of octreotide on the serum amylase changes and the clinical symptoms after ERCP

Basis of evaluation	Study group ($n = 599$)	Control group ($n = 600$)	Significance
Number of patients with serum amylase increase more than twice the normal limit	192 (32%)	216 (36%)	$p < 0.05$
Mean percentage increase in serum amylase levels 6 h after ERCP	392%	546%	$p < 0.01$
Clinical symptoms (fever and/or abdominal pain)	46 (5.9%)	48 (6%)	NS

TABLE 3
Frequency of serum amylase increase (more than twice the normal limit) after ERCP in subgroups of patients

Subgroups of patients Significance	Study group	Control group	
Patients with EST following ERCP	42/161 (26%)	64/189 (34%)	$p < 0.01$
Patients with chronic obstructive pancreatitis	12/108 (12%)	20/89 (22%)	$p < 0.01$
Patients with normal pancreatic duct	106/174 (61%)	110/177 (62%)	NS
Only bile duct opacification	38/136 (28%)	30/123 (24%)	NS

RESULTS

In an overall comparison, an increase in serum amylase activity more than twice the normal limit occurred in somewhat fewer patients in the study group. Also a smaller percentage increase in serum amylase levels 6 h after the ERCP was observed. As for the clinical symptoms following ERCP, such as abdominal pain and fever, no difference was found between the treated and the control groups (Table 2). When comparing the subgroups of patients, we found that the frequency of serum amylase increase was influenced by octreotide only after EST or in patients with chronic pancreatitis. In all the other cases, no significant difference was observed between the two groups (Table 3).

DISCUSSION

While somatostatin and octreotide inhibit pancreatic secretion, they also increase the sphincter of Oddi's basal pressure and the frequency of phasic wave contractions [11]. In patients subsequently undergoing EST after the ERCP, sphincterotomy allowed a free outflow of the contrast material. For this reason, the protective effect of octreotide could presumably not be counteracted by its effects on the sphincter of Oddi. In cases with chronic obstructive pancreatitis there is an outflow obstruction caused by the disease itself; therefore the sphincter tone increasing effect of octreotide seems to be a less prominent factor in the post-ERCP enzyme changes than its secretion inhibitory effect. In the other cases, the two effects of octreotide are thought to be counterbalanced.

CONCLUSION

On the basis of our multicentre study, we can conclude that long-acting somatostatin may diminish the amylase increase in the serum after ERCP in patients with chronic obstructive pancreatitis, or in those patients who subsequently undergo EST. The prophylactic use of octreotide during ERCP can be recommended in chronic pancreatitis and in cases of EST with special regard to high-risk patients.

REFERENCES

1. Arcidiacono R, Gamitta P, Rossi A, Grosso C, Bini M, Zanasi G. The use of a long-acting somatostatin analogue (octreotide) for prophylaxis of acute pancreatitis after endoscopic sphincterotomy. Endoscopy. 1994;26:715–18.
2. Binmöller KF, Harris AG, Dumas R, Grimaldi C, Delmont JP. Does the somatostatin analogue octreotide protect against ERCP induced pancreatitis? Gut. 1992;33:1129–33.
3. Bordas JM, Toledo V, Mondelo F, Rodes J. Prevention of pancreatic reactions by bolus somatostatin administration in patients undergoing endoscopic retrograde cholangiopancreatography and endoscopic sphincterotomy. Hormone Res. 1988;29:106–8.
4. Cicero GF, Laugier R, Sahel J, Manganero M, Sarles H. Effects of somatostatin on clinical, biochemical and morphological changes following ERCP. Ital J Gastroenterol. 1985;17:265–8.
5. Guelrud M, Mendoza S, Viera L, Gelrud D. Somatostatin prevents acute pancreatitis after pancreatic duct sphincter hydrostatic balloon dilatation in patients with idiopathic recurrent pancreatitis. Gastrointest Endosc. 1991;37:44–7.
6. Person B, Slezak P, Efendic S, Häggmark A. Can somatostatin prevent infection pancreatitis after ERCP? Hepatogastroenterology. 1992;39:259–61.
7. Testoni PA, Lella F, Bagnalo F, Buizza M, Colomba E. Controlled trial of different dosages of octreotide in the prevention of hyperamylasaemia induced by endoscopic papillosphincterotomy. Ital J Gastroenterol. 1994;26:431–6.
8. Sternlieb JM, Aronchick CA, Retig JN et al. A multicenter, randomized, controlled trial to evaluate the effect of prophylactic octreotide on ERCP-induced pancreatitis. Am J Gastroenterol. 1992;87:1561–6.

9. Tulassay Z, Papp J. The effect of long-acting somatostatin analogue on enzyme changes after endoscopic pancreatography. Gastrointest Endoscopy. 1991;37:48–50.

10. Tyden G, Nyberg B, Sonnenfeld T, Thulin L. Effect of somatostatin on hyperamylasemia following endoscopic pancreatography. Acta Chir Scand. 1986;530:43–5

11. Binmöller KF, Dumas R, Harris AG, Delmont JP. Effect of somatostatin analog octreotide on human sphincter of Oddi. Dig Dis Sci. 1992;37:773–7.

CELL INJURY AND PROTECTION OF THE PREMALIGNANT STATUS AND MALIGNANT DISEASES IN THE GASTROINTESTINAL TRACT

G Mózsik et al. Cell Injury and Cytoprotection in the GI Tract. 343–347.

GENETIC POLYMORPHISMS OF CYP1A1, CYP2E1, AND GSTM1 GENES: SUSCEPTIBILITY TO COLON CANCER

I. KISS* AND I. EMBER

Department of Preventive Medicine, University Medical School of Pécs, Szigeti st. 12, H-7643 Pécs, Hungary
*Correspondence

ABSTRACT

Cancer susceptibility is influenced by genetic polymorphisms of enzymes metabolising and detoxifying carcinogenic chemical compounds. Phenotypic and genetic differences in cytochrome P_{450} 1A1, 2E1 and GSTM1 enzymes often correlate with occurrence of certain cancers. Beside lung and bladder cancer, there is considerable evidence that colorectal tumours are also affected by these polymorphisms. We have examined the distribution of genotypes among non-familiar colon tumour patients and controls. There was a moderate effect of each polymorphism on colon cancer sensitivity alone, but the combination of the three high-risk alleles was significantly associated with increased risk of colon cancer (RR: 1.73, CI: 1.07–2.81).

Keywords: colon cancer, individual susceptibility, genetic polymorphism, CYP1A1, CYP2E1, GSTM1

INTRODUCTION

Application of molecular biological methods to epidemiology has given new possibilities for the epidemiologists to describe the predisposition for development of disease processes [1]. In recent years, the molecular epidemiology of cancer has expanded rapidly [2], developing new biomarkers for exact measurement of predisposing factors [3,4], giving early and precise diagnosis, evaluating the prognosis [5,6] and investigating the individual susceptibility. The latter points are where molecular epidemiology has an interest in common with the clinical oncologists and family physicians. The question of individual susceptibility to cancer used to involve hereditary cancers or well-defined syndromes with increased cancer incidence, and other differences in cancer occurence were ascribed to external factors. However, recently, numerous studies have suggested possible minor genetic differences for cancer susceptibility [7–9]. Genetic polymorphisms were described in oncogenes and enzymes of the cytochrome P_{450} system, which affect the occurence of certain cancer types. Since the cytochrome P_{450} enzymes are responsible for metabolism of carcinogenic chemicals, it is not surprising that changes in their activity can influence human carcinogenesis. Similarly, other detoxifying enzymes, such as glutathione-S transferases, might have a role in determining cancer susceptibility.

This paper was presented at the Symposium on 'Cell injury and protection in the gastrointestinal tract: from basic science to clinical perspectives', October 8–11, 1995, Pécs, Hungary.

Cytochrome P_{450} 1A1, responsible for aryl-hydrocarbon-hydroxylase activity, has been found to possess a polymorphic site, differing in a single base (A–G), causing a valin/isoleucin change in the enzyme [10]. Several studies have shown an association between the Val genotype and some cancers, while others found no differences [11,12]. Cytochrome P2E1 is an ethanol-inducible enzyme with more than 100 identified substrates [13]. One of its known polymorphisms is a DraI RFLP, located within intron 6 [14], which is associated with sensitivity to lung and other cancers [13]. GSTM1 is a member of μ family of glutathione-S transferase superfamilies. Almost 50% of Caucasian populations carry a homozygous deletion of this gene with lack of enzyme activity. Individuals with this 0 genotype are probably at higher risk for certain cancers [15,16].

In contrast to the hereditary cancers, the mentioned allelic differences generally cause moderate differences in cancer risks. Ethnic distribution of the alleles is also different, which makes the comparison of studies even more difficult and might be responsible for controversial results. According to our hypothesis, combined evaluation of the three polymorphisms will emphasize the small differences and gives a much better chance of identifying high-risk individuals. In our present study, we investigated the genetic polymorphisms of CYP1A1, CYP2E1 and GSTM1 genes on susceptibility to colon cancer, evaluating the results separately and in combination with each other.

MATERIALS AND METHODS

A total of 35 patients with non-familiar colon cancer, and 40 healthy controls were included in the study. Sterile anticoagulated blood was used to determine CYP1A1, CYP2E1 and GSTM1 genotype.

CYP1A1 polymorphism was determined by allele-specific polymerase chain reaction (PCR) with two downstream primers, differing in the last base: AAGACCTCC-CAGCGGGCAA**T**, AAGACCTCCCAGCGGGCAA**C**. Each sample was tested in two parallel reactions, using one of the downstream primers and the same upstream primers (GAAAGGCTGGGTCCACCCTCT). The reactions were carried out in a total volume of 20 μl, containing 1.5 mmol/L $MgCl_2$, 10 mmol/L Tris–HCl, pH 8.3, 2 μg/ml bovine serum albumin, 0.2 mmol/L each dNTP, 1 μmol/L each primer, 2 U Taq DNA polymerase, 30 cycles of 60 s at 94°C, 45 s at 59°C and 90 s at 72°C. After electrophoresis in parallel lanes of a 2% agarose gel, amplification was detected with the exactly matching primer only.

The DraI polymorphic site of CYP2E1 was investigated by a restriction fragment length polymorphism method combined with PCR. The surrounding 373-bp region was amplified in the previously described reaction mix, with TCGTCAGTTCCT-GAAAGCAGG and GAGCTCTGATGCAAGTATCGCA primers, 30 cycles of 60 s at 94°C, 60 s at 60°C and 60 s at 72°C. The amplification product was digested with excess amount of DraI, and electrophoresed in 2% agarose gel. In the case of the C allele, the undigested 373-bp DNA fragments, the D allele showed a 240- and a 133-bp fragment.

The GSTM1 genotype was tested by an amplification of a 273-bp sequence from the wild type gene in the presence of an internal control. GSTM1 primers were CTGCCCTACTTGATTGATGGG and CTGGATTGTAGCAGATCATGC; the internal control primers (GCAAACCACAATCGAATGCA and CTTTACTTCCT-TTGCCTCAG) amplified a CA-repeat marker on a chromosome 16q, with a length of 154–170 bp. The amplification took place in the same reaction mix, 30 cycles of 45 s at 94°C, 45 s at 59°C and 80 s at 72°C. The products were analysed on a 2% agarose gel. Absence of the 273-bp sequence indicated the homozygous deleted (null) genotype, and the assay did not differentiate between homozygous and heterozygous carriers of the normal gene.

For each type of PCR, 2 µl whole blood served as a template. The reaction components without Taq DNA polymerase and with the blood were heated to 94°C for 15 min followed by 10 min at 80°C. The Taq polymerase was then added and the 30 PCR cycles performed.

RESULTS

Table 1 shows the frequency of genotypes found among patients with colon tumours, while Table 2 contains the results for healthy controls. When analysed separately, the relative risks for the disease-associated alleles and colon cancer were as follows: GSTM1 0 genotype RR: 1.08, CI: 0.67–1.75; CYP1A1 Val allele RR: 1.19, CI: 0.68–2.05; CYP2E1 C allele RR: 1.11, CI: 0.68–1.82. The results suggest a positive, but not significant, association, the strongest being for the CYP1A1 polymorphism. The homozygous and heterozygous carriers of disease-associated alleles were treated as a single group because of the rare occurrence of homozygotes.

The combined analysis found no significant differences if the disease-associated alleles were grouped in pairs (data not shown) but a statistically significant difference was observed in comparing the number of individuals with disease-associated alleles for each investigated polymorphism. In the colon cancer group, 6 people had this genotype (GSTM1 0, CYP1A1 Val, CYP2E1 C) but only 2 individuals among controls. This is a significant association with RR: 1.73, CI: 1.07–2.81.

TABLE 1
Genotypes of patients with colon tumours ($n = 35$)

GSTM1	CYP1A1	CYP2E1
0: 17	Ile/Ile: 27	DD: 22
+: 18	Ile/Val: 7	CD: 11
	Val/Val: 1	CC: 2

TABLE 2
Genotypes of healthy controls ($n = 40$)

GSTM1	CYP1A1	CYP2E1
0: 18	Ile/Ile: 33	DD: 27
+: 22	Ile/Val: 7	CD: 12
	Val/Val: 0	CC: 1

DISCUSSION

It is widely accepted that genetic polymorphisms may affect cancer susceptibility. However, many studies have controversial results and conclusions about the significance of the investigated allelic distribution [17,18]. The allele frequencies among healthy individuals might be significantly different between populations and geographical areas. This makes the comparison of national studies difficult, and might be partly responsible for the differences. The actual role of allelic polymorphism may also differ, according to environmental and other genetic factors. On the other hand, the effect of some polymorphisms might be so small, that a very large population must be observed to be able to detect it. The immediate practical significance of these minor variations in cancer risk is also very low, since there is no way to define high-risk groups or individuals.

In order to eliminate these shortcomings, we combined the results of three genetic polymorphisms on colon cancer susceptibility. None of them alone was a significant risk factor, but, after combining the high-risk alleles, a significant positive association with colon cancer risk was found. Concerning the distribution of genotypes in normal indivuals, our results are consistent with most reports on European populations. However, investigations in Japan show quite different allelic distributions, and the application of our method to such populations has yet to be investigated.

Identifying high-risk individuals may help in prevention of malignant tumours. If someone, a successfully treated cancer patient or a family member, has the high-risk genotype, preventive measures should be taken seriously, regular cancer screenings should be performed, advice must be given to the patient on how to avoid high-risk activities, and continuous follow-up from the family physician is necessary. Of particular importance is the investigation of patients with precancerous lesions because the high-risk genotypes, together with carrying the disease-associated alleles of metabolising enzymes, carry a very high risk of subsequent tumour formation.

REFERENCES

1. McMichael AJ. Molecular epidemiology: new pathway or new travelling companion? Am J Epidemiol. 1994;140:1–11.
2. Perera FP. Molecular cancer epidemiology: a new tool in cancer prevention. J Natl Cancer Inst. 1987;78:887–98.
3. Perera FP, Weinstein IB. Molecular epidemiology and carcinogen-DNA adduct detection: new approaches to studies of human cancer causation. J Chron Dis. 1982;35:581–600.
4. Ember I, Raposa T, Varga Cs, Kiss I. Effect of different cytostatic protocols on oncogene expression in CBA/Ca mice. Anticancer Res. 1995;15:1285–8.
5. Kozma L, Kiss I, Szakáll Sz, Ember I. Investigation of c-myc oncogene amplification in colorectal cancer. Cancer Lett. 1994;81:165–9.
6. Kiss I, Ember I, Dezsényi E, Csécsei Gy. Activation of different oncogenes in malignant brain tumors. Cancer Detect Prev. 1993;17:97.
7. Taylor YA, Bell DA, Nagorney D. L-myc proto-oncogene alleles and susceptibility to hepatocellular carcinoma. Int J Cancer. 1993;54:927–30.
8. Zhong S, Wyllie AH, Barnes D, Wolf CR, Spurr NK. Relationship between GSTM1 genetic polymorphism and susceptibility to bladder, breast and colon cancer. Carcinogenesis. 1993;14:1821–4.
9. E Thelu MA, Zarski JP, Froissart B, Rachail M, Seigneurin JM. c-Ha-ras polymorphism in patients with hepatocellular carcinoma. Comparison of healthy subjects and alcoholic patients with cirrhosis. Gastroenterol Clin Biol. 1993;17:903–7.
10. Hayashi S, Watanabe J, Nakachi K, Kawajiri K. Genetic linkage of lung-cancer associated MspI polymorphisms with amino acid replacement in the heme binding region of the human cytochrome P450IaI gene. J Biochem. 1991;110:407–11.
11. Sivaraman L, Leathem MP, Yee Y, Wilkens LR, Lau AF, Le Marchand L. CYP1A1 genetic polymorphism and in situ colorectal cancer. 1994;54:3692–5.
12. Hirvonen A, Husgafvel-Pursiainen K, Karjalainen A, Anttila S, Vainio H. Point-mutational MspI and Ile-Val polymorphisms closely linked in the CYP1A1 gene: Lack of association with susceptibility to lung cancer in a Finnish population. Cancer Epid Biom Prev. 1992;1:485–9.
13. Rannung A, Alexandrie A-K, Persson I, Ingelman-Sundberg M. Genetic polymorphism of cytochromes P450 1A1, 2D6 and 2E1: Regulation and toxicological significance. J Occup Environ Med. 1995;37:25–36.
14. Uematsu F, Kikuchi H, Ohmachi T et al. Two common RFLPs of the human CYP2E gene. Nucl Acids Res. 1991;19:2803.
15. Lin HJ, Han C-Y, Bernstein DA, Hsiao W, Lin BK, Hardy S. Ethnic distribution of the glutathione transferase Mu 1-1 (GSTM1) null genotype in 1473 individuals and application to bladder cancer susceptibility. Carcinogenesis. 1994;15:1077–81.
16. Chenevix-Trench G, Young J, Coggan M, Board P. Glutathione-S-transferase M1 and T1 polymorphisms: susceptibility to colon cancer and age of onset. Carcinogenesis. 1995;16:1655–7.
17. Uematsu F, Kikuchi H, Motomiya M et al. Association between restriction fragment length polymorphism of the human cytochrome P450IIE1 gene and susceptibility to lung cancer. Jpn J Cancer Res. 1991;82:254–6.
18. Hirvonen A, Husgafvel-Pursiainen K, Anttila S, Karjalainen A, Vainio H. The human CYP2E1 gene and lung cancer: DraI and RsaI restriction fragment length polymorphisms in a Finnish study population. Carcinogenesis. 1993;14:85–8.

G Mózsik et al. Cell Injury and Cytoprotection in the GI Tract. 349–355.
© 1997 Kluwer Academic Publishers.

SERUM CAROTENOIDS AND MALIGNANT GASTROINTESTINAL DISEASES IN PATIENTS

Gy. RUMI[1], K. KOVÁCS[1], Z. MATUS[2], Gy. TÓTH[2], Á. VINCZE[1] AND Gy. MÓZSIK[1*]
[1]First Department of Medicine, and [2]Department of Chemistry, Medical University of Pécs, Hungary
*Correspondence

ABSTRACT

The serum levels of carotenoids (vitamin A, lutein, zeaxanthin, α- and β-cryptoxanthin, α- and β-carotene) were measured in healthy people and in patients with different malignant gastrointestinal diseases (21 colon, 13 stomach, 8 pancreas adenocarcinoma, 10 hepatocellular carcinoma). The serum levels of carotenoids were measured with high pressure liquid chromatography (HPLC). The sera of the patients were taken at the time of the diagnosis.

Results: The measurements indicated that:

1. The serum levels of vitamin A and zeaxanthin were significantly lower in all these groups but the extent of the decrease was different in patients with different types of gastrointestinal malignancy. The serum level of vitamin A in healthy subjects ($n = 16$) was 2.07 ± 0.209 μmol/L and in patients with gastrointestinal malignancies ($n = 52$) was 0.77 ± 0.078 μmol/L. The serum level of zeaxanthin in healthy subjects was 0.1435 ± 0.066 μmol/L and in those with malignancies was 0.042 ± 0.009 μmol/L.

2. There were no significant differences in the serum levels of other carotenoids in the examined group.

3. The serum levels of cholesterol, total protein, albumin and haemoglobin were in the normal range in these patients.

These results indicate that: (1) the carotenoids may be responsible nutritional factors in the development of different malignant diseases; and (2) this supposed role in carcinogenesis does not depend fully on vitamin A activity.

Keywords: retinoids, carotenoids, gastrointestinal malignancies, carcinogenesis

INTRODUCTION

It is a well known fact that retinoids affect the differentiation and proliferation of many cell types. Deficiency in dietary vitamin A leads to a clinical syndrome manifested as metaplasia of epithelial tissues, growth retardation and degeneration of reproductive organs [1]. Recently, several epidemiological investigations have noted an inverse relationship between vitamin A intake and risk for developing or progression of cancer [2,3]. The role of retinoids as chemopreventive agents has been examined in numerous in-vitro and in-vivo models. These studies have demonstrated that retinoids can suppress

This paper was presented at the Symposium on 'Cell injury and protection in the gastrointestinal tract: from basic science to clinical perspectives', October 8–11, 1995, Pécs, Hungary.

malignant transformation of cells in vitro, irrespective of whether the transformation is induced by ionizing radiation, chemical carcinogens or transforming polypeptides. Retinoids are potential chemopreventive agents, since they are involved in the general maintenance or enhancement of differentiation and cancer is a process in which loss of differentiation occurs [4]. Animals deficient in vitamin A are also more susceptible than non-deficient animals to chemical carcingens [5,6]. β-Carotene prevents the development of gastric mucosal erosions in rats treated with indomethacin [7].

To determine whether there is a relationship between carotenoids and human malignant diseases, we examined the changes in serum levels of carotenoids in patients with different types of gastrointestinal malignancy.

PATIENTS AND METHODS

A total of 51 patients with different types of gastrointestinal malignancy were examined. These patients were at different stages of disease; some of them had multiple metastasis. In spite of the heterogeneity of the patients, we did not classify them on the basis of the extent of disease because the aim of this investigation was to determine whether or not there is a correlation between the malignant disease and the serum carotenoid level. The patients were divided into smaller groups depending on the localization of their disease.

There were 21 patients with colon adenocarcinoma, 13 with gastric cancer, 10 with hepatocellular adenocarcinoma and 8 patients with pancreas adenocarcinoma. Blood (10 ml) was taken from the patients at the time of diagnosis.

The serum levels of the carotenoids were measured by the high pressure liquid chromatography (HPLC) method. We measured the serum levels of vitamin A, lutein, zeaxanthin, α- and β-cryptoxanthin and α- and β-carotene.

Preparation of samples for HPLC measurements: 2 ml of the serum sample was shaken with 2 ml of 96% ethanol for 2 min, then it was extracted with 3 ml of hexane being shaken for 2 min. The mixture was centrifuged for 5 min. As an internal standard, canthaxantin was added to the removed homogenous organic phase. Then it was evaporated to dryness in a vacuum and the residue was dissolved in 0.2 ml of 1:4 mixture of dichloromethane and methanol; 0.025 ml of this solution was injected.

The chromatographic system consisted of a gradient former Model 250 B (Gynkotec, Germany), HPLC pump Model 300 B Glenco injector (Gynkotec, Germany), and a time programmable UV-vis detector Model 166-2, equipped with gold chromatography software (Beckmann, USA). The column was 150×4.6 mm packed with Chromsil-C 0.186 mm not endcapped reversed phase packing.

The eluent was 3% (v/v) water in methanol (A), methanol (B) and 20% (v/v) dichloromethane in methanol. The flow rate was 1.5 ml/min. The gradient programme was 100% A 30 s to 100% B in 3 min, to 100% C in 4 min (linear steps). The time programme of wavelength was 325 nm for 3.5 min (detecting vitamin A), then 450 nm (detecting other carotenoids).

Quantification of HPLC peaks: the chromatograms were evaluated quantitatively by relating the peak areas of the individual compounds to that of canthaxantin used as an internal standard. The ratios of the molar extinctions of the authentic samples to that of canthaxantin were employed as correction factors of the detector signals. The results were given in µmol/L.

The results for 16 healthy persons were used as control values in the statistical analysis. The results were expressed as mean ± SEM. Two-paired Student's test and calculation of regression between some parameters were used for the statistical evaluation.

RESULTS

The serum level of vitamin A was highest in the healthy subjects, the levels of zeaxanthin, lutein and β-cryptoxanthin were about 10%, while the serum levels of α-cryptoxanthin, α- and β-carotene were about 1% of the vitamin A level (Figure 1).

The serum level of vitamin A was significantly lower in patients with gastrointestinal malignancy than in the control group. The reduction was different in patients with different types of GI malignancy. The smallest decrease was found in patients with gastric cancer; the largest was found in patients with colon adenocarcinoma (Figure 2). The serum level of lutein did not differ significantly from the control values (Figure 2).

The zeaxanthin level was also significantly lower in all these groups. It decreased most significantly in patients with adenocarcinoma; the smallest decrease was found in patients with gastric cancer (Figure 3). The serum levels of β-cryptoxanthin and β-

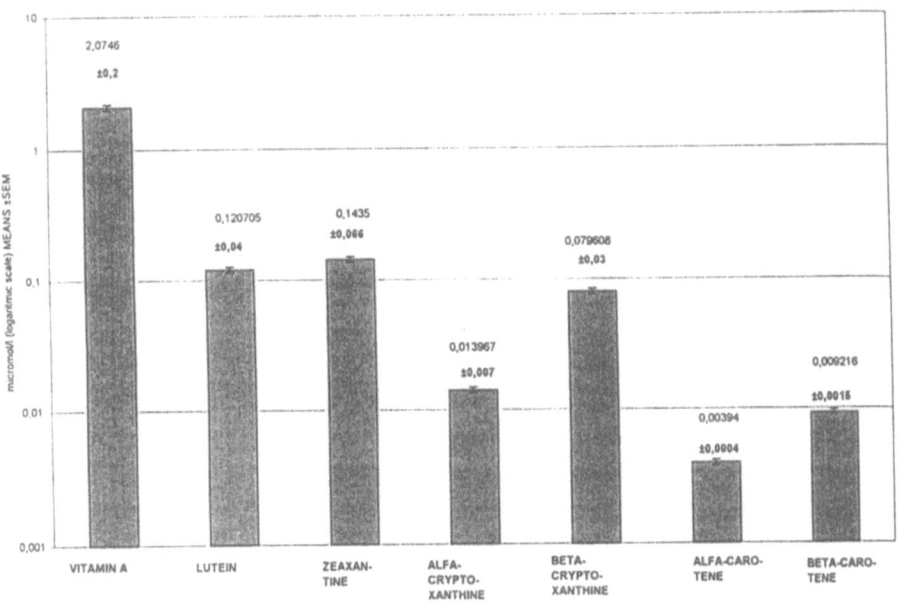

Figure 1. The serum retinoid levels in healthy subjects ($n = 16$)

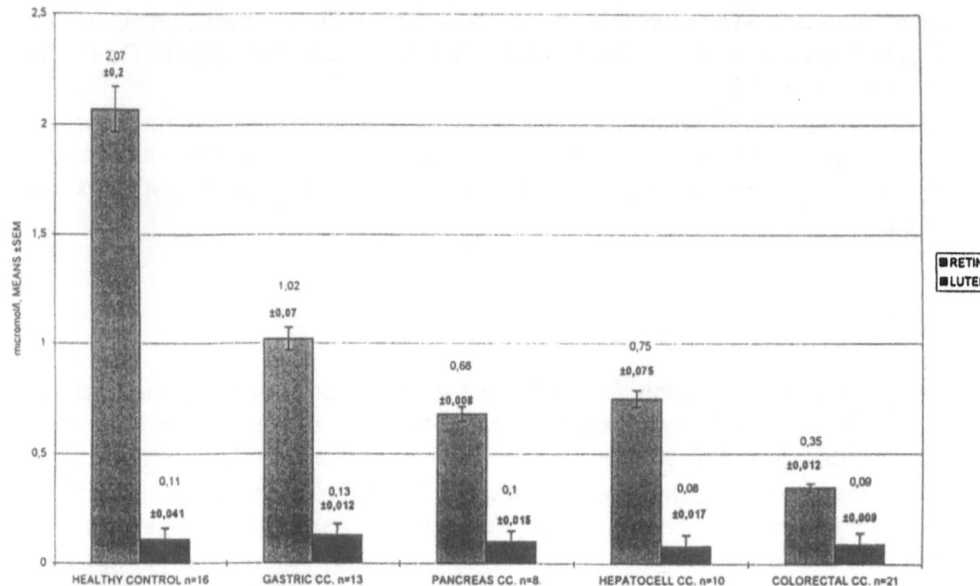

Figure 2. The serum retinol and lutein levels in patients with different types of gastrointestinal malignancies

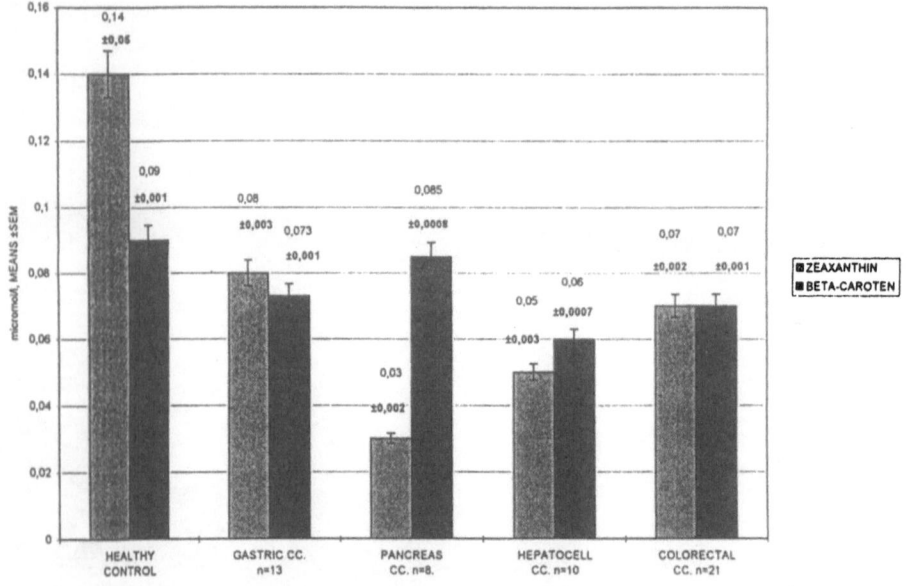

Figure 3. The serum zeaxanthin and β-carotene levels in patients with different types of gastrointestinal malignancies

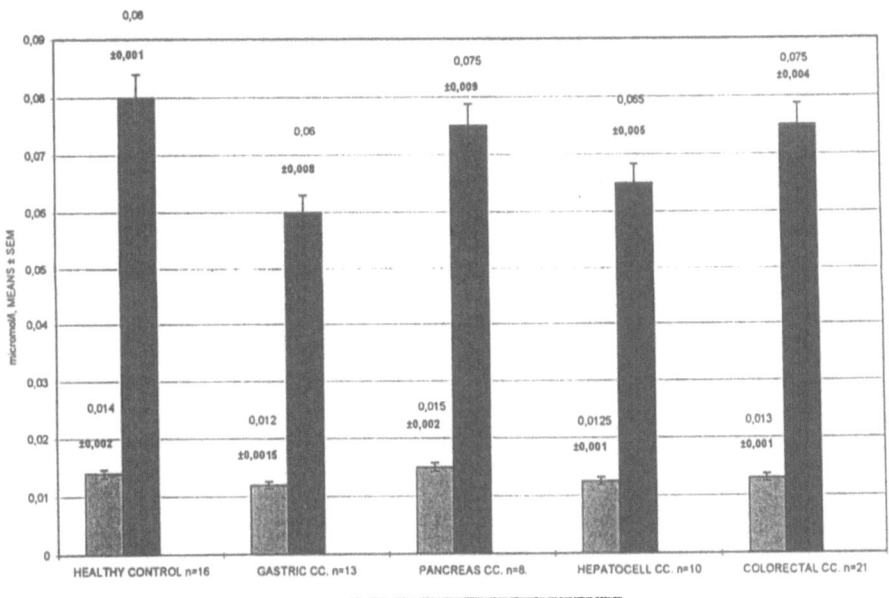

Figure 4. The serum α- and β-cryptoxanthin levels in patients with different types of gastrointestinal malignancies

carotene showed slight, but not significant, decreases (Figures 3 and 4). The α-cryptoxanthin and α-carotene levels did not differ significantly from the control values (Figures 3 and 4).

Vitamin A and carotenoids are fat-soluble compounds; therefore, the absorption of these materials is highly dependent on fat absorption. In the case of malnutrition or malabsorption, the serum carotenoid levels will also be lower than the normal values. To rule out this possibility, we calculated the correlation between serum vitamin A and cholesterol level. No correlation was found between these two parameters. Moreover, the examined patients had normal levels of serum cholesterol, albumin, total protein, and haemoglobin (5.03 ± 0.32 mmol/L, 38.5 ± 2.01 g/L, 68.42 ± 2.56 g/L and 128.76 ± 6.78 g/L, respectively).

A chromatogram from a healthy subject (Figure 5) and from a patient with colon adenocarcinoma (Figure 6) is demonstrated.

SUMMARY

In spite of the large amount of experimental data, the exact mechanism of action of carotenoids has not been found yet. It is most likely that different mechanisms of action exist. Part of the beneficial effects comes from the vitamin A activity; the remainder is the consequence of the structure and does not depend on vitamin A activity (zeaxanthin).

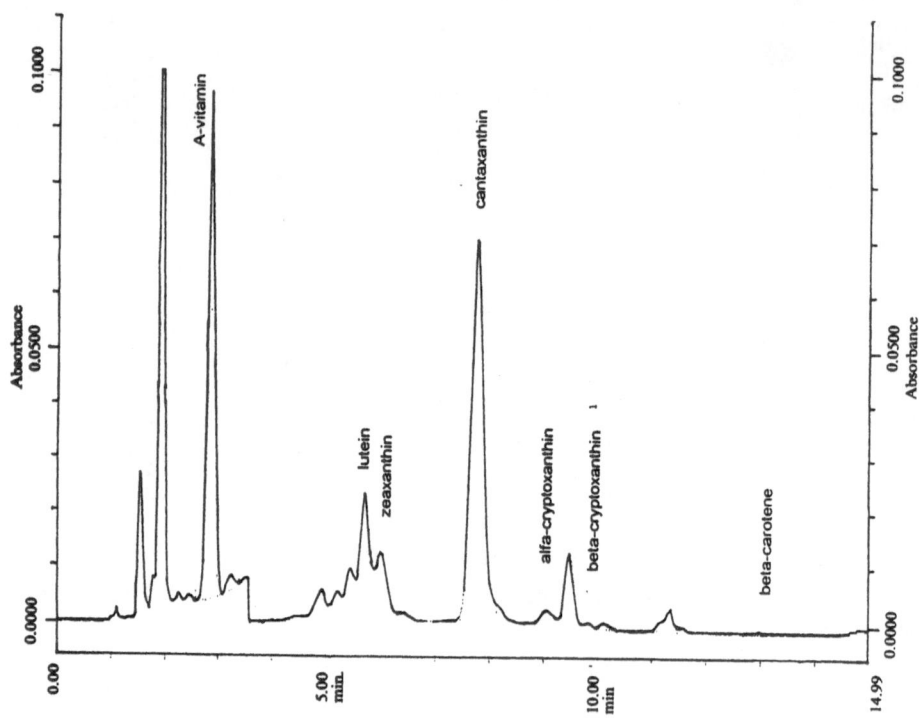

Figure 5. The chromatogram of a healthy subject

The retinoids may influence the effects of different enzymes, such as adenylate cyclase, ornithine decarboxylase, cytochrome P_{450}, glutathione reductase, etc. The polyunsaturated carbon chain has a good scavenger capacity. The carotenoids scavenge the oxygen free radicals, which may act to prevent the initiation phase of carcinogenesis [8]. On the other part only recently became possible to unifying the hypothesis, which involves the protein kinase C cascade system. Furthermore, they regulate the membrane functions, the growth functions and the genomic expression. The carotenoids can influence the immunological system too. There is good evidence that the antitumour activity of retinoids, as well as of cytokines, is at least partially mediated by inhibition of cell proliferation and by induction of cell differentiation.

Our results indicate that the carotenoids (and not only the retinoids which have vitamin A activity) may be responsible nutritional factors in the development of different malignant diseases. This suggested role in carcinogenesis does not depend entirely on the vitamin A activity.

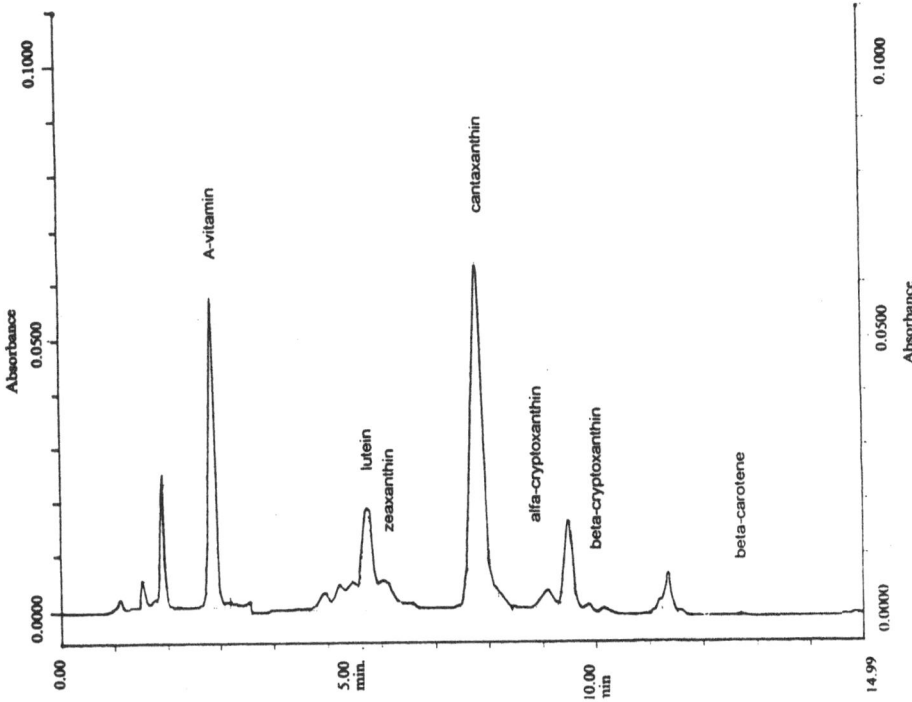

Figure 6. The chromatogram of a patient with colon adenocarcinoma

ACKNOWLEDGEMENTS

This study was supported by the Hungarian National Research Fund (OTKA TO 20098) and the Ministry of Welfare and Health (ETT-03660/93).

REFERENCES

1. Hicks RM. The scientific basis for regarding vitamin A and its analogs as anticarcinogenic agents. Proc Nutr Soc. 1983;43:83–93.
2. Mettlin C, Graham S, Swanson M. Vitamin A and lung cancer. Natl Cancer Inst. 1979;62:1435–8.
3. Bjelke E. Dietary vitamin A and lung cancer. Int J Cancer. 1975;15:561–5.
4. Moon RC, Iltri L. Retinoids and cancer. In: Sporn MB, Roberts AB, Goodman DS, eds. The Retinoids. Orlando, FL: Academic Press; 1984:327–71.
5. Rogers AE, Herndon BJ, Newberne PM. Induction by dimethylhydrazine of intestinal carcinoma in normal rats fed high and low levels of vitamin A. Cancer Res. 1973;33:1003–9.
6. Cohen SM, Wittenberg JF, Bryn GT. Effect of avitaminosis A and hypervitaminosis A on urinary bladder carcinogenesis of N-[4-(5-nitrofuril)-2-thozolil)] formamide. Cancer Res. 1976;36:2334–9.
7. Király Á, Sütő G, Vincze Á, Tóth Gy, Matus Z, Mózsik Gy. Correlation between the cytoprotective effect of beta-carotene and its gastric mucosal level in indomethacin treated rats with or without acute surgical vagotomy. In: Cell injury and protection in the gastrointestinal tract: from basic sciences to clinical perspectives. Acta Physiol Hungarica. 1992;80:213–18.
8. Lippman SM, Kessler JF, Meyskens FL Jr. Retinoids as preventive and therapeutic anticancer agents. Cancer Treat Rep. 1987;71:391–405.

INDEX